Physical Therapy Management of
Low Back Pain

A Case-Based Approach

Julia Chevan, PT, PhD, MPH, OCS
Professor of Physical Therapy
Springfield College
Springfield, MA

Phyllis A. Clapis, PT, DHSc, OCS
Associate Professor of Physical Therapy
American International College
Springfield, MA

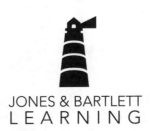

JONES & BARTLETT
LEARNING

World Headquarters
Jones & Bartlett Learning
5 Wall Street
Burlington, MA 01803
978-443-5000
info@jblearning.com
www.jblearning.com

Jones & Bartlett Learning books and products are available through most bookstores and online booksellers. To contact Jones & Bartlett Learning directly, call 800-832-0034, fax 978-443-8000, or visit our website, www.jblearning.com.

Substantial discounts on bulk quantities of Jones & Bartlett Learning publications are available to corporations, professional associations, and other qualified organizations. For details and specific discount information, contact the special sales department at Jones & Bartlett Learning via the above contact information or send an email to specialsales@jblearning.com.

Production Credits
Publisher: David D. Cella
Acquisitions Editor: Katey Birtcher
Managing Editor: Maro Gartside
Editorial Assistant: Teresa Reilly
Senior Production Editor: Renée Sekerak
Marketing Manager: Grace Richards
Manufacturing and Inventory Control Supervisor: Amy Bacus
Composition: Auburn Associates, Inc.
Photo Researcher: Sarah Cebulski
Cover Design: Kristin E. Parker
Cover Image: © Lightspring/ShutterStock, Inc.
Printing and Binding: Malloy, Inc.
Cover Printing: Malloy, Inc.

Some images in this book feature models. These models do not necessarily endorse, represent, or participate in the activities represented in the images.

Library of Congress Cataloging-in-Publication Data
Physical therapy management of low back pain : a case-based approach /
[edited by] Julia Chevan, Phyllis A. Clapis.
    p. ; cm.
 Includes bibliographical references and index.
 ISBN-13: 978-0-7637-7945-0 (alk. paper)
 ISBN-10: 0-7637-7945-8 (alk. paper)
 I. Chevan, Julia. II. Clapis, Phyllis A.
 [DNLM: 1. Low Back Pain—therapy—Case Reports. 2. Physical Therapy
Modalities—Case Reports. WE 755]

 617.5'6406—dc23
                                            2011042578
6048
Printed in the United States of America
16 15 14 13 12   10 9 8 7 6 5 4 3 2

Contents

Chapter 1: Low Back Pain in the United States 1
Julia Chevan, PT, PhD, MPH, OCS
Phyllis A. Clapis, PT, DHSc, OCS

Chapter 2: Meet Joe Lores 15
Julia Chevan, PT, PhD, MPH, OCS
Phyllis A. Clapis, PT, DHSc, OCS

Chapter 8: The Paris Approach **157**
Jeffrey A. Rot, PT, DHSc, OCS, MTC, FAAOMPT
James A. Viti, PT, MSc, DPT, OCS, MTC, FAAOMPT

Chapter 9: The Osteopathic Approach **191**
Maria Meigel, PT, DPT, CFMT, OCS

Chapter 10: Movement System Impairment Syndromes Approach **213**
Shirley Sahrmann, PT, PhD, FAPTA

Chapter 11: A Treatment-Based Classification Approach **247**
Paul E. Mintken, PT, DPT, OCS, FAAOMPT
Mark D. Bishop, PT, PhD

Julia Chevan, PT, PhD, MPH, OCS
Phyllis A. Clapis, PT, DHSc, OCS

Preface

Back pain, put simply, is a universal human problem for which there exists no magic bullet. There are many therapeutic options for patients and many practitioners who claim to have the answer to the conundrum of back pain. A quick search for treatment yields options that include surgery, injection, medication, exercise, and practitioners who range from physicians and physical therapists to acupuncturists and yoga teachers. The array of options can be confusing to both patient and provider. Within physical therapy, approaches to the problem of back pain are also numerous. As physical therapist educators, we are challenged by the task of introducing our students to the vast assortment of physical therapy approaches to lower back pain (LBP), some of which have sound scientific rationale and others that do not. Our goal in writing this book was to provide a resource on the models that are used in physical therapy to treat acute low back pain using the example of a single patient case. The book is intended primarily for students entering the profession of physical therapy but may also be of interest to practitioners trying to understand the array of intervention options used in physical therapy. Both students and clinicians are encouraged to further their knowledge in these approaches by reading the primary sources cited or by attending continuing education courses.

We are indebted to our own students who pushed us to pull all of this material into one text. These students always returned from their clinical experiences asking us to explain why two therapists in two different clinics would treat the same patient so differently. To those students we can finally say that we have some of the answers and they are in this book.

Acknowledgments

When I look up at the full moon, I know that the full moon is there. And I want only to focus my attention, my whole attention, on the presence of the full moon. So I take an in-breath and I say, "full moon." And then full moon suddenly reveals herself to me very clearly. There's only the full moon at that moment. And when I breathe out, I smile and say, "Thank you for being there." So, I and the full moon were very real in that moment. And I repeat, I do it two, three, four times, and my happiness increases all the time. I feel very alive in that moment.

—From a dharma talk by the Venerable Thich Nhat Hanh entitled "Be Like the Earth" given at Plum Village on July 23, 1996.

Thank you for being there:

Patricia, Saadya, and Nava, my family, the keepers of my heart

My friends and colleagues at Springfield College

Regina Kaufman, who inspires and critiques in the same breath

David Miller, a leader I am always following

Gail Stern and Esther Haskvitz, my fan club

Phyllis, for helping birth this baby and many others

—Julia Chevan

There are so many people who deserve my heartfelt thanks for helping this book come to fruition:

Thank you to my colleague and coeditor Julia Chevan for conceiving the idea for this book and for her expertise, professionalism, and sense of humor throughout the process. I can't imagine working with a better partner.

Thank you to each of the chapter authors. I have been honored to work with such brilliant clinicians and I am keenly aware that this project would not have been possible without their expertise.

Thank you to my students and colleagues at American International College who have inspired and supported me, especially Gail Stern and Sue Davis for their never-ending encouragement and enthusiasm.

A special thanks and dedication to my parents who are, quite simply, the greatest teachers I've ever had, and to my family for their daily love and support.

Finally, thank you to the individual pioneers of our profession who developed the models we have presented in this book. It is through their contributions that we have been able to so greatly impact the lives of our patients.

—Phyillis Clapis

About the Authors

Julia Chevan graduated with a BS degree in physical therapy from Boston University in 1985. Since that time, she has worked in a variety of clinical settings mostly focused on providing care for patients with orthopedic problems. In 1993 she joined the faculty of Springfield College where she now serves as Professor and Chair in the Department of Physical Therapy. Julia is a board-certified clinical specialist in orthopedic physical therapy through the American Board of Physical Therapy Specialties and has passed the credentialing examination with the McKenzie Institute. Her academic background includes advanced degrees in public health from the University of Massachusetts, in orthopedic physical therapy from Quinnipiac University, and a doctoral degree in health studies from Virginia Commonwealth University. Julia's research interests have drawn her into examining health services issues related to the care of persons with low back and neck pain. In addition to her professional life, Julia is the mother and soccer coach for two young children who can almost run faster than she can. She is the partner of Patricia Jung, a physical therapist of exceptional ability who can run as fast as anyone.

Phyllis A. Clapis has been practicing in the area of orthopedic physical therapy for over 25 years. She graduated with a BS degree in physical therapy from University of Connecticut in 1983 and received her Master's degree in orthopedic physical therapy from Quinnipiac University in 1994. In 2004 she received a doctorate in health science from the University of St. Augustine. She started her academic career in 1996 at American International College where she currently serves as an Associate Professor in the Division of Physical Therapy. Her teaching focus includes spinal and extremity orthopedic patient management as well as evidence-based physical therapy practice. Phyllis has been a board-certified specialist in orthopedic physical therapy through the American Board of Physical Therapy Specialties since 1994. She is a consultant at Mount Holyoke College and is a regular contributor to McKesson Clinical Reference System's *Sports Medicine Advisor* series. She resides in western Massachusetts with her family.

Contributors

Elaine Atkins, DProf, MA, MCSP owns a private practice in London, United Kingdom. She holds a doctorate in Professional Studies (Orthopaedic Medicine Education), is a Fellow of the Society of Orthopaedic Medicine and the programme leader for the MSc Orthopaedic Medicine.

Mark D. Bishop, PT, PhD is an Assistant Professor in the Department of Physical Therapy at the University of Florida in Gainsville, Florida.

Helen Clare, PhD, FACP, Dip Phy, Dip MDT is in private practice in Sydney, Australia and serves as Associated Academic Staff with Sydney University. She is a Fellow of the Austrialian College of Physiotherapists and an instructor, and the International Director of Education with the McKenzie Institute.

Emily Goodlad, MSc, MCSP is in private practice in Edinburgh, United Kingdom. She is a Fellow of the Society of Orthopaedic Medicine.

Jill Kerr, MSc, BSc, MCSP is in private practice in Edinburgh, United Kingdom. She is a Fellow of the Society of Orthopaedic Medicine and a course principal for the society's Diploma in Orthopaedic Medicine.

John Krauss, PT, PhD, OCS, FAAOMPT is an Associate Professor at Oakland University in Rochester, Michigan. Dr. Krauss received his Orthopedic Manipulative Therapy Certification through the International Seminar of Orthopedic Manipulative Therapy and completed an orthopedic residency training and received his Graduate Certificate in Orthopedic Manual Physical Therapy through Oakland University. He is a Fellow of the American Academy of Orthopedic Manual Physical Therapists.

Kenneth E. Learman, PT, PhD, OCS, COMT, FAAOMPT is an Associate Professor at Youngstown State University in Youngstown, Ohio. He is a Fellow of the American Academy of Orthopedic Manual Physical Therapists and is senior teaching faculty for Maitland-Australian Physiotherapy Seminars.

Maria Meigel, PT, DPT, CFMT, OCS is in private practice in Long Island, New York. She is a member of the teaching faculty at both Touro College and Stony Brook University. Dr. Meigel is a principal in Integrative Manual Therapy Solutions.

Paul E. Mintken, PT, DPT, OCS, FAAOMPT is an Assistant Professor in the physical therapy program at the University of Colorado in Denver, Colorado. He is a Fellow of the American Academy of Orthopedic Manual Physical Therapists and teaches for Evidence in Motion.

Donald K. Reordan, PT, MS, OCS, MCTA is in private practice in Jacksonville, Florida. He is a certified member of the Mulligan Concept Teachers Association and serves as the regional manager for the Mulligan Concept.

Jeffrey A. Rot, PT, DHSc, OCS, FAAOMPT is an Associate Professor at the University of St. Augustine at the St. Augustine, Florida campus. He is a Fellow of the American Academy of Orthopedic Manual Physical Therapists and teaches the S3 coursework for the University's Institute of Physical Therapy.

Shirley Sahrmann, PT, PhD, FAPTA is an Associate Professor of Physical Therapy and Neurology at Washington University School of Medicine, St. Louis, Missouri. She is a Fellow of the American Physical Therapy Association. Dr. Sahrmann is the director of the Movement Science Program at Washington University.

Christopher R. Showalter, PT, OCS, COMT, FAAOMPT, FABS is in private practice in New York. He is a Fellow of the American Academy of Orthopedic Manual Physical Therapists and is the clinical director for Maitland-Australian Physiotherapy Seminars.

James A. Viti, PT, MSc, DPT, OCS, MTC, FAAOMPT is an Assistant Professor at the University of St. Augustine in St. Augustine, Florida. He is a Fellow of the American Academy of Orthopedic Manual Physical Therapists and teaches full time in the entry-level and advanced studies programs.

Reviewers

Amy J. Bayliss, PT, DPT
Assistant Clinical Professor
Department of Physical Therapy
School of Health and Rehabilitation Sciences
Indiana University
Indianapolis, Indiana

Ronald De Vera Barredo, PT, DPT, EdD, GCS
Head, Department of Physical Therapy
Tennessee State University
Nashville, Tennessee

Rogelio Adrian Coronado, PT, CSCS, FAAOMPT
Doctoral Student
University of Florida
Gainesville, Florida

Paul-Neil Czujko, PT, DPT, OCS
Clinical Assistant Professor
Physical Therapy Program
Stony Brook University
Stony Brook, New York

Patricia M. King, PT, PhD, OCS, MTC
Associate Professor and Chair
Department of Physical Therapy

Introduction

In the United States, considerable resources are allocated to care related to back pain. Annual expenditures have been estimated to reach the sum of $86 billion per year.[1] Worse, the trend in dollars expended for spine problems, based on data from 1997–2006, indicates that we spend more money each year on care for this condition.[2] Despite the wide variety of treatment options available, the cost of work-related disability continues to rise.[3] For physicians, treatment of low back pain has remained a challenge since most patients with low back pain lack a specific pathoanatomic diagnosis.[4] The term "nonspecific low back pain" has been coined to describe these patients whose pain is of unknown origin.

Physical therapists have also been challenged by the treatment of patients with nonspecific low back pain. These patients make up the majority of an outpatient physical therapist's case load.[5] Some therapists are intimidated by the seemingly complex signs and symptoms that accompany patients with back pain while others pride themselves in being so-called "spine specialists."

Today, physical therapy interventions for low back pain are wide and varied, but that was not always the case. During World War I, the first physical therapists, better known then as reconstruction aides, provided simple treatments such as exercise, hydrotherapy, and massage to wounded veterans. Physical therapy was prescription-based; the physician examined the patient and provided the therapist with detailed orders for each intervention, including parameters for duration, frequency, and intensity. Physical therapists were not allowed to evaluate their patients and any form of independent thinking was viewed as a challenge to the authority of the physician. Most patients received the same treatment for the same diagnosis. The profession grew from one that was focused on polio and postwar injuries to one that provided intervention for multiple diseases ranging from cardiovascular and pulmonary conditions to neurology and orthopedic conditions.[6] The 1960s and 1970s heralded an era of growth in the area of orthopedic physical therapy and a growth in the approaches that therapists used for treating low back pain from physician-based approaches to approaches developed and tested by physical therapists.

During the prescription-based era of physical therapy, the primary form of exercise prescribed for patients with low back pain was "William's Flexion Exercises." These exercises, named after Dr. Paul C. Williams, were designed to both improve trunk stability while promoting flexibility of the hip flexors and the lumbar extensor muscles. According to Williams, the first rule for those who suffered from back pain was to reduce the lumbar lordosis to a minimum.[7] Williams' work in the U.S. was contrasted with the work being done by Dr. James Cyriax who opened a department of massage and manipulation at St. Thomas' Hospital in London in which methods of massage and manipulation were carried out by physiotherapists working under the auspices of orthopedic physicians.

In the early 1950s and 1960s, Freddy Kaltenborn, a Norwegian physical therapist developed an approach to manual therapy and back care treatment that was based on normalizing joint movement. Kaltenborn was not the only physical therapist working on a manual approach to back pain. As orthopedic physical therapy grew, the work of a number of these early manual therapists including Freddy Kaltenborn, Mariano Rocobado, and Geoffrey Maitland diffused into the United States.[8] In 1970, Cyriax, Kaltenborn, and an internationally representative group of therapists formed the International Federation of Orthopaedic Manipulative Therapists, bringing many schools of thought and approaches to manual therapy and spine treatment together in one association. In parallel, 1974 saw the founding of the Orthopaedic Section of the American Physical Therapy Association (APTA) in the United States, led by Stanley Paris. At this point, the astute student should note the parallel between the names we are mentioning in this brief history and the names associated with the models presented in subsequent chapters of this book.

The 1980s brought a paradigm shift to the treatment of LBP when Robin McKenzie, a New Zealand physical therapist, introduced the radical notion that extension, not flexion, was the preferred direction of movement for managing acute back pain. He suggested that excessive flexion was actually the cause of one's low back pain and that most back pain was caused by an accumulation of fluid in the disc. In terms of treatment, now physical therapists were either teaching patients how to reduce their lordosis or how to increase it. Ultimately in an era of prescription-based care, it was still the physician's call.

The 1980s also saw an expanded role for the U.S. physical therapist and the end to prescription-based physical therapy. In 1984, the APTA House of Delegates passed a motion that allowed physical therapists to evaluate and treat patients. This solidified physical therapy as a true profession, with its own defined body of knowledge and autonomy. With this newfound role came the ability to evaluate patients and render a diagnosis. The challenge, however, was to differentiate a diagnosis made by a physical therapist from one made by a physician. While the early definition of the term "diagnosis" took on many shapes, it was ultimately adopted by the APTA and is described in the *Guide to Physical Therapist Practice* as "both the process and the end result of evaluating examination data which the physical therapist organizes into defined clusters, syndromes, or categories to help determine prognosis (including plan of care) and the most appropriate intervention strategies." The key point here is that a diagnosis made by a physical therapist is meant to describe problems in terms of the disablement model in categories that guide treatment. The role and purpose of diagnosis by physical therapists was also clarified by Anthony Delitto and Lynn Snyder-Mackler[9] who stated:

> *The classic medical diagnosis can be defined as identifying a patient's disease by its signs, symptoms, and laboratory data, and the other general definition, which we believe to be synonymous with clinical classification, entails placing a label on clusters of clinical data.*

As a profession that has grown into more independent modes of practice and one in which therapists were writing prescriptions rather than just filling them, there was an increased emphasis on the development of diagnostic protocols. Academics and clinicians were being challenged to develop the theory and content for these protocols that were based on a gathering of patient signs and symptoms.[10]

While it was agreed upon that the diagnostic process was meant to guide treatment, there was still little evidence on what constituted appropriate care for treatment of LBP.[11] Clinicians were often using two types of diagnostic processes to guide treatment. One, based on a pathoanatomical model, and the other, which was considered newer, was based on a classification system that would allow the clinician to identify clusters of symptoms, signs, and characteristics of patients who responded to a specific treatment.[10,11] These diagnostic processes are the framework on which many of the approaches to LBP today are built, including a number that are presented in this book.

Years ago, an article appeared in the *Wall Street Journal* in which the writer, who had chronic knee pain, was examined by five different physical therapists and ultimately received five different treatment suggestions.[12] The author expressed some concern with the level of ambiguity amongst the therapists and concluded that "physical therapy is still as much art as science."[12] As a result of the article, our profession was scrutinized for the therapists' uncertainty and lack of agreement in managing the patient's knee symptoms.[13] There was little evidence that supported one treatment approach over the other. The general school of thought when the article was published was that the key to treating patellofemoral pain was to strengthen the vastus medialis obliquus (VMO). With the rise in evidence, we know today that VMO is not necessarily the optimal treatment strategy. The evidence-based practice movement has provided us with more scientific evidence of the impact of clinical interventions, more information on the validity of our tests and measures, and models that are based on sound scientific rationale. Given the current variety of approaches to treating back pain, what would we expect if the patient sought treatment for her low back pain? Would the patient be examined in a similar way by each of the therapists? Would the treatments be similar?

The answers to these questions are precisely what this book is about. We recruited therapists from around the world who are experts in their specified models. Our experts include Mulligan, McKenzie, and Paris certified therapists, along with many more. We selected models that were brought to our attention by our own students who, during their clinical experiences, are exposed to practice that is based both in evidence and in habit.

To write this book, each expert was provided with a hypothetical case of a patient named Joe Lores who had been experiencing LBP for 2 weeks as a result of an injury. We used the documentation template from the *Guide to Physical Therapy Practice*[14] as a means to structure the screening and examination, and to initially provide the same generic information to each therapist. This template was chosen for its ability to identify red flags that would indicate a need for immediate medical referral. Once given this basic examination information, the experts were asked what tests and measures they might require as part of their model's examination strategy. After this information was provided, each author determined a diagnosis, prognosis, and plan of care for the patient. Authors were asked to structure their work using a plan for examination and intervention that would be employed by a therapist working under the paradigm of that model's science and theory.

While this book is intended to serve as an introduction to each of the common approaches to management of low back pain, it is in no way exhaustive. It might be best to think of it as a primer, giving the reader a flavor for each approach, but not a comprehensive description of each one. We urge the reader to delve a little deeper into the information by reading the literature and attending continuing education courses that are specific to each model. Most importantly, we urge the reader to think critically about the information provided by any model or any guru claiming to have the "answer to low back pain." We are still looking. . . .

REFERENCES

1. Martin BI, Deyo RA, Mirza SK, et al. Expenditures and health status among adults with back and neck problems. *JAMA*. 2008;299(6):656–664.
2. Martin BI, Turner JA, Mirza SK, Lee MJ, Comstock BA, Deyo RA. Trends in health care expenditures, utilization, and health status among US adults with spine problems, 1997–2006. *Spine*. 2009;34(19):2077–2084.
3. Deyo RA, Cherkin D, Conrad D, Volinn E. Cost, controversy, crisis: low back pain and the health of the public. *Annu Rev Public Health*. 1991;12:141–156.
4. Deyo RA. Diagnostic evaluation of LBP: reaching a specific diagnosis is often impossible. *Arch Intern Med*. 2002;162(13):1444–1447.
5. Jette AM, Davis KD. A comparison of hospital-based and private outpatient physical therapy practices. *Phys Ther*. 1991;71(5):366–375.
6. Moffat M. The history of physical therapy practice in the United States. *Journal of Physical Therapy Education*. 2003;17(3):15–25.
7. Williams PC. Lesions of the lumbosacral spine: chronic traumatic (postural) destruction of the intervertebral disc. *J Bone Joint Surg*. 1937;29:690–703.
8. Paris SV. In the best interests of the patient. *Phys Ther*. 2006;86(11):1541–1553.
9. Delitto A, Snyder-Mackler L. The diagnostic process: examples in orthopedic physical therapy. *Phys Ther*. 1995;75(3):203–211.
10. Rose SJ. Musing on diagnosis. *Phys Ther*. 1988;68(11):1665.
11. Van Dillen LR, Sahrmann SA, Norton BJ, et al. Reliability of physical examination items used for classification of patients with low back pain. *Phys Ther*. 1998;78(9):979–88.
12. Miller L. One bum knee meets five physical therapists. *Wall Street Journal*. September 22, 1994:B1, B6.
13. Craik R. A tolerance for ambiguity. *Phys Ther*. 2001;81(7):1292–1294.
14. American Physical Therapy Association. *Interactive Guide to Physical Therapist Practice*. Alexandria, VA: American Physical Therapy Association; 2003. http://guidetoptpractice.apta.org/.

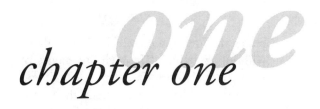

chapter one

Low Back Pain in the United States

Julia Chevan, PT, PhD, MPH, OCS
Phyllis A. Clapis, PT, DHSc, OCS

INTRODUCTION

Low back pain (LBP) is extraordinarily common. Think about it; have you ever felt some pain or a twinge in your back? It is a rare person who has not had at least one episode of LBP by the time he or she reaches the age of 50. One commonly used estimate cites that 80% of adults will have an episode of LBP at some point in their lives. Because of its high rate of occurrence, LBP accounts for a substantial portion of outpatient care and is one of the most frequent complaints among all adults who see healthcare practitioners. The condition has created a tremendous economic and social burden on society and on our medical care system.

In this chapter we will give a brief overview of the scope of the problem of LBP in the general population. As healthcare providers we need to understand not only care at the individual level, but also the population implications of LBP and LBP care. The topics that will be summarized include the prevalence of LBP, healthcare utilization for LBP, the status of diagnostics, outcomes and outcome measures, medical community approaches, and policy issues. All of these topics impact on decisions about individual care in the clinic and on our ability as physical therapists to treat patients in the most efficacious manner achieving the best outcomes.

PREVALENCE OF LOW BACK PAIN

LBP is defined as "pain localized below the line of the twelfth rib and above the inferior gluteal folds, with or without leg pain."[1] The high prevalence of LBP is one of the principal reasons that it is a priority area for research and the subject of many academic and lay texts. Published measures of the prevalence of LBP vary due to the differing definitions of LBP proffered by surveys and researchers, the different populations studied, and the range of methodologies that may be used in studying prevalence.[1,2]

Prevalence is a measure of the rate of all persons who have a condition at a specified point in time in a given population. Prevalence rates are dependent upon several factors related to the condition being considered. These factors include the duration of the condition and the impact of treatment on the condition. For LBP one might see a differentiation if the distinction was made between an acute episode, which is typically of short duration, as opposed to a chronic condition, which can endure for years. A number of different types of prevalence rates are typically measured when trying to understand the epidemiology of any condition. Lifetime prevalence is a measure of the number of persons who have a condition during the course of their lifetime. Annual prevalence is a measure of the number of persons who have a condition during the course of a year. Period prevalence is a measure of the number of persons who have a condition during a specified time period. Finally, point prevalence is a measure of the number of persons who have a condition at a single specific point in time.

Loney and Stratford[2] examined the methodologies used in studying LBP prevalence in a broad-based review of the quality of published prevalence studies. These authors attributed much of the differences in prevalence statistics to methodological differences among the studies. A great deal of the variation in prevalence rates was related to the definitions for the duration of LBP used by previous researchers. These definitions ranged from LBP lasting several days in some studies to LBP lasting at least 2 weeks in others. Those studies that used a definition of LBP with a shorter duration tended to report higher prevalence rates than those that used a definition incorporating greater time duration. In addition, differences in prevalence rates among studies were found based on the age range of the population studied. Younger adults (20–35 years) had lower prevalence rates, rates rose in the middle ages (40–60 years), and then rates dropped after the age of 60.

Deyo and Tsui-Wu[3] published an oft-cited study that used the National Health and Nutrition Examination Survey II (NHANES II) data and its definition of LBP to determine lifetime prevalence, point prevalence, and care-seeking patterns for LBP. In the NHANES II survey, LBP was defined as "pain in your back on most days for at least 2 weeks." The lifetime prevalence of LBP was 14% and the point prevalence was 6.8%. Among demographic subgroups, prevalence rates were found to be similar for males and females but different by race, with Caucasians (14%) having a higher lifetime prevalence of LBP than African Americans (11%). When level of educational attainment was considered it was found that the less education a person reported the higher the prevalence of LBP. Individuals with less than a high school degree had the highest lifetime prevalence of LBP at 17%. Those individuals who had a high school degree had a lifetime prevalence of 14% and those with a college degree had a lifetime prevalence of 11%. In the United States regional differences were evident for LBP prevalence with the highest prevalence in the western states (15%) and the lowest in the northeastern states (11%). In a follow-up study in 2006 that also used data from national surveys, Deyo[4] and colleagues found that 26% of adults have had a bout of LBP when asked about their previous three-months health status. Again, as education level declined and income level declined, rates of back pain increased.

Additional estimates of the prevalence of LBP in the United States come from two published studies of care seeking conducted using a random sample of residents of North Carolina.[5,6] The benefit of these two studies is that one was focused on acute LBP while the other dealt with chronic LBP. Chronic LBP was defined as functionally limiting back pain that lasted for more than 3 months or that produced 25 occurrences in 1 year, while acute severe LBP was back pain that was functionally limiting for at least 1 day. The 1-year period prevalence of acute severe LBP was 8%. The prevalence was higher among adults aged 35–39 and higher among Caucasian persons. The 1-year period prevalence of chronic LBP was 4%.

Prevalence studies and prevalence data are useful as they identify the size and the scope of the LBP problem and help to clarify the population that may require the provision of health services. LBP is a problem that is wide in its scope, having an impact on a large proportion of the population in the United States

RISK FACTORS FOR LOW BACK PAIN

In most prevalence studies the analysis of demographic or even clinical subgroups does not extend beyond bivariable descriptions of prevalence. This means we know the rate of LBP by educational attainment, we believe it to be higher among those with less education, but since there are so many factors involved we can't be sure that educational attainment is truly related to developing LBP. The development of multivariable models makes possible identification of subgroups at risk for back pain or back pain care. The introduction of control variables allows multivariable models to identify more clearly associated risk factors.

Reisbord and Greenland[7] studied LBP prevalence in relation to demographic characteristics using these multivariable techniques. The authors' intent was to develop a model for the prediction of LBP. In this study, the data source was the RAND Health Insurance Experiment and the survey definition of LBP was "frequent back pain during the 12 months prior to the interview." The demographic variables investigated included age, gender, race, education, occupation, physical demand of the occupation, income, and marital status. In the univariate analysis the authors found that all of the variables except race had a significant association with back pain. The prevalence of LBP was 4% higher among women than men. The multivariable modeling produced three identifiable subgroups for demographic profiles and prevalence. The high prevalence group comprised persons 50–64 years old and no longer married. The intermediate prevalence group was made up of persons 35–49 years old and no longer married and married persons with a high school education or less, regardless of age. Finally, the low prevalence group consisted of persons who were married with greater than a high school education and 18–34 year old persons who were no longer married regardless of level of education. The most important predictors for LBP prevalence in this analysis were education, gender, and marital status.

Studies of risk factors for LBP have also demonstrated that a key factor in risk is occupation and physical load/demand placed on the body. In Reisbord and Greenland's[7] model, income, occupation, and demand were factors shown to be intermediate to education, gender, and marital status. This study was not only unique in the use of multivariable analysis but also in the finding that demographics may play a more important predictive role than physical attributes.

Heistaro et al.[8] examined 20 years of data from a series of surveys conducted in Finland. The 20 years enabled these researchers to examine the stability of prevalence rates in relation to demographic and social characteristics and behavioral risk factors for LBP. The authors used statistical models to analyze the change in prevalence rates over time for subgroups divided by age and gender. Back pain was most prevalent among persons with lower levels of education, with lower levels of income, with blue-collar occupations, and with jobs that required heavier physical workloads. These prevalence rates were relatively stable over the 20 years of the study, though the strongest and most time-stable determinant of LBP in this study was level of education.

Education level is a demographic factor that deserves attention on its own because it plays an important role as a determinant not only of back pain prevalence, but it has also been found to be a predictor of the outcomes of back pain episodes and the outcomes of care for episodes of back pain.[9] A review of the evidence of the relationship between level of education and measures of back pain prevalence found that low educational status was associated with increased back pain prevalence in at least 16 separate studies. Education level, according to the authors' analysis, had a stronger effect on the duration and recurrence of back pain than it did with the actual onset of back pain. Five hypotheses were postulated to explain the relationship between education level and LBP. The hypotheses were based on the premise that education level may also be linked to socioeconomic status or other risk factors that occur in the presence of lower education levels. The hypotheses incorporated a profile of persons with lower education levels that included more toxic and hazardous living environments, more life stressors, more physically demanding occupations, compromised "health stock," and differential access to and differential use of health services. The authors urged for more rigorous methodology in future studies to adjust for confounding factors such as level of education and to develop a model accounting for multiple factors. It seems evident that social determinants play a crucial role in the occurrence of LBP and that LBP prevalence has an inverse relationship with measures of higher socioeconomic status.

LOW BACK PAIN AND RECURRENCE

LBP can be described as a condition in which pain and accompanying disability typically decrease rapidly within 1 month. Most individuals who are off of work due to LBP are able to return within a month.[10] Improvement from the condition continues for 3 months. After the 3-month point, levels of pain, disability, and return to work remain constant with pain and disability, both at low levels for up to 12 months following onset. Finally, the risk of at least one recurrence of LBP within a year was estimated as a range from 66–84%. From this analysis, LBP could be characterized as a condition that for most people has a good prognosis since its impact is time-limited and improvement is imminent. However, the analysis also shows that LBP is a condition that likely will recur.

Von Korff et al.[11] examined the outcomes of back pain among patients enrolled in a health maintenance organization (HMO) who sought care from primary care physicians. In this study 1,128 patients participated in an interview 1 year after initially seeing a physician for back pain. Outcomes measured by the researchers included pain, disability, and depression. Patients were divided into two groups based on previous occurrences of back pain. At the 1-year follow up, both groups reported high levels of back pain in the month prior to the phone interview (69% and 82%). Poor outcomes in terms of persistence of pain and disability were associated with being female and having a lower level of education. This study suggests that the good prognosis of LBP may only be apparent if analysis is undertaken within a short timeframe after the initial onset.

Carey et al.[12] also examined the likelihood of recurrence after an episode of acute LBP. Subjects in the study were enrolled through a care provider and interviewed at 6 and 22 months after the initial visit to the provider. Over one-half of the 921 subjects identified as being at risk had a recurrence of LBP. The level of recurrence rose from the 6-month to the 22-month interviews. Predictors for recurrence included a history of more episodes of back pain and a higher level of disability.

Most studies that examine recurrence are restricted to follow-up periods of 1 year's time or shorter. Enthoven, Skargren, and Oberg[13] extended the time period of follow up to 5 years to understand the long-term clinical course of persons with LBP. These authors surveyed a cohort of subjects who had participated in a prospective study on treatment by chiropractors and physical therapists. In this study, the researchers found that overall 63% of the subjects reported two or more recurrences or a continuous episode of daily pain at the 5-year point. In addition they found that 32% of their subjects reported seeking care during the 6 months prior to the survey. In summary, there is evidence that repeated episodes are common with LBP and that they often occur within 5 years of the first episode.

DISABILITY DUE TO LOW BACK PAIN

LBP results in a significant burden to society and to the individual due to the disability that is often a consequence of these conditions. Among chronic conditions reported in the U.S. National Health Survey, back pain is the most frequent cause of limitation for persons less than 45 years old.[14] Fanuele et al.[15] examined the impact of spine disorders and comorbidities on physical function. Functional status was measured using the Physical Component

Summary (PCS) derived from the SF-36 Questionnaire. The mean PCS score for subjects in this study was 30, which was lower than 50, the mean for the general U.S. population. Persons with greater numbers of comorbidities tended to have lower PCS scores; in this sample, 46% of the patients had at least one comorbidity. When subjects who had only a spine condition and no comorbidity were analyzed, the mean PCS was 32.

As with prevalence, demographic variables play a role as determinants of disability for persons with LBP. Deyo and Tsui-Wu[16] found that disability due to LBP was most strongly correlated with education level. Hurwitz and Morgenstern[17] found that the correlates of disability due to back pain included age, gender, race, education, marital status, employment status, presence of comorbidities, weight, and traumatic onset of back problem. Men, unemployed individuals, and persons with other disabling conditions were most likely to report a disabling back problem. Disabling back conditions were most common in the 35–54-year-old groups and among those with less than a high school degree.

Disability is an important outcome of LBP since it potentially results in a reduction of people available for the workforce. Recognizing the impact of disability, Rizzo et al.[18] investigated the labor productivity losses associated with back pain. The authors used models to examine the probabilities of being employed and of missing workdays. Having back pain among older age cohorts resulted in a lower probability of being employed and increased the risk of incurring a disability day. When the models were translated into lost earnings the results for loss of employment were an average of $1,106 annually for men and $725 annually for women. The results for disability days were an average of $124 annually for men and $48 annually for women. At an aggregated level these figures result in annual productivity losses due to back pain of 28 billion in 1996 dollars.

HEALTHCARE UTILIZATION DUE TO LOW BACK PAIN

Rates of provider utilization for spine-related pain vary by provider type. The utilization rate for persons with LBP ranges from 39–85% for care sought from any category of healthcare provider. Rates of physician utilization are the highest of any provider followed by rates of chiropractic utilization and rates of PT utilization.

Utilization rates vary by the country in which a study was conducted and by the nature of the sample. By country, rates reflect healthcare patterns that are specific to the health services systems in place. The U.S. utilization rate of 85% of all persons with LBP having seen any provider[3] is the rate most often used to represent a national standard. However, in studies based on a population in North Carolina a utilization rate of 40% from all persons with LBP was reported.[6]

Feuerstein, Marcus, and Huang[19] demonstrated that trends in overall utilization rates in the United States are stable by using a 10-year period of time. The rate of utilization for outpatient treatment for LBP was 4.5 per 100 population. Among those who received care, the proportion of physician care increased from 64–74% and the proportion of PT care increased from 5–9% in the 10-year period.

Only two studies have examined rates of multiple provider utilization and the factors that influence multiple provider use. Sundararajan et al.[20] examined the combination of using a physician and a chiropractor. Twenty-one percent of subjects saw more than one provider and this was associated with being referred by the initial provider seen, disease severity, and type of provider first seen. Côté et al.[21] provided data on many provider types but only conducted a detailed analysis of the physician and chiropractor combination. These authors found that utilization of this combination of providers was associated with increasing age, lower levels of educational attainment, lower income levels, and worse general health and health-related quality of life scores.

Medical Care

LBP is not a true pathology but rather a symptomatic complaint that encompasses a number of diagnostic entities. Physicians account for the largest proportion of healthcare utilization due to LBP, with 59% of all persons with LBP seeing a physician.[3] At least 2% of all ambulatory care visits to physicians are related to LBP, accounting for 13 million visits on an annual basis.[4,22] Encounters with physicians have been analyzed by two published studies.[23,24]

Cypress[23] published a study examining patient encounters with physicians among persons whose principal complaint was back symptoms. Among persons with back symptoms 61% were treated by primary care physicians while the remainder were seen by specialty physicians. Most persons visiting physicians due to LBP were aged 25–64 (70%) and the highest visit rate was found among males aged 45–64 years. Services ordered or provided by the physicians were both diagnostic and therapeutic in nature. Among diagnostic services, physicians offered a physical exam, X-ray, blood pressure check, and clinical lab tests most often. Among the therapeutic interventions, physicians most often prescribed drugs, provided medical counseling, and referred to physical therapy. Study results were representative of a national snapshot of ambulatory care offered in physician offices for LBP.

Hart et al.[24] conducted a follow-up study on physician office visits for LBP. Persons aged 25–44 made the largest number of visits. Women made more visits than men. Among the racial and ethnic groups identified, African Americans and Hispanics had the highest rates of visits per thousand persons. The most common source of payment for visits was commercial insurance. In an analysis of the content of care provided, these authors concurred with Cypress in finding that the therapeutic intervention of choice for physicians was prescribing drugs followed by medical counseling. Again, physicians conducted physical examinations and used X-ray in diagnosis.

Physician care for LBP is quite varied and is greatly dependent upon physician specialty.[25] Orthopedists are more likely to order X-rays; physiatrists are more likely to order exercise; osteopathic physicians use more spinal manipulation. Nonetheless, guidelines on the management of acute LBP have clarified the medical nonsurgical approach to mechanical conditions affecting the spine.[26,27] The guidelines and more recently published review articles[26–29] have reiterated that medical care should revolve around conservative care, counseling, and education. Conservative care in this context refers directly to the care provided through physical therapy for LBP and includes manipulative and exercise approaches to the problem.

Physical Therapy Care

LBP is a disorder that has tremendous impact on service provision in physical therapy. Given this impact it is surprising that only three studies have examined physical therapy utilization among persons with LBP.[30-32] These three studies examined the patterns of utilization, the nature of therapy provided, and its cost.

Freburger, Carey, and Holmes[30] studied physician referrals to physical therapy, specifically among persons with spine disorders. Thirty-eight percent of the sample was referred to physical therapy (PT). Need-based characteristics of the patient, specifically physician diagnosis, were positively associated with PT referral, as was education level, with more educated patients more likely to be referred. Older persons and men were less likely to be referred to PT.

In terms of utilization, LBP is the most frequent primary reason a person seeks care from PT.[31] PTs tend to use a combination of interventions in treating LBP rather than relying on any single modality or tool.[31] The interventions most commonly employed by PTs include therapeutic exercise, education, spinal mobilization, and physical modalities.[31-33]

Freburger et al.[30] conducted a study to identify determinants of PT use or care seeking for persons with spine disorders. Using the data from the National Spine Network they found that education level and healthcare payment attributes explained the greatest amount of variation in PT use. The demographic characteristics associated with PT use included being female and being over 50 years of age. Persons who had PT were also more likely to be receiving workers' compensation and be in litigation. The results of their study are key in identifying that there are issues of disparities in access to physical therapy.

Mielenz et al.[32] examined utilization of PT among persons with acute LBP in North Carolina. The likelihood of being treated by a PT was influenced by a person having a greater level of disability and by the provider first seen for an episode of LBP. Persons who saw orthopedic surgeons were most likely to be treated by a PT while persons who saw chiropractors were least likely. Demographic characteristics associated with utilization were similar to those found by Freburger et al.[30]

OUTCOMES MEASUREMENT IN LOW BACK PAIN

With the need for physical therapy established by epidemiologic measures and patients pursuing a course of therapy for symptom resolution, physical therapists need to consider the issues of measurement and, in particular, measurement of outcomes due to LBP. In later chapters, readers will learn about the types of measures used during patient examination by therapists employing the manual therapy approaches in this book. The chapter authors most often use impairment-based measures such as range of motion, strength, or symptom response to provocative movements, as tools of measurement for the patient examination. These measures aid the therapist in determining a diagnosis and in assessing the prognosis, scope, and severity of the patient's problem. In Chapter 11, we draw the reader's attention to the Treatment-Based Classification (TBC) model, which relies on both impairment-based measures and two specific outcome/survey style measures to determine the appropriate intervention and to ascertain prognosis. The measures outlined in Chapter 11, the Fear-Avoidance Beliefs Questionnaire (FABQ) and the

Pain Catastrophizing Scale (PCS) are of use to therapists who wish to understand more about the impact of a patient's pain on daily life and function. In Chapter 11, the reader will learn about the implications of scores on the FABQ and the PCS for treatment decision making and how they fit into clinical prediction rule use.

Outcome measures enable the therapist to assess the impact of the condition, in this case LBP, on the patient's daily activities. Outcome measures may be used to ascertain impact on function at both an initial visit and then as a measure of the effect of an intervention on a patient later in the course of an episode of care. By using an outcome measure at multiple points during an episode of patient care, the therapist can understand and document the impact of interventions on function, quality of life, activities of daily living, and instrumental activities of daily living.

The outcomes measures we present here are all self-administered, condition specific, and commonly used for research and clinical efforts in the area of LBP. The three questionnaires are the Modified Oswestry Disability Questionnaire,[34,35] the Roland Morris Disability Questionnaire,[36] and the Quebec Back Pain Disability Scale.[37] We suggest the therapist select an outcome measure that is appropriate to the patient, that has valid measurement qualities, and that is brief and easy to use. The instruments we present here meet these criteria. While a therapist can certainly elect to use generic health status or health-related quality-of-life instruments, we only selected outcomes measures that are condition specific to LBP. A brief overview of each instrument follows for the patient case presented in the next chapter; we give data using the Modified Oswestry Disability Questionnaire,[35] but any of these three outcomes measures are suitable to clinical practice.

The first iteration of the Oswestry Disability Questionnaire was developed at an orthopaedic hospital in Oswestry, a town in Shropshire, England, in the latter part of the 1970s.[34] The Oswestry contains 10 sections that describe pain and its impact on a number of daily living activities. Each section is scored from 0 to 5 with higher values indicating more severe activity limitations due to LBP. The Oswestry has been modified with the question about sex life replaced by a question related to home/work function.[35] This replacement from the original questionnaire was made since many patients were unwilling to respond to the sex life question in the clinic. Scoring and interpretation of the modified questionnaire are the same as with the original questionnaire. The Oswestry score calculated from the tool represents the sum of all the values from each of the 10 sections as a percentage out of 50 or the total possible points a patient could have scored if the patient does not answer all the questions. The Oswestry has been reported to have high test-retest reliability. The Oswestry value for minimal detectable change has been reported as 10.5 points.[38]

The Roland Morris Disability Questionnaire was originally published in 1983 and has since been translated into 36 languages and is used widely for LBP outcomes.[36] The scale is made up of 24 statements. The patient is asked to read each statement and make a mark next to any statements that are true about his/her pain. The scoring ranges from 0, which is indicative of no LBP disability, to 24, which indicates severe LBP disability.

The Quebec Back Pain Disability Scale was developed in Canada and published in the mid-1990s as a tool for clinicians to use for the measurement of "functional disability."[37] The scale comprises 20 items that are scored using Likert-style scoring that ranges from 0, "not difficult at all," to 5, "unable to do." A patient's total score is the sum of each of the item scores with higher scores indicating more severe limitation.

SUMMARY

Based on the presentation in this chapter, the therapist should have some understanding of the broader issues that surround LBP care. With this knowledge the therapist can now consider how each patient fits into the picture of the clinical care continuum. In the remaining chapters we explore a single patient on this continuum that has been referred to a physical therapist. The patient is demographically typical of persons with LBP. We will present the patient, his clinical signs and symptoms, and his scores on the outcomes measures. In subsequent chapters we will analyze several models of care a physical therapist may use in the process of examination and intervention for LBP.

REFERENCES

1. Woolf AD, Pfleger B. Burden of major musculoskeletal conditions. *Bull World Health Organ.* 2003;81(9):646–656.
2. Loney PL, Stratford PW. The prevalence of low back pain in adults: a methodological review of the literature. *Phys Ther.* 1999;79(4):384–396.
3. Deyo RA, Tsui-Wu YJ. Descriptive epidemiology of low-back pain and its related medical care in the United States. *Spine.* 1987;12(3):264–268.
4. Deyo RA, Mirza SK, Martin BI. Back pain prevalence and visit rates: estimates from U.S. national surveys, 2002. *Spine.* 2006;31(23):2724–2727.
5. Carey TS, Evans A, Hadler N, Kalsbeek W, McLaughlin C, Fryer J. Care-seeking among individuals with chronic low back pain. *Spine.* 1995;20(3):312–317.

6. Carey TS, Evans AT, Hadler NM, et al. Acute severe low back pain. A population-based study of prevalence and care-seeking. *Spine*. 1996;21(3):339–344.

7. Reisbord LS, Greenland S. Factors associated with self-reported back-pain prevalence: a population-based study. *J Chronic Dis*. 1985;38(8):691–702.

8. Heistaro S, Vartiainen E, Heliövaara M, Puska P. Trends of back pain in eastern Finland, 1972–1992, in relation to socioeconomic status and behavioral risk factors. *Am J Epidemiol*. 1998;148(7):671–682.

9. Dionne CE, Von Korff M, Koepsell TD, Deyo RA, Barlow WE, Checkoway H. Formal education and back pain: a review. *J Epidemiol Community Health*. 2001;55(7):455–468.

10. Pengel LH, Herbert RD, Maher CG, Refshauge KM. Acute low back pain: systematic review of its prognosis. *BMJ*. 2003;327(7410):323.

11. Von Korff M, Deyo RA, Cherkin D, Barlow W. Back pain in primary care. Outcomes at 1 year. *Spine*. 1993;18(7):855–862.

12. Carey TS, Garrett JM, Jackman A, Hadler N. Recurrence and care seeking after acute back pain: results of a long-term follow-up study. North Carolina Back Pain Project. *Med Care*. 1999;37(2):157–164.

13. Enthoven P, Skargren E, Oberg B. Clinical course in patients seeking primary care for back or neck pain: a prospective 5-year follow-up of outcome and health care consumption with subgroup analysis. *Spine*. 2004;29(21):2458–2465.

14. Kelsey JL, White AA, Pastides H, Bisbee GE. The impact of musculoskeletal disorders on the population of the United States. *J Bone Joint Surg Am*. 1979;61(7):959–964.

15. Fanuele JC, Birkmeyer NJ, Abdu WA, Tosteson TD, Weinstein JN. The impact of spinal problems on the health status of patients: have we underestimated the effect? *Spine*. 2000;25(12):1509–1514.

16. Deyo RA, Tsui-Wu YJ. Functional disability due to back pain. A population-based study indicating the importance of socioeconomic factors. *Arthritis Rheum*. 1987;30(11):1247–1253.

17. Hurwitz EL, Morgenstern H. Correlates of back problems and back-related disability in the United States. *J Clin Epidemiol*. 1997;50(6):669–681.

18. Rizzo JA, Abbott TA, Berger ML. The labor productivity effects of chronic backache in the United States. *Med Care*. 1998;36(10):1471–1488.

19. Feuerstein M, Marcus SC, Huang GD. National trends in nonoperative care for nonspecific back pain. *Spine J*. 2004;4(1):56–63.

20. Sundararajan V, Konrad TR, Garrett J, Carey T. Patterns and determinants of multiple provider use in patients with acute low back pain. *J Gen Intern Med*. 1998;13(8):528–533.

21. Côté P, Cassidy JD, Carroll L. The treatment of neck and low back pain: who seeks care? who goes where? *Med Care*. 2001;39(9):956–967.

22. Cherry DK, Burt CW, Woodwell DA. National Ambulatory Medical Care Survey: 2001 summary. *Adv Data*. 2003;(337):1–44.

23. Cypress BK. Characteristics of physician visits for back symptoms: a national perspective. *Am J Public Health*. 1983;73(4):389–395.

24. Hart LG, Deyo RA, Cherkin DC. Physician office visits for low back pain. Frequency, clinical evaluation, and treatment patterns from a U.S. national survey. *Spine*. 1995;20(1):11–19.

25. Cherkin DC, Deyo RA, Wheeler K, Ciol MA. Physician views about treating low back pain. The results of a national survey. *Spine*. 1995;20(1):1–9.

26. Bigos S, Bowyer O, Braen G, et al. *Acute Low Back Problems in Adults*. Clinical Practice Guideline No. 14. AHCPR Publication No. 95-0642. Rockville, MD: Agency for Health Care Policy and Research, Public Health Service, U.S. Department of Health and Human Services. December; 1994.

27. Chou R, Qaseem A, Snow V, et al. Diagnosis and treatment of low back pain: a joint clinical practice guideline from the American College of Physicians and the American Pain Society. *Ann Intern Med.* 2007;147(7):478–491.
28. Atlas SJ, Deyo RA. Evaluating and managing acute low back pain in the primary care setting. *J Gen Intern Med.* 2001;16(2):120–131.
29. Deyo RA, Weinstein JN. Low back pain. *N Engl J Med.* 2001;344(5):363–370.
30. Freburger JK, Carey TS, Holmes GM. Management of back and neck pain: who seeks care from physical therapists? *Phys Ther.* 2005;85(9):872–886.
31. Jette AM, Smith K, Haley SM, Davis KD. Physical therapy episodes of care for patients with low back pain. *Phys Ther.* 1994;74(2):101–110.
32. Mielenz TJ, Carey TS, Dyrek DA, Harris BA, Garrett JM, Darter JD. Physical therapy utilization by patients with acute low back pain. *Phys Ther.* 1997;77(10):1040–1051.
33. Li LC, Bombardier C. Physical therapy management of low back pain: an exploratory survey of therapist approaches. *Phys Ther.* 2001;81(4):1018–1028.
34. Fairbank JC, Couper J, Davies JB, O'Brien JP. The Oswestry Low Back Pain Disability Questionnaire. *Physiotherapy.* 1980;66(8):271–273.
35. Fritz JM, Irrgang JJ. A comparison of a modified Oswestry Low Back Pain Disability Questionnaire and the Quebec Back Pain Disability Scale. *Phys Ther.* 2001;81(2):776–788.
36. Roland M, Morris R. A study of the natural history of back pain. Part I: development of a reliable and sensitive measure of disability in low-back pain. *Spine.* 1983;8(2):141–144.
37. Kopec JA, Esdaile JM, Abrahamowicz M, et al. The Quebec Back Pain Disability Scale. Measurement properties. *Spine.* 1995;20(3):341–352.
38. Davidson M, Keating JL. A comparison of five low back disability questionnaires: reliability and responsiveness. *Phys Ther.* 2002;82(1):8–24.

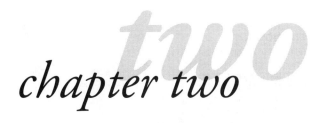

chapter two

Meet Joe Lores

Julia Chevan, PT, PhD, MPH, OCS
Phyllis A. Clapis, PT, DHSc, OCS

Joe Lores represents a typical patient seen in a physical therapy clinic with acute low back pain. This chapter provides the reader with the basic history and examination findings from Joe's first day at the clinic.

BACKGROUND

The patient/client management model from the *Guide to Physical Therapist Practice*[1] provides an ideal prototype to structure the data from our patient's presentation. The patient/client management model (Figure 2–1) contains five elements. These elements lead the therapist through a process that results in selection of the most appropriate intervention for the patient and that incorporates and assures that outcomes are evaluated and measured. For Joe, we documented initial history and examination data on a template that was based on the patient/client management model (Figure 2–2). We used a pain diagram (Figure 2–3) to show the location of Joe's symptoms. In an effort to consider the anticipated goals and outcomes of Joe's care, we used the Oswestry Disability Questionnaire as a measure of his functional limitations and limitations in activities of daily living (Figure 2–4). In later chapters of this book you will find Joe's examination data embellished by the information requested from each chapter author, in a manner consistent with the model being described. The additional data requested was provided by the two text authors (Chevan and Clapis) using the patient/client model and then documented, either in narrative form or on a documentation template provided by the chapter author.

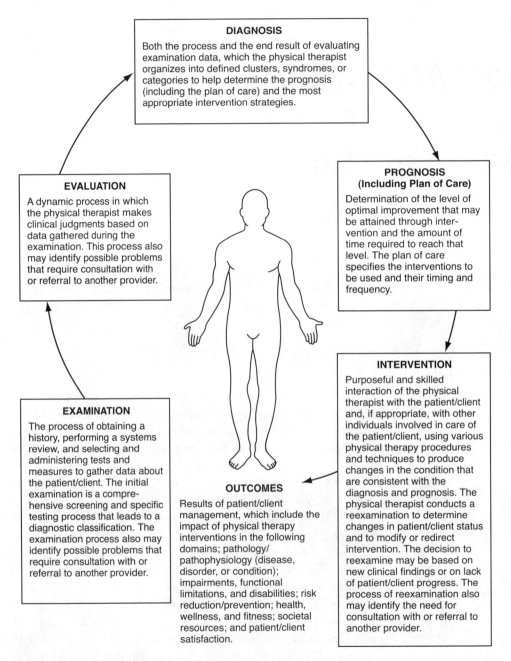

DIAGNOSIS
Both the process and the end result of evaluating examination data, which the physical therapist organizes into defined clusters, syndromes, or categories to help determine the prognosis (including the plan of care) and the most appropriate intervention strategies.

EVALUATION
A dynamic process in which the physical therapist makes clinical judgments based on data gathered during the examination. This process also may identify possible problems that require consultation with or referral to another provider.

PROGNOSIS
(Including Plan of Care)
Determination of the level of optimal improvement that may be attained through intervention and the amount of time required to reach that level. The plan of care specifies the interventions to be used and their timing and frequency.

EXAMINATION
The process of obtaining a history, performing a systems review, and selecting and administering tests and measures to gather data about the patient/client. The initial examination is a comprehensive screening and specific testing process that leads to a diagnostic classification. The examination process also may identify possible problems that require consultation with or referral to another provider.

OUTCOMES
Results of patient/client management, which include the impact of physical therapy interventions in the following domains; pathology/pathophysiology (disease, disorder, or condition); impairments, functional limitations, and disabilities; risk reduction/prevention; health, wellness, and fitness; societal resources; and patient/client satisfaction.

INTERVENTION
Purposeful and skilled interaction of the physical therapist with the patient/client and, if appropriate, with other individuals involved in care of the patient/client, using various physical therapy procedures and techniques to produce changes in the condition that are consistent with the diagnosis and prognosis. The physical therapist conducts a reexamination to determine changes in patient/client status and to modify or redirect intervention. The decision to reexamine may be based on new clinical findings or on lack of patient/client progress. The process of reexamination also may identify the need for consultation with or referral to another provider.

Figure 2–1 Patient/Client Management model. *Source:* Reprinted from *Interactive Guide to Physical Therapist Practice,* 2003, with permission of the American Physical Therapy Association. This material is copyrighted, and any further reproduction or distribution is prohibited.

EXAMINATION

History and Systems Review

Joe is a 40-year-old male who lives in Springfield, Massachusetts. He is of Hispanic descent and speaks and understands Spanish and English. Joe has worked full time as a self-employed plumber since graduating from technical school 14 years ago. He was married at age 23 and became divorced 5 years ago. He currently owns his own home and lives with his 13-year-old son Joey. Joe describes himself as generally healthy, having stopped smoking 11 years ago. He usually drinks one or two cans of beer every day after coming home from work. Although he participated on the varsity wrestling team in high school, he does not exercise regularly. At age 35 Joe was diagnosed with hypertension, for which he is currently taking medication. Additional medical history includes a fractured left clavicle in 1985 and arthroscopic knee surgery in 1986. His family medical history includes heart disease, diabetes, and cancer.

Joe's back pain came on approximately 2 weeks ago, nearly 1 year from the date of his initial back injury, which resolved on its own within a week. Joe was installing a sink, and while bent over, felt immediate pain on the right side of his lower back. He continued to work, but as the day went on the pain travelled into his right buttock. Three days later he saw his primary care physician who ordered an X-ray (which was negative for fracture) and prescribed Flexeril, a muscle relaxant, which he takes at night. He also takes a nonsteroidal anti-inflammatory drug twice daily for pain relief.

In terms of the systems review, Joe had cardiovascular and spinal range of motion impairments. The cardiovascular impairment is related to his blood pressure, which is elevated and being monitored by his physician. The spinal range of motion impairment is presumed to be related to his back pain, the reason he pursued physical therapy. Joe's height and weight corresponded to a body mass index of 28, which is considered overweight. Joe reported that he learned best through pictures and demonstration.

Tests and Measures

Posture: Joe presented with no significant postural deformities. His pelvis was level and his lumbar lordosis was slightly reduced. Both patellae were "frog eyed," meaning they were pointed outward.

Range of Motion: Active and passive movements were assessed. Actively, Joe presented with a 50% loss in flexion and extension, with both movements increasing his symptoms. Sidebending to the right and rotation to the left were also slightly limited, with both movements also increasing symptoms.

Left side bending and right rotation were pain free and range of motion was full. Passive extension was tested in prone, revealed a 25% limitation, and was painful. Flexion in supine (knees to chest) was full yet elicited pain.

Neurological Exam: Joe presented with no neurological deficits. Sensation, myotomal strength, and reflexes were within normal limits.

Palpation: There was palpable fullness in the right lumbar paravertebrals. There was also visible and palpable muscle guarding in the right lower back region.

Joe scored 42% on the Modified Oswestry Disability Questionnaire.[2] This reflects a moderate degree of disability. Accordingly, Joe's greatest difficulties are in sitting, a task that he can only do for less than 10 minutes due to his pain level, and in lifting. It is notable that for Joe, all the tasks of the Oswestry are affected by his current bout of low back pain (LBP). Therapists using the Oswestry for an initial measure and goal development should do so with consideration for the minimum clinically important difference, which has been calculated as a six-point change.[2]

EVALUATION

Evaluation is a process in which the therapist renders a clinical judgment based on the data gathered. Since the data we have presented thus far is only partially completed, the evaluation is limited to classifying Joe into one of the "Musculoskeletal Preferred Practice Patterns" from the *Guide to Physical Therapist Practice*.[1] Thus, Joe is classified into Pattern 4F: "Impaired Joint Mobility, Motor Function, Muscle Performance, Range of Motion, and Reflex Integrity Associated with Spinal Disorders."[3]

THE NEXT STEPS

Further data is needed to complete the picture of Joe in the patient/client management model. This data includes additional information in his history and additional tests and measures. Our hypothesis in writing this textbook is that although all the theories and models used in musculoskeletal physical therapy have some commonalities, they differ not only in intervention choices but also in examination schema. As a result, we have structured Joe's exam so that each chapter author will need to lay out the examination in accordance to their specific model. In the next chapters the student should take note of how the examination leads into a process of evaluation, a resultant diagnosis, the determination of a prognosis, and the selection of interventions.

DOCUMENTATION TEMPLATE FOR PHYSICAL THERAPIST PATIENT/CLIENT MANAGEMENT

Outpatient Form 1, Page 1

Today's Date: _____
Patient ID#: _____

Outpatient History
American Physical Therapy Association

1 Name:

Lores
a Last

Joseph   *S*
b First   c MI   d Jr/Sr

2 Street Address: *99 Mulberry Street*

Springfield   *MA*   *01109*
City   State   Zip

3 Date of Birth: Month [1][0] Day [1][2] Year [1][9][7][1]

4 Sex: a ☒ Male   b ☐ Female

5 Are you: a ☒ Right-handed   b ☐ Left-handed

6 Type of Insurance: a ☒ Insurer   *HMO Blue (Blue Cross Blue Shield)*
b ☐ Workers' Comp c ☐ Medicare d ☐ Self-pay e ☐ Other

7 Race:
a ☐ American Indian or Alaska Native
b ☐ Asian
c ☐ Black or African American
d ☒ Hispanic or Latino
e ☐ Native Hawaiian or Other Pacific Islander
f ☐ White

8 Ethnicity:
a ☒ Hispanic or Latino
b ☐ Not Hispanic or Latino

9 Language:
a ☒ English understood
b ☐ Interpreter needed
c ☒ Language you speak most often: *English*

10 Education:
a Highest grade completed (Circle one): 1 2 3 4 5 6 7 8 9 10 11 12
b ☒ Some college / technical school
c ☐ College graduate
d ☐ Graduate school / advanced degree

SOCIAL HISTORY

11 Cultural/Religious: Any customs or religious beliefs or wishes that might affect care?
No

12 With whom do you live:
a ☐ Alone
b ☐ Spouse only
c ☐ Spouse and otherts)
d ☒ Child (not spouse)   *Joey, age 13*
e ☐ Other relative(s) (not spouse or children)
f ☐ Group setting
g ☐ Personal care attendant
h ☐ Other:

13 Have you completed an advance directive? a ☐ Yes b ☒ No

14 Who referred you to the physical therapist?
Medical doctor

15 Employment/Work (Job/School/Play)
a ☒ Working full-time outside of home
b ☐ Working part-time outside of home
c ☐ Working full-time from home
d ☐ Working part-time from home
e ☐ Homemaker f ☐ Student g ☐ Retired h ☐ Unemployed
i Occupation: *Plumber*

LIVING ENVIRONMENT

16 Does your home have:
a ☐ Stairs, no railing
b ☒ Stairs, railing
c ☐ Ramps
d ☐ Elevator
e ☐ Uneven terrain
f ☐ Assistive devices (eg, bathroom): _____
g ☐ Any obstacles:

17 Do you use:
a ☐ Cane
b ☐ Walker or rollator
c ☐ Manual wheelchair
d ☐ Motorized wheelchair
e ☒ Glasses, hearing aids
f ☐ Other:
_____

18 Where do you live:
a ☒ Private home
b ☐ Private apartment
c ☐ Rented room
d ☐ Board and care / assisted living / group home
e ☐ Homeless (with or without shelter)
f ☐ Long-term care facility (nursing home)
g ☐ Hospice
h ☐ Other: _____

19 GENERAL HEALTH STATUS
a Please rate your health:
(1) ☐ Excellent (2) ☒ Good (3) ☐ Fair (4) ☐ Poor
b Have you had any major life changes during past year? (eg, new baby, job change, death of a family member) (1) ☐ Yes (2) ☒ No

20 SOCIAL/HEALTH HABITS
a Smoking
(1) Currently smoke tobacco? (a) ☐ Yes 1. ☐ Cigarettes: # of packs per day___
2. ☐ Cigars/Pipes: # per day___
(b) ☒ No

(2) Smoked in past? (a) ☒ Yes Year quit: [7][9][9][9] (b) ☐ No

b Alcohol
(1) How many days per week do you drink beer, wine, or other alcoholic beverages, on average? *5-7*
(2) If one beer one glass of wine, or one cocktail equals one drink, how many drinks do you have on an average day? *1-2*

c Exercise
Do you exercise beyond normal daily activities and chores?
(a) ☐ Yes Describe the exercise: _____
1. On average, how many days per week do you exercise or do physical activity? _____
2. For how many minutes, on an average day? _____
(b) ☒ No

21 FAMILY HISTORY (Indicate whether mother, father, brother/sister, aunt/uncle, or grandmother/grandfather, and age of onset if known)
a Heart disease: *Father*
b Hypertension: *Father*
c Stroke: _____
d Diabetes: *Mother*
e Cancer: *Father*
f Psychological: _____
g Arthritis: _____
h Osteoporosis: _____
i Other: _____

Figure 2–2 Documentation template for physical therapist patient/client management. *Source:* Reprinted from *Interactive Guide to Physical Therapist Practice,* 2003, with permission of the American Physical Therapy Association. This material is copyrighted, and any further reproduction or distribution is prohibited.

DOCUMENTATION TEMPLATE FOR PHYSICAL THERAPIST PATIENT/CLIENT MANAGEMENT
Outpatient Form , Page 2

22 MEDICAL/SURGICAL HISTORY

a Please check if you have ever had:

(1) ☐ Arthritis
(2) ☒ Broken bones/ fractures *Clavicle, 1985*
(3) ☐ Osteoporosis
(4) ☐ Blood disorders
(5) ☐ Circulation/vascular problems
(6) ☐ Heart problems
(7) ☒ High blood pressure
(8) ☐ Lung problems
(9) ☐ Stroke
(10) ☐ Diabetes/ high blood sugar
(11) ☐ Low blood sugar/ hypoglycemia
(12) ☐ Head injury

(13) ☐ Multiple sclerosis
(14) ☐ Muscular dystrophy
(15) ☐ Parkinson disease
(16) ☐ Seizures/epilepsy
(17) ☐ Allergies
(18) ☐ Developmental or growth problems
(19) ☐ Thyroid problems
(20) ☐ Cancer
(21) ☐ Infectious disease (eg, tuberculosis, hepatitis)
(22) ☐ Kidney problems
(23) ☐ Repeated infections
(24) ☐ Ulcers/stomach problems
(25) ☐ Skin diseases
(26) ☐ Depression
(27) ☐ Other: _____

b Within the past year, have you had any of the following symptoms? (Check all that apply)

(1) ☐ Chest pain
(2) ☐ Heart palpitations
(3) ☐ Cough
(4) ☐ Hoarseness
(5) ☐ Shortness of breath
(6) ☐ Dizziness or blackouts
(7) ☐ Coordination problems
(8) ☐ Weakness in arms or legs
(9) ☐ Loss of balance
(10) ☐ Difficulty walking
(11) ☒ Joint pain or swelling *knees*
(12) ☐ Pain at night

(13) ☐ Difficulty sleeping
(14) ☐ Loss of appetite
(15) ☐ Nausea/vomiting
(16) ☐ Difficulty swallowing
(17) ☐ Bowel problems
(18) ☐ Weight loss/gain
(19) ☐ Urinary problems
(20) ☐ Fever/chills/sweats
(21) ☐ Headaches
(22) ☐ Hearing problems
(23) ☐ Vision problems
(24) ☐ Other: _____

c Have you ever had surgery? (1) ☒ Yes (2) ☐ No
If yes, please describe, and include dates:

	Month	Year
Knee arthroscope	1 1	1 9 8 6
	☐☐	☐☐☐☐
	☐☐	☐☐☐☐

For men only: d Have you been diagnosed with prostate disease?
(1) ☐ Yes (2) ☒ No

For women only:
Have you been diagnosed with:
e Pelvic inflammatory disease?
(1) ☐ Yes (2) ☐ No
f Endometriosis?
(1) ☐ Yes (2) ☐ No
g Trouble with your period?
(1) ☐ Yes (2) ☐ No

h Complicated pregnancies or deliveries?
(1) ☐ Yes (2) ☐ No
i Pregnant, or think you might be pregnant?
(1) ☐ Yes (2) ☐ No
j Other gynecological or obstetrical difficulties?
(1) ☐ Yes (2) ☐ No
If yes, please describe:

23 CURRENT CONDITION(S)/CHIEF COMPLAINT(S)

a Describe the problem(s) for which you seek physical therapy:
Right sided low back pain and right buttock pain

	Month	Year
b When did the problem(s) begin (date)? *Started 2 weeks ago*
c What happened? *Installing a sink, when putting the sink in he felt a sudden pain*
d Have you ever had the problem(s) before?
(1) ☒ Yes
(a) What did you do for the problem(s)? *Rested, took Tylenol*
(b) Did the problem(s) get better?
1. ☒ Yes 2. ☐ No
(c) About how long did the problem(s) last? *One week*
(2) ☐ No

23 Current Condition(s)/Chief Complaint(s) (continued)

e How are you taking care of the problem(s) now? _____
Saw MD. taking medication
f What makes the problem(s) better? _____
Lying down, rest
g What makes the problem(s) worse? _____
Sitting, bending, many tasks at work, getting up from sitting, lifting
h What are your goals for physical therapy? _____
Get rid of the pain; be able to work pain-free
i Are you seeing anyone else for the problem(s)? (Check all that apply)

(1) ☐ Acupuncturist
(2) ☐ Cardiologist
(3) ☐ Chiropractor
(4) ☐ Dentist
(5) ☐ Family practitioner
(6) ☐ Internist
(7) ☐ Massage therapist
(8) ☐ Neurologist
(9) ☐ Obstetrician/gynecologist

(10) ☐ Occupational therapist
(11) ☐ Orthopedist
(12) ☐ Osteopath
(13) ☐ Pediatrician
(14) ☐ Podiatrist
(15) ☒ Primary care physician
(16) ☐ Rheumatologist
Other: _____

24 FUNCTIONAL STATUS/ACTIVITY LEVEL (Check all that apply)

a ☐ Difficulty with locomotion/movement:
(1) ☐ Bed mobility
(2) ☐ Transfers (such as moving from bed to chair, from bed to commode)
(3) ☐ Gait (walking)
(a) ☐ On level (c) ☐ On ramps
(b) ☐ On stairs (d) ☐ On uneven terrain
b ☐ Difficulty with self-care (such as bathing, dressing, eating, toileting)
c ☒ Difficulty with home management (such as household chores, shopping, driving/transportation, care of dependents)
d ☒ Difficulty with community and work activities/integration
(1) ☒ Work/school *Plumber tasks*
(2) ☐ Recreation or play activity

25 MEDICATIONS

a Do you take any prescription medications? (1) ☒ Yes (2) ☐ No
If yes, please list: *Lotensin. Flexeril*

b Do you take any nonprescription medications? (Check all that apply)

(1) ☒ Advil/Aleve
(2) ☐ Antacids
(3) ☐ Ibuprofen/ Naproxen
(4) ☐ Antihistamines
(5) ☐ Aspirin

(6) ☐ Decongestants
(7) ☐ Herbal supplements
(8) ☐ Tylenol
(9) ☐ Other: _____

c Have you taken any medications previously for the condition for which you are seeing the physical therapist?
(1) ☐ Yes (2) ☒ No If yes, please list:

26 OTHER CLINICAL TESTS Within the past year, have you had any of the following tests? (Check all that apply)

a ☐ Angiogram
b ☐ Arthroscopy
c ☐ Biopsy
d ☐ Blood tests
e ☐ Bone scan
f ☐ Bronchoscopy
g ☐ CT scan
h ☐ Doppler ultrasound
i ☐ Echocardiogram
j ☐ EEG (electroencephalogram)
k ☐ EKG (electrocardiogram)
l ☐ EMG (electromyogram)

m ☐ Mammogram
n ☐ MRI
o ☐ Myelogram
p ☐ NCV (nerve conduction velocity)
q ☐ Pap smear
r ☐ Pulmonary function test
s ☐ Spinal tap
t ☐ Stool tests
u ☐ Stress test (eg, treadmill, bicycle)
v ☐ Urine tests
w ☒ X-rays
x ☐ Other: _____

Figure 2–2 Documentation template for physical therapist patient/client management (continued).

**DOCUMENTATION TEMPLATE FOR
PHYSICAL THERAPIST PATIENT/CLIENT MANAGEMENT**
Systems Review

	Not Impaired	Impaired		Not Impaired	Impaired
CARDIOVASCULAR/PULMONARY SYSTEM	☐	☒	**MUSCULOSKELETAL SYSTEM**		

CARDIOVASCULAR/PULMONARY SYSTEM

Blood pressure: _135/85_

Edema: _None noted_

Heart rate: _68_

Respiratory rate: _12_

Patient's blood pressure controlled by medication and diet

INTEGUMENTARY SYSTEM ☒ ☐

Integrity
Pliability (texture): _Normal_
Presence of scar formation: _None noted_
Skin color: _Normal_
Skin integrity: _Normal_

MUSCULOSKELETAL SYSTEM

Gross Range of Motion ☐ ☒

Gross Strength ☒ ☐

Gross Symmetry ☐ ☐
Standing: _Grossly symmetrical_
Sitting: _Grossly symmetrical_
Activity specific: _____

Other: _____

Height _5' 10"_

Weight _195 lbs_

NEUROMUSCULAR SYSTEM

Gross Coordinated Movements
Balance ☒ ☐
Gait ☒ ☐
Locomotion ☒ ☐
Transfers ☒ ☐
Transitions ☒ ☐
Motor function (motor control, motor learning) ☒ ☐

COMMUNICATION, AFFECT, COGNITION, LEARNING STYLE

Communication (eg, age-appropriate) ☒ ☐

Orientation x 3 (person/place/time) ☒ ☐

Emotional/behavioral responses ☒ ☐

Learning barriers:
☒ None
☐ Vision
☐ Hearing
☐ Unable to read
☐ Unable to understand what is read
☐ Language/needs interpreter
☐ Other: _____

Education needs:
☒ Disease process
☐ Safety
☐ Use of devices/equipment
☒ Activities of daily living
☒ Exercise program
☐ Other: _____

How does patient/client best learn? ☒ Pictures ☐ Reading ☐ Listening ☒ Demonstration ☐ Other:

Figure 2–2 Documentation template for physical therapist patient/client management (continued).

DOCUMENTATION TEMPLATE FOR
PHYSICAL THERAPIST PATIENT/CLIENT MANAGEMENT
Tests and Measures

KEY TO TESTS AND MEASURES:

1 Aerobic Capacity/Endurance
2 Anthropometric Characteristics
3 Arousal, Attention, and Cognition
4 Assistive and Adaptive Devices
5 Circulation (Arterial, Venous, Lymphatic)
6 Cranial and Peripheral Nerve Integrity
7 Environmental, Home, and Work (Job/School/Play) Barriers
8 Ergonomics and Body Mechanics
9 Gait, Locomotion, and Balance
10 Integumentary Integrity
11 Joint Integrity and Mobility
12 Motor Function (Motor Control and Motor Learning)
13 Muscle Performance (Including Strength, Power, and Endurance)

14 Neuromotor Development and Sensory Integration
15 Orthotic, Protective, and Supportive Devices
16 Pain
17 Posture
18 Prosthetic Requirements
19 Range of Motion (Including Muscle Length)
20 Reflex Integrity
21 Self-Care and Home Management (Including Activities of Daily Living and Instrumental Activities of Daily Living)
22 Sensory Integrity
23 Ventilation and Respiration/Gas Exchange
24 Work (Job/School/Play), Community, and Leisure Integration or Reintegration (Including Instrumental Activities of Daily Living)

NOTES:

Posture

In standing: Iliac crestis. ASIS and PSIS all even

Lumbar lordosis is slightly reduced

Frog eyed patellae

Active ROM

Flexion 50%   increases symptoms

Extension 50% increases symptoms

Side bend right 75%   increases symptoms

Side bend left 100%

Rotation left   80%

Rotation right 100%

Passive ROM

Prone extension 75% increases symptoms

Supine flexion 100% increases symptoms

Neurologic Screen

Sensation testing by dermatome is bilateral normal

Reflexes are bilateral symmetrical with 2+ Patellar and Achilles

Strength by myotome level is bilateral normal

SLR is negative

Palpation

Increased fullness noted in right paravertebral region

Marked muscle guarding on right

Figure 2–2 Documentation template for physical therapist patient/client management (continued).

DOCUMENTATION TEMPLATE FOR
PHYSICAL THERAPIST PATIENT/CLIENT MANAGEMENT
Evaluation

PREFERRED PHYSICAL THERAPIST PRACTICE PATTERNS^SM

DIAGNOSIS:

Musculoskeletal Patterns

- ☐ A: Primary Prevention/Risk Reduction for Skeletal Demineralization
- ☐ B: Impaired Posture
- ☐ C: Impaired Muscle Performance
- ☐ D: Impaired Joint Mobility, Motor Function, Muscle Performance, and Range of Motion Associated With Connective Tissue Dysfunction
- ☐ E: Impaired Joint Mobility, Motor Function, Muscle Performance, and Range of Motion Associated With Localized Inflammation
- ☒ F: Impaired Joint Mobility, Motor Function, Muscle Performance, Range of Motion, and Reflex Integrity Associated With Spinal Disorders
- ☐ G: Impaired Joint Mobility, Muscle Performance, and Range of Motion Associated With Fracture
- ☐ H: Impaired Joint Mobility, Motor Function, Muscle Performance, and Range of Motion Associated With Joint Arthroplasty
- ☐ I: Impaired Joint Mobility, Motor Function, Muscle Performance, and Range of Motion Associated With Bony or Soft Tissue Surgery
- ☐ J: Impaired Motor Function, Muscle Performance, Range of Motion, Gait, Locomotion, and Balance Associated With Amputation

Neuromuscular Patterns

- ☐ A: Primary Prevention/Risk Reduction for Loss of Balance and Falling
- ☐ B: Impaired Neuromotor Development
- ☐ C: Impaired Motor Function and Sensory Integrity Associated With Nonprogressive Disorders of the Central Nervous System—Congenital Origin or Acquired in Infancy or Childhood
- ☐ D: Impaired Motor Function and Sensory Integrity Associated With Nonprogressive Disorders of the Central Nervous System—Acquired in Adolescence or Adulthood
- ☐ E: Impaired Motor Function and Sensory Integrity Associated With Progressive Disorders of the Central Nervous System
- ☐ F: Impaired Peripheral Nerve Integrity and Muscle Performance Associated With Peripheral Nerve Injury
- ☐ G: Impaired Motor Function and Sensory Integrity Associated With Acute or Chronic Polyneuropathies
- ☐ H: Impaired Motor Function, Peripheral Nerve Integrity, and Sensory Integrity Associated With Nonprogressive Disorders of the Spinal Cord
- ☐ I: Impaired Arousal, Range of Motion, and Motor Control Associated With Coma, Near Coma, or Vegetative State

Cardiovascular/Pulmonary Patterns

- ☐ A: Primary Prevention/Risk Reduction for Cardiovascular/Pulmonary Disorders
- ☐ B: Impaired Aerobic Capacity/Endurance Associated With Deconditioning
- ☐ C: Impaired Ventilation, Respiration/Gas Exchange, and Aerobic Capacity/Endurance Associated With Airway Clearance Dysfunction
- ☐ D: Impaired Aerobic Capacity/Endurance Associated With Cardiovascular Pump Dysfunction or Failure
- ☐ E: Impaired Ventilation and Respiration/Gas Exchange Associated With Ventilatory Pump Dysfunction or Failure
- ☐ F: Impaired Ventilation and Respiration/Gas Exchange Associated With Respiratory Failure
- ☐ G: Impaired Ventilation, Respiration/Gas Exchange, and Aerobic Capacity/Endurance Associated With Respiratory Failure in the Neonate
- ☐ H: Impaired Circulation and Anthropometric Dimensions Associated With Lymphatic System Disorders

Integumentary Patterns

- ☐ A: Primary Prevention/Risk Reduction for Integumentary Disorders
- ☐ B: Impaired Integumentary Integrity Associated With Superficial Skin Involvement
- ☐ C: Impaired Integumentary Integrity Associated With Partial-Thickness Skin Involvement and Scar Formation
- ☐ D: Impaired Integumentary Integrity Associated With Full-Thickness Skin Involvement and Scar Formation
- ☐ E: Impaired Integumentary Integrity Associated With Skin Involvement Extending Into Fascia, Muscle, or Bone and Scar Formation

PROGNOSIS: _____

_____
_____
_____
_____
_____
_____
_____
_____
_____

Figure 2–2 Documentation template for physical therapist patient/client management (continued).

**DOCUMENTATION TEMPLATE FOR
PHYSICAL THERAPIST PATIENT/CLIENT MANAGEMENT**
Plan of Care

Plan of Care

American Physical
Therapy Association

Anticipated Goals: _____
_____
_____
_____
_____

Expected Outcomes: _____
_____
_____
_____

Interventions: _____
_____
_____
_____
_____

**Frequency of Visits/Duration
of Episode of Care:**
_____
_____
_____

Education (including safety, exercise, and disease information): _____
_____
_____

Who was educated? ☐ Patient/client ☐ Family (name and relationship): _____
How did patient/family demonstrate learning:
☐ Patient/client verbalized understanding
☐ Family/significant other verbalized understanding
☐ Patient/client demonstrated correctly
☐ Demonstration was unsuccessful (describe): _____
_____
_____

Discharge Plan: _____
_____
_____
_____
_____
_____
_____
_____
_____
_____
_____

Figure 2–2 Documentation template for physical therapist patient/client management (continued).

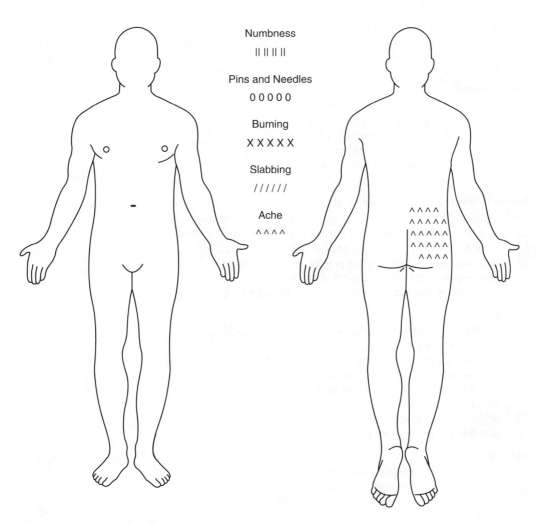

Figure 2–3 Joe's pain diagram.

This questionnaire has been designed to give your therapist information as to how your back pain has affected your ability to manage in everyday life. Please answer every question by placing a mark in the one box that best describes your condition today. We realize you may feel that 2 of the statements may describe your condition, but please mark only the box that most closely describes your current condition.

Pain Intensity
- ❑ I can tolerate the pain I have without having to use pain medication.
- ❑ The pain is bad, but I can manage without having to take pain medication.
- ❑ Pain medication provides me with complete relief from pain.
- ☑ Pain medication provides me with moderate relief from pain.   Value: 3
- ❑ Pain medication provides me with little relief from pain.
- ❑ Pain medication provides has no effect on my pain.

Personal Care (eg, Washing, Dressing)
- ❑ I can take care of myself normally without causing increased pain.
- ❑ I can take care of myself normally, but it increases my pain.
- ☑ It is painful to take care of myself, and I am slow and careful.
- ❑ I need help, but I am able to manage most of my personal care.
- ❑ I need help everyday in most aspects of my care.
- ❑ I do not get dressed, wash with difficulty, and stay in bed.

Lifting
- ❑ I can lift heavy weights without increased pain.
- ❑ I can lift heavy weights, but it causes increased pain.
- ❑ Pain prevents me from lifting heavy weights off the floor, but I can manage if the weights are conveniently positioned (eg, on a table).
- ☑ Pain prevents me from lifting heavy weights, but I can manage light to medium weights if they are conveniently positioned.   Value: 3
- ❑ I can lift only very light weights.
- ❑ I cannot lift or carry anything at all.

Walking
- ❑ Pain does not prevent me from walking any distance.
- ☑ Pain prevents me from walking more than 1 mile.   Value: 1
- ❑ Pain prevents me from walking more than ½ mile.
- ❑ Pain prevents me from walking more than ¼ mile.
- ❑ I can only walk with crutches or a cane.
- ❑ I am in bed most of the time and have to crawl to the toilet.

Sitting
- ❑ I can sit in any chair as long as I like.
- ❑ I can only sit in my favorite chair as long as I like.
- ❑ Pain prevents me from sitting for more than 1 hour.
- ❑ Pain prevents me from sitting for more than ½ hour.
- ☑ Pain prevents me from sitting for more than 10 minutes.   Value: 4
- ❑ Pain prevents me from sitting at all.

Figure 2–4 Modified Oswestry Low Back Pain Questionnaire: Joe Lores.

Standing

❏ I can stand as long as I want without increased pain.
❏ I can stand as long as I want, but it increases my pain.
☑ Pain prevents me from standing more than 1 hour.   Value: 2
❏ Pain prevents me from standing more than ½ hour.
❏ Pain prevents me from standing more than 10 minutes.
❏ Pain prevents me from standing at all.

Sleeping

❏ Pain does not prevent me from sleeping well.
☑ I can sleep well only by using pain medication.   Value: 1
❏ Even when I take pain medication, I sleep less than 6 hours.
❏ Even when I take pain medication, I sleep less than 4 hours.
❏ Even when I take pain medication, I sleep less than 2 hours.
❏ Pain prevents me from sleeping at all.

Social Life

❏ My social life is normal and does not increase my pain.
❏ My social life is normal, but it increases my level of pain.
☑ Pain prevents me from participating in more energetic activities (eg, sports dancing).   Value: 2
❏ Pain prevents me from going out very often.
❏ Pain has restricted my social life to my home.
❏ I have hardly any social life because of my pain.

Traveling

❏ I can travel anywhere without increased pain.
☑ I can travel anywhere, but it increases my pain.   Value: 1
❏ My pain restricts my travel over 2 hours.
❏ My pain restricts my travel over 1 hour.
❏ My pain restricts my travel to short necessary journeys under ½ hour.
❏ My pain prevents all travel except for visits to the physician/therapist or hospital.

Employment/Homemaking

❏ My normal homemaking/job activities do not cause pain.
❏ My normal homemaking/job activities increase my pain, but I can still perform all that is required of me.
☑ I can perform most of my homemaking/job duties, but pain prevents me from performing more physically stressful activities (eg, lifting, vacuuming).   Value: 2
❏ Pain prevents me from doing anything but light duties.
❏ Pain prevents me from doing even light duties.
❏ Pain prevents me from performing any job or homemaking chores.

Modified Oswestry Score = 3+2+3+1+4+2+1+2+1+2 = 21/50

42%

Figure 2–4 Modified Oswestry Low Back Pain Questionnaire: Joe Lores (continued).

REFERENCES

1. American Physical Therapy Association. Guide to Physical Therapist Practice. *Phys Ther*. 1997;77:1163–1650.
2. Fritz JM, Irrgang JJ. A comparison of a modified Oswestry Low Back Pain Disability Questionnaire and the Quebec Back Pain Disability Scale. *Phys Ther*. 2001;81(2):776–788.
3. American Physical Therapy Association. *Interactive Guide to Physical Therapist Practice*. Alexandra, VA: American Physical Therapy Association, 2003. Available at http://guideto practice.apta.org.

chapter three

The Cyriax Approach[*]

Elaine Atkins, DProf, MA, MSCP, Cert FE
Jill Kerr, MSc, BSc, MCSP
Emily Goodlad, MSc, MCSP

The "Cyriax" approach is based on the work of Dr. James Cyriax (1904–1985), a physician who for many years served as Honorary Consultant to the Department of Physical Medicine, St. Thomas' Hospital, London, United Kingdom. The approach is often acknowledged as the cornerstone of both orthopaedic physical therapy and medical nonsurgical treatment of disorders of the musculoskeletal system. Cyriax developed this approach in the 1920s and 1930s. He advocated a systematic examination to test the function of soft tissue and to determine a diagnosis. His three tenets of examination, which still form the basis of the Cyriax approach, are:

1. *All pain has a source.*
2. *The treatment must reach the source.*
3. *All treatment must benefit the lesion.*

Students can learn about the Cyriax approach and continuing education opportunities on the website of the Society of Orthopaedic Medicine, www.somed.org, which is based in London, United Kingdom. The American Association of Orthopaedic Medicine also provides information and educational programs on the approach: www.aaomed.org.

---

[*]Material from this chapter has been adapted from Atkins E, Kerr J, Goodlad E. *A Practical Approach to Orthopaedic Medicine.* 3rd ed. Edinburgh, England: Churchill Livingstone; 2010.

BACKGROUND

The Cyriax approach sits as a springboard for clinical reasoning in musculo-skeletal practice, with the intention of integrating other approaches to widen the clinician's individual practice and experience. We do not present it here dogmatically as the best or only way. Similar to other practitioners, we draw from many approaches for patient management, from our clinical experience, and from the best available evidence to guide, inform, and justify our practice.

The assessment procedures used in the Cyriax approach are based on the principle of "selective tension." That is, normal tissue will function painlessly whereas abnormal tissue will not. Active movements are used to assess range and the patient's willingness to move, allowing for the evaluation of the level of pain and irritability, and/or the identification of "yellow flags."[1] Resisted tests are used to test muscle, tendon, and the attachments to bone. Passive movements test range, but most importantly allow for the assessment of "end-feel," an important concept in the approach that allows for the identification of a so-called capsular or non-capsular pattern and forms part of clinical reasoning towards diagnosis.

The capsular pattern of a joint is denoted by pain and limitation of movement in a fixed proportion. It is usually associated with synovial joints and indicates that "arthritis" is present; be it inflammatory, traumatic, or degenerative. Each joint has its own defined capsular pattern and the non-capsular pattern is, simply, anything other than the capsular pattern. The non-capsular pattern could indicate a possible ligamentous lesion, bursitis, disc derangement, loose body, meniscal tear, or other mechanical disorder.

At the spinal joints the capsular pattern is represented by the spine as a whole, and for the lumbar spine the capsular pattern is limitation of extension; equal limitation of side flexions and usually full flexion. Lumbar rotations are not routinely tested within the Cyriax approach since there is no appreciable rotation[2] and are therefore not noted in the capsular pattern.

Capsular pattern of the lumbar spine

Limitation of extension
Equal limitation of side flexions
Usually full flexion

The non-capsular pattern in the lumbar spine involves a combination of limited and or painful movements but in different proportions. The pattern is normally asymmetrical (e.g., painful limited forward flexion and right-side flexion) with full range of left-side flexion and pain at end range of extension only. In the lumbar spine a non-capsular pattern is more usually associated with mechanical derangements that, with consideration of other factors, may usually be treated in musculoskeletal practice.

Cyriax's original premise was that "the great preponderance of lumbar disorders are attributable to disc lesions"[2] and subjective and objective signs were devised to establish whether the lesion was "nuclear," "annular," "mixed," or "sciatica associated with a large disc displacement" to guide treatment. However, as musculoskeletal practice has developed, practitioners have become less confident in the pathology or pathologies underlying nonspecific low back pain (LBP), believing that it could arise from many conditions.[3] Models classified on the basis of symptoms and signs rather than pathoanatomy have become more useful clinically to guide treatment choices in the management of non-specific LBP and these have now become the subject of scrutiny.[4,5] Building on Cyriax's classification based on symptoms and signs, Figure 3–1 outlines the four clinical models that guide the application of the approach.

For the patient classified as having signs and symptoms consistent with model 1, traction is the treatment of choice for a lumbar lesion of gradual onset. However, manipulation can be applied, providing there are no contraindications, since, if successful, the response is quicker. Manipulative techniques may be modified and applied as mobilizing techniques using manual distraction forces. Manipulation is the treatment of choice for patients with lumbar lesions of sudden onset, classified as model 2, provided there are no contraindications to treatment. Manipulation is also the treatment of choice for patients classified as model 3, as it can achieve immediate results. If manipulation fails or is only partially successful, traction may be applied.

For model 4 patients, treatment is aimed at relieving pain. The more peripheral the symptom, the less likely manipulation is to be successful. Manipulation should not be attempted if the neurological deficit is severe and progressing, but other modalities (e.g., traction and mobilization) may provide pain relief. A caudal epidural of corticosteroid and local anaesthetic may be indicated.[2,6-8] Alternatively, spontaneous recovery is likely and may be awaited, with suitable reassurance and/or analgesia being given to the patient.

Model 1—The lumbar lesion of gradual onset

Factors from the subjective examination

- Central, bilateral, or unilateral pain (ideally not referred below the knee)
- Gradual onset
- Patient cannot recall the exact mode and time of onset
- May be precipitated by a period of prolonged flexion

Factors from the objective examination

- Non-capsular pattern of pain and limitation of movement
- May have increased pain on side flexion towards the painful side
- No neurological signs

Model 2—The lumbar lesion of sudden onset

Factors from the subjective examination

- Central, bilateral, or unilateral pain (ideally not referred below the knee)
- Sudden onset
- Patient can recall the exact mode and time of onset

Factors from the objective examination

- Non-capsular pattern of pain and limitation of movement
- May have increased pain on side flexion away from the painful side
- No neurological signs

Model 3—The lumbar lesion of mixed onset

Factors from the subjective examination

- Central, bilateral, or unilateral pain (ideally not referred below the knee)
- Patient may recall the exact mode and time of onset, but the initial pain settles
- Sometime later (hours or days) a gradual onset of pain occurs

Factors from the objective examination

- Non-capsular pattern of pain and limitation of movement
- No neurological signs

Model 4—The lumbar lesion presenting with referred leg symptoms

Factors from the subjective examination

- Initial presentation of central or unilateral back or buttock pain, followed by referred leg pain (the central pain usually ceasing or diminishing, see below)
- Sudden or gradual onset
- Often part of a history of increasing, worsening episodes, therefore usually a progression of the above models
- Patient may or may not recall the exact time and mode of onset
- Patient may complain of root symptoms (i.e., paraesthesia felt in a segmental distribution)

Factors from the objective examination

- Non-capsular pattern of pain and limitation of movement reproducing back and/or leg symptoms
- Root signs may be present (i.e., sensory changes, muscle weakness, absent or reduced reflexes; consistent with the nerve root(s) involved)

Figure 3–1 The four clinical models of the Cyriax Approach.

Overview of the Examination

In this section a commentary will be provided to explain the clinical reasoning associated with the Cyriax examination procedure. The commentary follows the following headings used by Cyriax, which include observation, history (subjective examination), inspection, state at rest, and examination by selective tension (objective examination).

Figure 3–2 is a table of the "red flags" for the possible presence of serious pathology that should be listened for and identified throughout the examination. In isolation, many of the flags may have limited significance but it is for the clinician to consider the general profile of the patient and to decide whether contraindications to treatment exist and/or whether onward referral is indicated.

Observation

A general observation of the patient's face, posture, and gait will alert the examiner to the seriousness of the condition. Patients in acute pain will

---

Red flags: Lumbar Spine

- Young: Under 20
- Elderly: First episode over 55
- Violent trauma
- Past medical history of malignancy
- Constant progressive pain
- Cauda equina syndrome
- Unremitting night pain
- Systemically unwell
- Unexplained weight loss
- Drug abuse and HIV
- Long-term systemic steroid use
- Widespread neurological signs and symptoms
- Gait disturbance
- Thoracic pain
- Persisting severe restriction of lumbar flexion
- Associated abdominal pain
- Osteopenic/osteoporotic

Figure 3–2 Red flags: Lumbar spine. *Source:* ©2010 Elaine Atkins, Jill Kerr, and Emily Goodlad. Published by Elsevier Ltd.

generally look tired. They may have adopted an antalgic posture of flexion or lumbar scoliosis, which is generally indicative of an acute locked back, possibly due to a disc lesion. A lumbar lateral shift is pathognomic of a disc lesion.[9] Patients may not be able to sit during the examination due to discomfort from this particular posture. Their gait may be uneasy with steps taken cautiously, obviously wary of provoking twinges of pain by sudden movements or pain on weight-bearing. Foot drop may be evident on walking, indicating involvement of the L4 nerve root affecting the tibialis anterior muscle.

History (Subjective Examination)

There is a close relationship between signs and symptoms from the lumbar spine, sacroiliac joint, and hip joint. The history will help with the differential diagnosis but conditions at each of these areas can coexist.

The *age, occupation, sports, hobbies,* and *lifestyle* of the patient may give an indication of provoking mechanisms. Often the incident precipitating the episode of back pain may be relatively minor, or factors predisposing to the event may have been continuing for some time. Patients will require advice and guidance on the management of their back condition to prevent chronicity.

Many occupations involve flexion activities, for instance the prolonged flexion of the office worker who sits all day, or the repeated and prolonged flexion of the brick-layer. These activities stress the intervertebral joint and patients engaged in these activities require advice about changing postures to minimize the stress inflicted by work. Patients should receive advice about manual handling in their place of work. The vibration of motor vehicle driving may have an influence, as well as the sitting posture involved, which is known to increase intradiscal pressure.[10]

In patients with chronic LBP, emotional, environmental, and industrial factors may influence pain perception, while monotony or dissatisfaction at work or home is relevant as well.[10] Enquiry should be made about the possibilities of secondary gain factors relating to disability, or the presence of psychological or social stresses that might predispose the patient to chronic pain disorders.[11]

The *site* of the pain will give an indication of its origin. Lumbar pain is generally localized to the back and buttocks or felt in the limb in a segmental pattern. Sacroiliac pain may be unilateral, felt in the buttock, or more commonly in the groin, and occasionally referred into the leg. The hip joint may produce an area of pain in the buttock consistent with the L3 segment, pain in the groin, or pain referred down the anteromedial aspect of the thigh and leg to the medial aspect of the ankle.

Dural pain is multisegmental and may be central or bilateral. Pressure on the dural nerve root sleeve will be referred segmentally to the relevant dermatome. Pressure on the nerve root will refer pain to the relevant limb with accompanying symptoms of paraesthesia at the distal end of the dermatome.

The *spread* of pain will not only give an indication of its origin, but also the severity or irritability of the lesion. Generally, the more peripherally the pain is referred, the greater the source of irritation. A mechanical lesion due to a displaced lumbar disc produces central or unilateral back or buttock pain. If the pain shifts into the leg, it generally ceases or is reduced in the back. Pain of nonmusculoskeletal origin does not follow this pattern and serious lesions produce an increasing spreading pain, with pain in the back remaining as severe as that felt peripherally.

The *onset* and *duration* of the pain can guide the choice of treatment. In very general terms, a sudden onset of pain may respond to manipulation, while a gradual onset of pain may respond better to traction.

The nature and mode of onset are important. The patient may remember the exact time and mode of onset that may have involved a flexed and rotated posture. Even if the patient reports a gradual onset of pain, a minor traumatic incident some time before the onset of back pain or the maintenance of a sustained flexion posture may have been sufficient to provoke the symptoms.

The gradual onset of degenerative osteoarthrosis is common in the zygapophyseal joints and hip joints, while a subluxation of the sacroiliac joint can occur with a sudden onset. Serious pathology develops insidiously.

If trauma is involved, the exact nature of the trauma should be ascertained and any possible fracture eliminated. Direct trauma may produce soft tissue contusions, while fracture may involve the spinous process, transverse process, pars interarticularis, vertebral body, or vertebral end-plate. Compression fractures of the vertebral body are common in those falling from a height, horse riders, etc., and involve the vulnerable cancellous bone of the vertebral body.[12] Hyperflexion injuries may cause ligamentous lesions or involve the capsule of the zygapophyseal joint, while hyperextension injuries compress the zygapophyseal joints. Both forces can injure the intervertebral disc.

The *symptoms* and *behavior* need to be considered. The behavior of the pain will give an indication of the irritability of the patient's condition and provide clues to differential diagnosis. Serious pathologies of the spine, including fractures, tumors, or infections are relatively rare, accounting for less than 1% of all medical cases seen for spinal assessment. The clinician must remain alert to clinical indicators that need more extensive investigation than the basic clinical examination.[13]

The pattern of all previous episodes of back pain should be ascertained; as with disc lesions, a pattern of gradually worsening and increasing episodes of pain usually emerges.[1]

The typical pattern of pain from disc herniation is usually one of a central pain that moves laterally. As the pain moves laterally, the central pain usually ceases or reduces. A gradually increasing central pain accompanied by an increasing leg pain is indicative of serious pathology and this pain is usually not altered by either rest or activity.

The daily pattern of pain is important and typically a disc lesion produces either a pattern of pain that is better first thing in the morning after rest, becoming worse as the day goes on, or since the disc imbibes water overnight, the patient may experience increased pain on weight-bearing first thing in the morning due to increased pressure on sensitive tissues. Patients can sleep reasonably well at night, as they are usually able to find a position of ease, but may be woken as they turn.

Mechanical pain can cause an on/off response through compression or distortion of pain-sensitive structures. This can involve the annulus itself or structures in the vertebral canal. The patient with a disc lesion usually complains of pain on movement easing with rest. Changing pressures in the disc affect the pain and it tends to be worse with sitting and stooping postures than when standing or lying down. In an acute locked back, small movements can create exquisite "twinging" pain.

Herniated disc material may produce an inflammatory response resulting in chemical pain. Chemical pain is characteristically a constant ache associated with morning stiffness. Sharper pain can also be associated with chemical irritation as the nerve endings become sensitized and respond to a lower threshold of stimulation. It is important to differentiate mechanical back pain from inflammatory arthritis and sacroiliac joint lesions through consideration of other factors, since they also produce pain associated with early-morning stiffness.

Radicular pain is generally a severe lancinating pain, often burning in nature, which is felt in the distribution of the dermatome associated with the nerve root. Sciatica is commonly associated with lumbar disc pathology and will occur if the L4–L5, S1, or S2 nerve roots are involved. If the higher levels are involved, pain will similarly be referred into the relevant segment.

The language used by patients to describe the quality of their pain will indicate the balance between the physical and emotional elements of their pain.

The other symptoms described by the patient provide evidence for differential diagnosis, contraindications to treatment and the severity or irritability of the lesion.

An increase in pressure through coughing, sneezing, laughing, or straining can increase the back pain and this is the main dural symptom. Paraesthesia is usually felt at the distal end of the dermatome and is a symptom of nerve root compression. Confirmation of this is made through the objective compression signs of muscle weakness, altered sensation, and reduced or absent reflexes.

Specific questions must be asked concerning pain or paraesthesia in the perineum and genital area as well as bladder and bowel function. The presence of any of these symptoms indicates compression of the S4 nerve root and indicates immediate referral for surgical opinion. Manipulation is absolutely contraindicated in these cases, since a worsening of the situation could lead to irreversible damage to the cauda equina.

Bilateral sciatica with objective neurological signs and bilateral limitation of straight leg raise suggest a massive central protrusion compressing the cauda equina through the posterior longitudinal ligament, with possible rupture of the ligament.[14] It is an absolute contraindication to manipulation for the reason mentioned previously.

Questioning the patient about *other joint involvement* will indicate whether inflammatory arthritis exists or if there is a tendency towards degenerative osteoarthrosis.

The *past medical history* and the patient's current general health will help to eliminate possible serious pathology, past or present. An unexplained recent weight loss may be significant in systemic disease or malignancy. Visceral lesions can refer pain to the back (e.g., kidney, aortic aneurysm, or gynecological conditions). Infections should be obvious, with an unwell patient showing a fever. Malignancy can affect the lumbar and pelvic region but the pattern of the pain behavior does not generally fit that of musculoskeletal origin. Past history of primary tumor may indicate secondaries as a possible cause of back pain. Serious conditions produce an unrelenting pain; night pain is usually a feature and is responsible for the patient looking tired and ill.

Any ongoing conditions and treatment should be established as well as other previous or current musculoskeletal problems with previous episodes of the current complaint, any treatment given, and the outcome of treatment.

The *medications* taken by the patient will indicate their current medical state as well as alerting the examiner to possible contraindications to treatment. Anticoagulant therapy and long-term oral steroids are contraindications to manipulation. It is useful to know what analgesics are being taken and how frequently to give an indication of the severity of the condition. It can also be used as an objective marker for progression of treatment, with the need for less analgesia indicating a positive improvement. If patients are currently taking antidepressant medication, this may indicate their emotional state and possibly exclude them from manipulation. Care is needed in making this decision, however, since antidepressants can be used in low doses as an adjunct to analgesics in back pain.

Inspection

The patient should be adequately undressed down to underwear and in a good light. A general inspection from behind, each side, and in front will reveal any bony deformity. The general spinal curvatures are assessed as well as the level of the shoulders, inferior angles of the scapulae, buttock and popliteal creases, the position of the umbilicus, and the posture of the feet.

Any structural or acquired scoliosis is noted. Small deviations can be noted by assessing the distance between the waist and the elbow in the standing position. In hyperacute back pain, the patient may be fixed in a flexed posture and unable to stand upright, and any attempt to do so produces twinges of pain.

The level of the iliac crests, the posterior, and anterior superior iliac spine gives an overall impression of leg length discrepancy or pelvic distortion. If these are considered relevant, they can be investigated further.

Color changes and swelling would not be expected in the lumbar spine unless there has been a history of direct trauma. Any marks on the skin, lipomas, "faun's beards" (tufts of hair), birthmarks, or café-au-lait spots may indicate underlying spinal bony or neurological defects.[12,15] An isolated "orange-peel" appearance of the skin that is tough and dimpled may indicate spondylolisthesis at that level.[12] Patients with LBP often apply a hot water bottle to the area, which produces an erythematous skin reaction called erythema ab igne (redness from the fire). Swelling is not usually a feature, but muscle spasm may give the appearance or impression of swelling, especially to the patient.

Muscle wasting may not be obvious if the onset of LBP is recent. Chronic or recurrent episodes of pain may show wasting in the calf muscles or possibly the quadriceps or gluteal muscles.

Palpation may be conducted to assess changes in skin temperature and sweating suggestive of autonomic involvement. In standing, the lumbar spine is palpated for a "shelf" that would indicate spondylolisthesis.

State at Rest

Before any movements are performed, the state at rest is established to provide a baseline for subsequent comparison.

Examination by Selective Tension (Objective Examination)

The suggested sequence for the objective examination is found in Exhibit 3–1. A "Star Diagram" (Figure 3–3) can be used as convenient shorthand for recording the active movement findings of the objective examination. The diagram is explained more fully in Atkins et al.[1] and is shown in the filled in examination form for Joe (Figure 3–4). Active movements are tested in the lumbar spine since, in common with the other spinal regions and shoulders, it can be a focus for "emotional" symptoms. The active movements indicate the "willingness" to perform the movements as well as determining the presence of the capsular or non-capsular pattern. End-feel is not routinely assessed since the information gathered from the active movements is generally sufficient.

Look for apprehension, guarding, or exaggerated movements. An important finding is the non-capsular pattern, usually presenting as an asymmetrical limitation of lumbar movements and indicating a mechanical lesion. The presence of the capsular pattern indicates arthritis and is typically found in degenerative osteoarthrosis of the more mature spine.

Gastrocnemius is assessed for objective signs of nerve root compression. Testing the muscle group against gravity in standing is convenient at this point, in terms of sequence, before lying the patient down.

In supine lying, other joints are eliminated from the examination to confirm that the site of the lesion is in the lumbar spine. Passive flexion and medial and lateral rotation are conducted at the hip to assess the hip joint for the capsular pattern or other hip pathology. The sacroiliac joint is screened using three provocative tests and the FABER test. To limit these tests to the hip and sacroiliac joint it may be necessary to place the patient's forearm under the lumbar spine to increase the lordosis and to stabilize the spine. If the lesion in the lumbar spine is very irritable, it may not be possible to conduct these tests adequately.

The straight leg raise is applied passively to each leg in turn, keeping the knee straight. If positive, this may be interpreted as a dural sign, or as an indicator of neural tension affecting the L4, L5, S1, S2 nerve roots. It is an important clinical test for assessing nerve root tension due to a disc lesion

Exhibit 3–1 Cyriax objective examination sequence (main nerve roots involved are indicated in bold)

Articular Signs
- Active lumbar extension
- Active lumbar right side flexion
- Active lumbar left side flexion
- Active lumbar flexion
- Resisted plantar flexion, gastrocnemius: S1, **S2**

Supine Lying
- Passive hip flexion
- Passive hip medial rotation
- Passive hip lateral rotation
- Sacroiliac joint shear tests
- FABER test
- Straight leg raise: L4, L5, S1, S2

Resisted Tests for Objective Neurological Signs and Alternative Causes of Leg Pain
- Resisted hip flexion, psoas: **L2**
- Resisted ankle dorsiflexion, tibialis anterior : **L4**
- Resisted big toe extension, extensor hallucis longus: **L5**, S1
- Resisted eversion, peroneus longus and brevis: **L5**, **S1**, S2

Skin Sensation
- Big toe only: L4
- First, second, and third toes: L5
- Lateral two toes: S1
- Heel: S2

Reflexes
- Knee reflex: L2, L3, L4
- Ankle reflex : S1, S2
- Plantar response

Prone Lying
- Femoral stretch test: L2, L3, L4
- Resisted knee extension, quadriceps: L2, L3, **L4**
- Resisted knee flexion, hamstrings: **L5**, S1, S2
- Static contraction of the glutei: **L5**, S1, S2

Palpation
- Spinous processes for pain, range, and end-feel

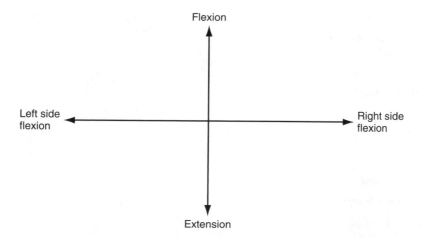

Figure 3–3 Star diagram to record active lumbar movements. *Source:* ©2010 Elaine Atkins, Jill Kerr, and Emily Goodlad. Published by Elsevier Ltd.

when back or leg pain is usually produced at 30° and 40°.[16,17] Increased pain on the addition of neck flexion incriminates the dura mater.

The normal range of movement for the straight leg raise is between 60 and 120°, with movement being limited by tension in the hamstrings. The range of the straight leg raise should be consistent with the range of lumbar flexion, which is also limited to a certain degree by tension in the hamstrings.

The patient is assessed for root signs and alternative causes of pain by the selective application of resisted tests. Objective signs of muscle weakness, altered skin sensation, and absent or reduced reflexes will indicate compression of a nerve root.

The plantar response is assessed by stroking up the lateral border of the sole of the foot and across the metatarsal heads. The normal response is flexor with flexion of the big toe. The Babinski reflex (or Babinski sign) is extension of the big toe. The extensor plantar response is indicative of an upper motor neuron lesion, although this is not likely to occur with lumbar lesions since the spinal cord ends at approximately the level of the L1–L2 disc.

The femoral stretch test (prone knee bending) is applied to assess the dura mater and the L2–L4 dural nerve root sleeves. The knee is passively flexed and, if positive, pain is usually produced at approximately 90°. A sensitizing component of hip extension can be added. Pain is usually felt in the back and the

Name (M/F): *Joe Lores (M)*

OBSERVATION: face, posture, and gait
(note any abnormalities):

Nil to note.

SUBJECTIVE EXAMINATION:

Age/DOB:

40 year old, 10/12/1971

Occupation:

Plumber, manual worker and still working

Sports, Hobbies, Lifestyle:

No hobbies, lives with 13-year-old son

Site & Spread: *Right-sided low back pain spreading into the right buttock.*

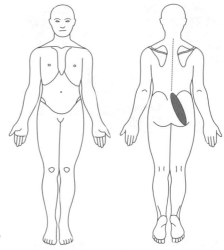

Onset: sudden, gradual, or insidious: *Sudden onset.*

Mechanism of injury: *Installing a sink at work when felt a sudden pain in right lumbar region when lowering sink into position.*

Duration: *Started 2 weeks ago, has seen the General Medical Doctor and been prescribed medication.*

Is it getting better/worse or staying the same? *There was improvement over the first week, although the pain was initially only in back and now has spread to the right buttock. Pain not improved over the 2nd week.*

Any investigations or interventions?

Symptoms:

Description of pain: *Ache*

VAS: At best *2/10*   At worst *6/10*

S4/Bladder or Bowel: *Normal function*

P&Ns or numbness draw on body chart: *None*

Edge/ Aspect? *N/A*

Cough/ Sneeze: *Pain not affected*

Behavior:

Constant/intermittent? *Constant in back and intermittent in buttock.*

Aggravated by: *Sitting (can only sit for 10 mins), bending, many work tasks, lifting, sitting to standing, standing for extended periods, walking limited to 1 mile*

Eased by: *Lying down and rest, medication.*

Night pain: *Sleeping well if taken medication*

24 hour pattern: *Best first thing in morning with pain 2/10 but bit stiff. Worse as the day goes on, at worst in evening after a full day's work.*

Figure 3–4 Cyriax proforma for lumbar spine assessment. *Source:* ©2010 Elaine Atkins, Jill Kerr, and Emily Goodlad. Published by Elsevier Ltd.

Past Medical History:

Previous back problems with outcome/treatment and investigations: *2002 had low back pain from a lifting injury, settled in a week with rest and Tylenol.*

Previous malignancy, major operations or illnesses: *Nothing major but had a fractured clavicle in 1985, a knee arthroscopy in 1986.*

General Health Checklist:

Diabetes; epilepsy; recent unexplained weight loss; heart; **high blood pressure**; visceral disease, fever, high cholesterol; rheumatoid arthritis; osteoarthritis; osteoporosis; smoker; other—including relevant family history.

Joint pain in last year—stiff right knee occasionally swollen. Has had arthroscopy. Functionally able to squat; semi-squat and kneel. Does not appear to be directly relevant to current episode.

Medications:

Analgesics: (how much and are they working)

Anti-inflammatories: *Advil*

Anticarcinogenics:

Antidepressants:

Muscle relaxants: *Flexeril*

Steroids:

Others: *Lotensin (hypertension)*

Recreational drugs:

Clinical impression prior to objective testing:

No red flags, mild to moderately severe and irritable back pain, no neurological symptoms, sudden onset, clear SI joints and hips. Probable mechanical lumbar problem.

INSPECTION:

Bony deformities: *Symmetry, no shift or scoliosis, slight flattening of the lumbar lordosis.*

Color changes: *Nil to note*

STATE AT REST: *Pain 4/10 on VAS*

Wasting: *Nil to note*

Swelling: *No swelling but spasm over right paravertebral muscles*

Figure 3–4 Cyriax proforma for lumbar spine assessment (continued).

OBJECTIVE EXAMINATION

Active Lumbar Movements: on star diagram

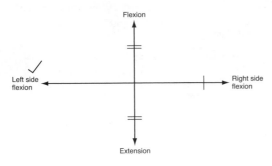

Myotomes in Supine:

Resisted hip flexion (L2/3) *Power 5 normal*

Resisted ankle dorsiflexion (L4) *Power 5 normal*

Resisted big toe extension (L5) *Power 5 normal*

Resisted ankle eversion (S1) *Power 5 normal*

Reflexes:

Knee jerk (L2/3) *Symmetrical and normal*

Ankle jerk (L5/S1) *Symmetrical and normal*

Babinski for plantar response? *Symmetrical and normal*

Sensation: Dermatomes, L3, L4, L5, S1, S2- *all equal and normal*

DIAGNOSIS:

Nonspecific Low Back Pain - Clinical model 2

TREATMENT PLAN:

Manipulation; exercises; advice.

Gastrocnemius Power (S1/2): *Power 5/normal*

Clear Hips:

	Left	**Right**
Passive flexion:	*Equal bilaterally and painfree, normal end feel*	
Passive Medial rotation:	*Equal bilaterally and painfree, normal end feel*	
Passive Lateral rotation:	*Equal bilaterally and painfree, normal end feel*	

Clear Sacroiliac Joints:

	Left	**Right**
Shear tests	*All pain free*	*All pain free*
Faber test	*Pain free*	*Pain free*

Straight Leg Raise (L & R): *Equal and pain free*

Femoral Nerve Stretch: *Equal and painfree*

Myotomes in Prone:

Resisted knee extension (L2/3) *Power 5 normal*

Resisted knee flexion (L5/S1) *Power 5 normal*

Gluteal contraction (S1/S2) *Power 5 normal*

Palpation of Spinous Processes: Tender over *L4/5 centrally and unilaterally over right side L4/5, spasm over the right paravertebral muscles.*

Any Additional Tests: *None applicable*

Figure 3–4 Cyriax proforma for lumbar spine assessment (continued).

test is limited by tension in the quadriceps. If positive unilaterally it implicates the nerve roots, if positive bilaterally the dura mater is at fault.

The remaining resisted tests for the quadriceps and hamstrings are conducted in prone lying. A static contraction of the gluteal muscles is performed to assess for muscle bulk and palpation is conducted, using the ulnar border of the hand on the spinous processes, for pain, range of movement, and end-feel.

Any other tests can be added to this basic routine examination of the lumbar spine, including repeated, combined, and accessory movements and neural tension testing as appropriate.

If serious pathology is suspected, further tests and specialist investigations will need to be implemented. From the examination the patient is categorized into a clinical model and a treatment plan prepared.

APPLICATION OF THE CYRIAX MODEL TO JOE LORES

Examination

Joe was examined using a form that is consistent with the Cyriax approach (Figure 3–4) employing the previously mentioned tests and measures.

Evaluation

The key findings for the evaluation of Joe's condition from a Cyriax approach include:

- Sudden recent onset mechanical right-sided back pain
- Limited referral of pain into right buttock
- Varying from mild (2) to moderate (6) severity and irritability of pain (i.e., subacute). This is drawn from the VAS scales,[18] medications being taken, and the aggravates and eases information
- Limited lumbar movements in a non-capsular pattern
- The hip and sacroiliac joint were cleared as a source of pain
- No neurological symptoms or signs
- Tender on palpation of L4–L5 spinous processes
- No red flags—as outlined in Figure 3–2
- No yellow flags as still working and motivated
- No suspicious features or contraindications to treatment

Diagnosis

By linking the key examination findings to the Cyriax clinical models provided previously, Joe fits best into clinical model 2 (Figure 3–1).

Intervention

A treatment plan is developed based on the individual patient's presentation and needs, with the principle aim of reducing pain towards the achievement of full function. The treatment of choice for a patient fitting model 2 is manipulation, however, if the technique was painful and or induced muscle spasm, then another technique would be applied or another approach would be used.

The limited side flexion is *toward* the painful side. Anecdotally, in the Cyriax approach, if side flexion away from the painful side is the more painful side flexion, manipulation is more likely to be effective. This is not a hard and fast rule though, and there is no evidence that "side flexion towards" would not respond to manipulation.

The Cyriax approach to Joe's treatment will therefore focus on manipulation. Additional support for the use of manipulation for patients with pain of recent onset, with minimal pain referral, and no neurological signs is provided by Chou[19] and Herbert.[20] Education, self-care advice, and an appropriate exercise program will also be provided as part of the care package and additional treatment approaches may be used if necessary to enhance recovery.

It is not possible to produce a definitive list of all contraindications to lumbar manipulation and the primary aim of the assessment is to screen for the "red flags" listed in Figure 3–2 and to establish the diagnosis of mechanical pain, within a clinical model suitable for manipulation. The principal contraindications to lumbar manipulation are as follows:

- Absence or withdrawal of patient consent
- Signs and symptoms of cauda equina syndrome, including S4 symptoms of saddle anaesthesia, sacral sensory loss, and signs of bladder or bowel dysfunction
- Bilateral sciatica from the same level with bilateral limitation of straight leg raise and bilateral objective neurological signs—indicative of a large central prolapse threatening the cauda equina
- Severe or progressive neurological deficit and hyperacute pain—both are too irritable for manipulation

- Suspicious features indicating tumor—constant, progressive, nonmechanical pain
- Upper motor neuron lesion (e.g., spinal cord compression, CVA)
- Inflammatory arthritis
- History of trauma with possible fracture
- Anticoagulant therapy/blood clotting disorders due to risk of intraspinal bleeding
- Psychosocial "yellow flags"
- Caution in first trimester of pregnancy

Joe does not appear to have any contraindications to manipulation.

Joe's symptoms are right sided, referring from the right lumbar region to the right buttock, and this will guide the selection of techniques and his body positioning. Cyriax advocated the use of rotation manipulation techniques and, specifically, the "distraction technique" as the first step to treat unilateral lumbar pain.[2] The rotation techniques are nonspecific and often referred to as "gross" (i.e., there is no attempt to localize the treatment to a specific level). The reasoning for this has been provided by Cyriax who posited that when a series of spinal joints are moved to end range, the normal joints move freely, whereas the "blocked" or hypomobile joint does not. Therefore the final overpressure falls on the hypomobile joint.[6] The rotation techniques are always performed with the patient lying on the painless side, painful side uppermost.

Informed consent is always gained first. This would include the warning of some after-treatment soreness since around half of people treated with manual therapy might expect minor adverse events,[21] and especially after the first treatment.[22]

Joe would be reassessed after each technique and the protocol would be adjusted, depending on the response. His VAS and range of movement would be used to determine improvement, as well as his functional activities between appointments. As mentioned previously, Joe's intervention plan would include education, advice, and exercise as part of usual care.

The terms "hyperacute" and "subacute" each have a specific meaning in the Cyriax approach that is relevant for treatment selection. They are not necessarily linked to time from initial onset. Hyperacute pain is severe pain associated with severe irritability, muscle spasm, and twinges. Subacute pain is associated with mild to moderate pain and irritability.

In Joe's case, the pain is mild to moderate, and moderately irritable (i.e., subacute but not hyperacute). A distraction manipulation technique would be the appropriate first technique to try but would only proceed if the positioning and application to end range did not induce increased pain or spasm. Although instructions for techniques described for Joe's intervention plan are provided below, it is recommended that a course in orthopaedic medicine is attended before they are applied in clinical practice. For all the rotation techniques the bed should be as low as is comfortable for the operator.

Distraction technique

Position the patient in side lying with the painful side uppermost (Figure 3–5). Flex the upper hip and knee with the knee just resting over the side of the bed to assist the rotational stress. Extend the lower leg. Pull the underneath shoulder firmly through such that the uppermost shoulder is positioned backwards and the pelvis positioned forwards. Stand behind the patient at waist level and place one hand over the greater trochanter, point-

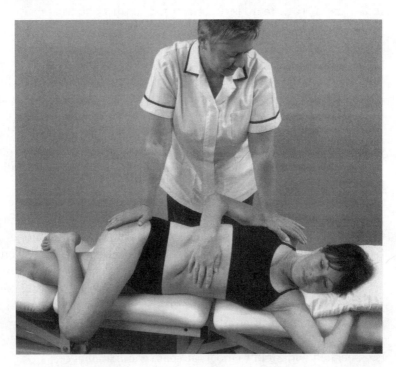

Figure 3–5 Distraction technique. *Source:* ©2010 Elaine Atkins, Jill Kerr, and Emily Goodlad. Published by Elsevier Ltd.

ing outwards. Put your other hand comfortably on the patient's uppermost shoulder with your fingers pointing away from your other hand. Apply rotation with the hand on the greater trochanter until the pelvis lies just forwards of the midline and the patient's waist is upwards. Apply pressure equally through both hands to impart a distraction force; you will see the patient's waist crease stretch out as you lean through your arms. Keep your arms straight as you apply a minimal amplitude, high velocity thrust once all of the slack has been taken up.

If on reassessment the VAS is reduced and range of movement increases then the technique can be repeated. If there is no change, and the treatment itself was comfortable, it is still worth attempting the technique again, before abandoning it to move onto another.

As mentioned previously, the distraction technique is appropriate to try as the first technique. Beyond that, there is not an order of efficacy for the rotation manipulation techniques as such and there are many that could be selected in the various texts on the Cyriax approach. The practitioner's experience in applying the techniques and patient specific factors may have an influence on technique selection. The comparable signs are assessed after every technique and the next technique is chosen based on the outcome. As long as a technique is gaining an increase in range and/or a decrease in pain, it can be repeated. Improvement may reach a plateau or the feedback from the patient may become unclear. Only professional judgement will reliably dictate when treatment should be stopped in each treatment session and the advice would always be to err on the side of caution, especially in the earlier stages of acquiring manipulative skill.

Two additional rotation manipulation techniques will now be described by way of examples.

Short-lever rotation manipulation technique–pelvis forwards

Position the patient in supine, lying with the hips and knees flexed (crook lying, see Figure 3–6). Ask the patient to lift and rotate the hips so that they are lying with the painful side uppermost and the shoulders relatively flat. Position the legs as for the "distraction technique." Stand in front of the patient with one hand fixing the patient's shoulder while the other is placed with the heel of the hand on the blade of the ilium, with the forearm horizontal and your fingers pointing back towards you. Apply pressure through the hand on the ilium in a horizontal direction towards you to achieve a rotational strain. Apply a minimal amplitude, high velocity thrust once all the

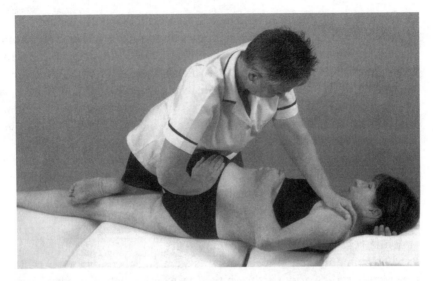

Figure 3–6. Short-lever rotation manipulation technique—pelvis forwards. *Source:* ©2010 Elaine Atkins, Jill Kerr, and Emily Goodlad. Published by Elsevier Ltd.

slack has been taken up. If you find it difficult to apply the thrust with your hand against the ilium, slide your hand towards you to place your forearm against the bone to give you improved leverage.

Short-lever rotation manipulation technique pelvis backwards[2,6]

Position the patient in side lying with the painful side uppermost (Figure 3–7). Take the lower arm behind the patient and place the upper arm into elevation, resting in front of the patient's face. Extend the upper leg and flex the hip and knee of the lower leg. The shoulder will now be positioned forwards and the pelvis backwards. Stand behind the patient; place one hand on the scapula to give a little distraction to take up the slack. Place the other hand on the front of the pelvis with your forearm horizontal and pointing back towards you. Apply a minimal amplitude, high velocity thrust once all of the slack is taken up.

Joe's symptoms may centralize to be more localized to the spine itself, albeit completely central or a short unilateral pain. In this instance a central manipulation technique may be applied and the following "unilateral extension thrust" is described as an example.

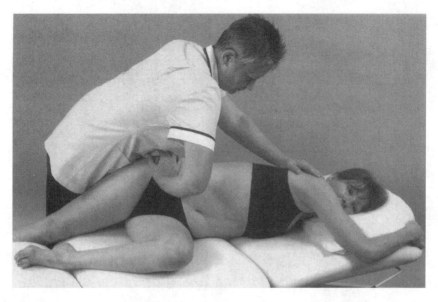

Figure 3–7 Short-lever rotation manipulation technique—pelvis backwards. *Source:* ©2010 Elaine Atkins, Jill Kerr, and Emily Goodlad. Published by Elsevier Ltd.

Unilateral extension thrust technique[2,6]

Position the patient in prone lying, stand on the painful side and palpate the spinous process to locate the painful level (Figure 3–8). Place the ulnar border of the hand over the transverse process at the tender level on the side furthest away from you. The pisiform should be adjacent to the spinous process and the pressure is applied through the paravertebral muscles for patient comfort. Stand close to the bed with your knees hooked onto the edge to enable you to lean over the patient. Apply pressure down onto the transverse process through arms as straight as possible, directing the pressure back towards your own knees. Apply a minimal amplitude, high velocity thrust once all of the slack is taken up by lifting and dropping your head between your shoulders.

Returning to the possibility that the distraction manipulation technique might increase Joe's pain and produce spasm as it is applied, it would be abandoned. It is possible that an alternative technique, such as the short-lever pelvis backwards manipulation technique described previously, could be more comfortable, but if it is clear that the pain is too irritable then a technique known as the "pretzel" could be more suitable and would be used in preference as a mobilising technique.

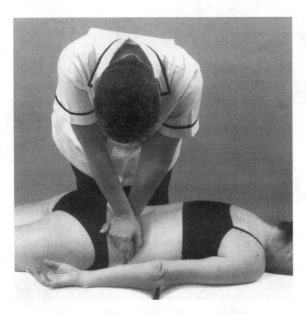

Figure 3–8 Unilateral extension thrust technique. *Source:* ©2010 Elaine Atkins, Jill Kerr, and Emily Goodlad. Published by Elsevier Ltd.

The pretzel positioning can also be adapted as a strong rotation manipulation for subacute back pain; we need to be clear that it is being used for hyperacute pain here and is applied in the manner described below.

The "Pretzel" technique[2,6]

For hyperacute pain, each step is conducted individually using a gentle, pain-free mobilization (usually in the midrange), constantly monitoring for improvement before progressing to the next step. Progression through the steps is made cautiously and steadily and may take 5 or 10 minutes to achieve in the very irritable state. The end of range will not necessarily be reached before proceeding to the next step. The technique should not aggravate the pain and the patient should be firmly and comfortably supported throughout. This is not a manipulation as such and any other mobilizing modality may be applied at each stage. It may be useful for correcting a lateral shift.[2]

- Stand on the patient's painless side with the patient in supine lying. Flex the knees and cross the good leg over the bad (Figure 3–9).

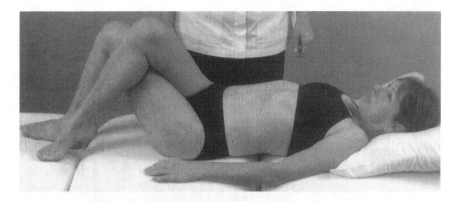

Figure 3–9 "Pretzel" technique: Starting position with knees flexed and "good" leg placed over the "bad." *Source:* ©2010 Elaine Atkins, Jill Kerr, and Emily Goodlad. Published by Elsevier Ltd.

- Flex both hips (Figure 3–10).
- Place your knee that is furthest from the patient's head at the patient's waist to act as a pivot point. Place your hands on the patient's knees and side flex the lumbar spine to gap the affected side (Figure 3–11).
- Rotate the pelvis towards you until the patient's knees are resting on your thigh (Figure 3–12).

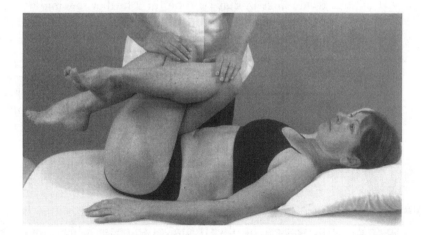

Figure 3–10 "Pretzel" technique: Both hips flexed. *Source:* ©2010 Elaine Atkins, Jill Kerr, and Emily Goodlad. Published by Elsevier Ltd.

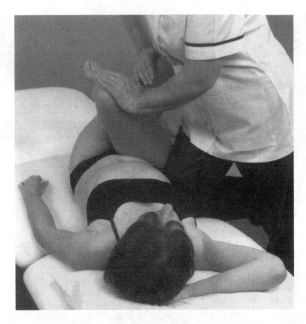

Figure 3–11 "Pretzel" technique: Spine side-flexed around pivot of caudal knee placed in patient's waist. *Source:* ©2010 Elaine Atkins, Jill Kerr, and Emily Goodlad. Published by Elsevier Ltd.

- Continue to mobilize in that position for a further few minutes, ensuring that the technique remains comfortable and the patient relaxed. Help the patient back to the starting position and review the comparable signs and symptoms.

By way of a summary, the flowchart in Figure 3–13 shows a typical treatment approach for clinical model 2. In the case of Joe, if his symptoms are too acute for manipulation, mobilizations using the stages of the pretzel would be appropriate until the pain is subacute and the flowchart steps may then be applied as described previously.

Prognosis

Joe might experience some after-treatment soreness, which can arise within the first 24 hours and can take up to 72 hours to settle.[21] This type of clinical model 2 presentation usually responds quickly to manipulation.[14] However

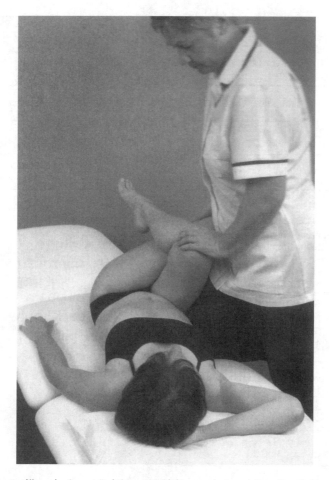

Figure 3–12 "Pretzel" technique: Pelvis rotated forwards to rest patient's knees against thigh. *Source:* ©2010 Elaine Atkins, Jill Kerr, and Emily Goodlad. Published by Elsevier Ltd.

this is his second episode of pain and, typically, each episode may be a little worse than the one before,[1] arguably requiring more sessions of treatment. Complete recovery in two to three sessions would be expected.[14]

Supportive Evidence

It is generally accepted from the scientific data produced to date that spinal manipulation has shown short-term benefits of improvement in pain, move-

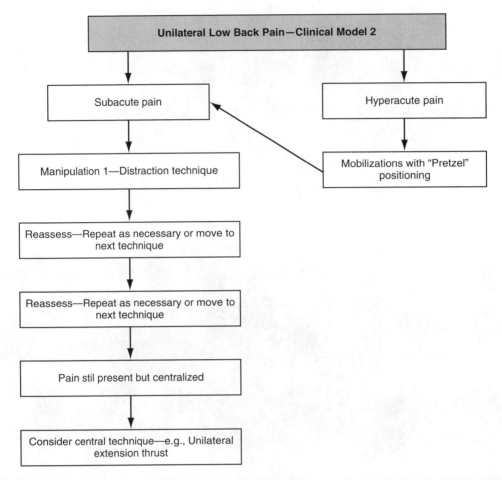

Figure 3–13 Flowchart of a typical treatment approach for a patient classified as Cyriax clinical model 2. *Source:* ©2010 Elaine Atkins, Jill Kerr, and Emily Goodlad. Published by Elsevier Ltd.

ment, and functional ability. Waddell et al.[23] reviewed the evidence relating to LBP for the Royal College of General Practitioners, which guided the Clinical Standards Advisory Group (CSAG) audit towards the development of guidelines for the management of acute LBP. A system of diagnostic triage was introduced on which to base management. The guidelines have continued to be presented as a patient booklet, *The Back Book*,[24] to promote the recommendations of the guidelines on a wider scale. For simple acute back pain, the advice is given to avoid bed rest and to stay active, and manipulation is upheld as providing short-term improvement in pain and activity levels.

Waddell[25] reported on the evidence for manipulation that showed positive results of good short-term symptomatic relief for patients with back pain of less than 4–6 weeks' duration and without nerve root pain. It was suggested that manipulation may also be effective in recurrent attacks.

A review conducted by Nadler[26] found that the benefit from manipulation was more marked in the earlier stages of a painful episode; although the limit of the time period for "earlier" is unclear.

Bogduk[27] conducted an evidence review of prevailing approaches to the management of chronic LBP and found manipulation to be slightly more effective than sham therapy but not more effective than other forms of care. This hints at the importance of patient selection prior to manipulation however, and the more chronic model is not recommended as "ideal" for manipulation in the orthopaedic medicine approach.

The UK BEAM trial[28] declared that relative to "best care" in general practice, manipulation followed by exercise achieved a moderate benefit at 3 months and a small benefit at 12 months; spinal manipulation achieved a small to moderate benefit at 3 months and a small benefit at 12 months; and exercise achieved a small benefit at 3 months but not 12 months. On the face of it, the trial does provide support for the benefit of manipulation, but although the trial set out with large numbers, a significant percentage of patients was lost to follow up and the criticism was made that it was hard to establish whether it was the "hands-on" effect or the effect of manipulation itself that led to the improvement.

An analysis of cost effectiveness drawn from the trial concluded that manipulation alone probably gives better value for money than manipulation followed by exercise.

Oliphant[29] conducted a review and concluded that there was evidence that spinal manipulation has a beneficial effect on pain, straight leg raising, range of motion, size of disc herniation, and neurological symptoms. Relating to the safety of manipulation, Oliphant also provided the estimate that lumbar manipulation is 37,000–148,000 times safer than nonsteroidal anti-inflammatory drugs (NSAIDs) and 55,500–444,000 times safer than surgery for the treatment of lumbar disc herniation. The same review produced the calculation that cauda equina syndrome is 7,400–37,000 times more likely to occur as a complication of surgery than from spinal manipulation.

A review conducted by Williams et al.[30] concluded that there was some evidence that manipulation also improved psychological outcomes more than mobilization. They recommend that more trials should include psychological markers in their studies and that there may be a case for comparing manipulation with cognitive behavioral therapy. Chou et al.,[19] when reviewing the evidence of nonpharmacologic therapies for acute and chronic LBP, concurred that there is good evidence for spinal manipulation and cognitive behavioral therapy for LBP of less than four weeks.

Based on empirical evidence, and especially that passed on from the clinical experience of Cyriax, for selected patients, when manipulation works it works quickly.[14] This concept may have positive implications for reducing the overall cost of the management of LBP of recent onset. The long-term benefits of manipulation remain unknown, although if the aim of manipulation is to expedite recovery in the early stages, these are of little significance. There is insufficient evidence to support or to refute the use of manipulation for chronic LBP (i.e., back pain of over three months' duration).

As mentioned previously, the principal aim of manipulation, and for all early treatment programs, is to prevent the development of chronic back pain. Childs et al.[31] set out to determine if patients who do not receive manipulation for their LBP are at an increased risk of worsening disability, compared to patients who receive manipulation. Seventy patients received manipulation and exercise and 61 patients were assigned to an exercise group without manipulation. The study found that those in the latter group were eight times as likely to experience a worsening in disability than those in the manipulation group. The importance of patient selection was emphasized.

How manipulation works continues to be a topic of debate. There is a growing body of evidence that the neurophysiologic mechanisms are the reason manipulation is successful and not the traditional biomechanical theory.[32,33] Herbert[32] explains that, when applied, spinal manipulative forces increase afferent discharge; depress the motoneuron pool; cause changes in the motor activity such as reflexive muscle activation; and decrease resting electromyographic signal intensity, as well as reducing pain perception in response to standard stimulus. So collectively the manipulation has an effect on the central nervous system by gating of the nociception at the spinal cord by stimulation of the mechanoreceptors, direct stimulation of a spinal reflex to alter muscle activity, or stimulation of pain centres in the brain.

The nonspecific neurophysiological effects such as treatment expectation and placebo also have a powerful influence on pain perception.

Bialosky[33] conducted a small, randomized controlled trial primarily to assess the immediate effects of manipulation on thermal pain perception in patients with chronic LBP. The secondary aim was to determine whether the resulting hypoalgesia was a local effect and if the psychological influences were associated with the changes in pain perception. They found that inhibition of temporal summation in participants with LBP associated with manipulation was greater than the changes observed in response to riding a bike or performing extension exercises. This inhibition appeared to be local, as it was observed only in the lower extremity, and psychological factors were not strongly associated with the resultant inhibition of temporal summation. These findings suggest that manipulation may work through a neurophysiological mechanism rather than a biomechanical mechanism.

The success of manipulation depends on the selection of suitable patients and indiscriminate manipulation will produce unsatisfactory results.[31] Support for the characteristics of clinical model 2 are provided through consideration of the following authors' ideas. Flynn et al.[34] presented five markers for manipulation as the treatment of choice that were listed as: no symptoms distal to the knee; duration of symptoms < 16 days; lumbar hypomobility (of individual segments); fear-avoidance beliefs questionnaire > 19; hip internal rotation > 35 degrees. However, Ebell[35] states the five-item rule is limited because it requires the patient to complete a survey and requires the physician to assess hypomobility. He proposes a validated simpler two-item rule including symptom duration of less than 16 days and no symptoms distal to the knee. In the Cyriax approach, clinical model 2 expands on Ebell's proposal but those two factors lie at the heart of the model.

Orthopaedic medicine spinal manipulation techniques aim to reduce the signs and symptoms of a lumbar lesion. In terms of expectations of treatment outcomes, the ideal patient for manipulation has, in summary:

- Mainly central or short unilateral back or buttock pain (the more distal the pain, the less likely manipulation is to succeed)
- Recent onset of pain, preferably within the last 6 weeks
- History of sudden onset of pain; the patient recalls the exact time and mode of onset
- Non-capsular pattern on examination
- No red flags
- Pain increased by side flexion away from the painful side
- No objective neurological signs
- No suspicious features or contraindications to manipulation

SUMMARY

The Cyriax approach uses a systematic procedure to examine joint pain. The principle of selective tension underlies the physical exam. In acute LBP, there are four clinical models to which patients are classified with intervention proceeding from out of the classification. Joe Lores fit the Cyriax model 2, which was a mechanical lesion of sudden onset that is treated by manipulation. The art of sequencing and selecting appropriate manipulative techniques has been demonstrated as a key component of treatment under the Cyriax approach.

REFERENCES

1. Atkins E, Kerr J, Goodlad E. *A Practical Approach to Orthopaedic Medicine: Assessment, Diagnosis and Treatment.* 3rd ed. Edinburgh, Scotland: Churchill Livingstone; 2010.
2. Cyriax J, Cyriax P. *Illustrated Manual of Orthopaedic Medicine.* London, England: Butterworths; 1993.
3. Kent PM, Keating JL, Buchbinder R. Searching for a conceptual framework for nonspecific low back pain. *Manual Therapy.* 2009;14:387–396.
4. McCarthy CJ, Arnall FA, Strimpakos N, et al. The bio-psycho-social classification of nonspecific low back pain: a systematic review. *Physical Therapy Reviews.* 2004;9:17–30.
5. Shäfer A, Hall T, Briffa K. Classification of low-back related leg pain—a proposed pathomechanism-based approach. *Manual Therapy.* 2009;14:222–230.
6. Cyriax J. *Textbook of Orthopaedic Medicine.* Vol 2. 11th ed. London, England: Baillière Tindall; 1984.
7. Vroomen P, de Krom M, Slofstra P, et al. Conservative treatment of sciatica: a systematic review. *Journal of Spinal Disorders.* 2000;13(6):463–469.
8. Boswell M, Trescot A, Datta S, et al. Interventional techniques: evidence-based practice guidelines in the management of chronic spinal pain. *Pain Physician.* 2007;10:7–111.
9. Porter RW. Pathology of symptomatic lumbar disc protrusion. *Journal of the Royal College of Surgeons of Edinburgh.* 1995;40:200–202.
10. Osti OL, Cullum DE. Occupational low back pain and intervertebral disc degeneration—epidemiology, imaging and pathology. *Clinical Journal of Pain.* 1994;10:331–334.
11. Swezey R. Pathophysiology and treatment of intervertebral disk disease. Rheumatic Disease. *Clinics of North America.* 1993;19:741–757.
12. Hartley A. *Practical Joint Assessment: Lower Quadrant.* 2nd ed. London, England: Mosby; 1995:188.
13. Sizer P, Brismée J, Cook C. Medical screening for red flags in the diagnosis and management of musculoskeletal spine pain. *Pain Practice.* 2007;7(1):53–71.
14. Cyriax J. *Textbook of Orthopaedic Medicine.* 8th ed. London, England: Baillière Tindall; 1982.
15. Hoppenfeld S. *Physical Examination of the Spine and Extremities.* Philadelphia, PA: Appleton Century Crofts; 1976.
16. Supik LF, Broom MJ. Sciatic tension signs and lumbar disc herniations. *Spine.* 1994;19:1066–1068.
17. Jönsson B, Strömqvist B. The straight leg raising test and the severity of symptoms in lumbar disc herniation. *Spine.* 1995;20:27–30.

18. Jenson MP, Chen C, Brugger A. Interpretation of Visual Analogue Scale ratings and change scores: a reanalysis of two clinical trials of postoperative pain. *The Journal of Pain.* 2003;4(7):407–414.

19. Chou R, Huffman LH. Non Pharmacologic therapies for acute and chronic low back pain: A review of the evidence for an American Pain Society/American College of Physicians Clinical Practice Guidelines. *Annals of Internal Medicine.* 2007;147(7):492–504.

20. Herbert J, Koppenhaver S, Fritz J, et al. Clinical prediction for success of interventions for managing low back pain. *Clinics in Sports Medicine.* 2008;27(3):463–479.

21. Carnes D, Mars TS, Mullinger B, et al. Adverse events and manual therapy: a systematic review. *Manual Therapy.* 2010;15:355–363.

22. Rubinstein SM, Leboeuf-Yde C, Knolo DL, et al. The benefits outweigh the risks for patients undergoing chiropractic care for neck pain: a prospective, multicenter, cohort study. *Journal of Manipulative and Physiological Therapeutics.* 2007;30(6):408–418.

23. Waddell G, Feder G, McIntosh A, et al. *Low back pain evidence review.* London, England: Royal College of General Practitioners; 1996.

24. Roland M, Waddell G, Klaber Moffett J, et al. *The Back Book.* 2nd ed. Norwich, England: Stationery Office; 2002.

25. Waddell G. *The Back Pain Revolution.* Edinburgh, Scotland: Churchill Livingstone; 2004.

26. Nadler SF. Non pharmacologic management of pain. *Journal of the American Osteopathic Association.* 2004;104(11 suppl 8):6–12.

27. Bogduk N. Management of chronic low back pain. *Medical Journal of Australia.* 2004;180(2):79–83.

28. UK BEAM Trial Team. United Kingdom back pain exercise and manipulation randomised trial: effectiveness of physical treatments for back pain in primary care. *British Medical Journal.* 2004;329(7479):1377.

29. Oliphant D. Safety of spinal manipulation in the treatment of lumbar disc herniation: a systematic review and risk assessment. *Journal of Manipulative and Physiological Therapeutics.* 2004;27(3):197–210.

30. Williams N, Hendry M, Lewis R, et al. Psychological response in spinal manipulation (PRISM): a systematic review of psychological outcomes in randomised controlled trials. *Complementary Therapies in Medicine* 2007;15:271–283.

31. Childs JD, Flynn TW, Fritz JM. A perspective for considering the risks and benefits of spinal manipulation in patients with low back pain. *Manual Therapy.* 2006;11:316–320.

32. Herbert J, Koppenhavers S, Fritz J, et al. Clinical prediction for success of interventions for managing low back pain. *Clinics in Sports Medicine* 2008;27(3) 463–479.

33. Bialosky JE, Bishop MD, Robinson ME, et al. Spinal manipulative therapy has an immediate effect on thermal pain sensitivity in people with low back pain: A randomized controlled trial. *Physical Therapy.* 2009;89(12):1292–1303.

34. Flynn T, Fritz J, Whitman J, et al. A clinical prediction rule for classifying patients with low back pain who demonstrate short-term improvement with spinal manipulation. *Spine.* 2002;27(24):2835–2843.

35. Ebell M. Predicting benefit of spinal manipulation for low back pain. *American Family Physician* 2009;79(4):318–319.

Cyriax Proforma for Lumbar Spine Assessment

Source: Elaine Atkins, Jill Kerr, and Emily Goodlad

Name (M/F):

OBSERVATION: face, posture, and gait (note any abnormalities):

SUBJECTIVE EXAMINATION:

Age/DOB:

Occupation:

Sports, Hobbies, Lifestyle:

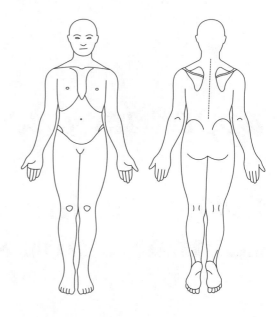

Site & Spread:

Onset: sudden, gradual, or insidious:

Mechanism of injury:

Duration:

Is it getting better/worse or staying the same?

Any investigations or interventions?

Symptoms:
Description of pain:

VAS: At best   At worst

S4/Bladder or Bowel:

P&Ns or numbness draw on body chart:

Edge/Aspect?

Cough/Sneeze:

Behavior:
Constant/intermittent?

Aggravated by:

Eased by:

Night pain:

24 hour pattern:

Past Medical History:

Previous back problems with outcome/treatment and investigations:

Previous malignancy, major operations or illnesses:

Medications:

Analgesics: (how much and are they working)

Anti-inflammatories:

Anticarcinogenics:

Antidepressants:

General Health Checklist:

Diabetes; epilepsy; recent unexplained weight loss; heart; high blood pressure; visceral disease, fever, high cholesterol; rheumatoid arthritis; osteoarthritis; osteoporosis; smoker; other—including relevant family history.

Muscle relaxants:

Steroids:

Others:

Recreational drugs:

Clinical impression prior to objective testing:

INSPECTION:

Bony deformities:

Color changes:

Wasting:

Swelling:

STATE AT REST:

OBJECTIVE EXAMINATION

Active Lumbar Movements: on star diagram

Flexion

Left side flexion ←————————→ Right side flexion

Extension

Gastrocnemius Power (S1/2):
Clear Hips:

	Left	Right
Passive flexion:		
Passive Medial rotation:		
Passive Lateral rotation:		

Clear Sacroiliac Joints:

	Left	Right
Shear tests		
Faber test		

Straight Leg Raise (L & R):

Myotomes in Supine:

Resisted hip flexion (L2/3)

Resisted ankle dorsiflexion (L4)

Resisted big toe extension (L5)

Resisted ankle eversion (S1)

Femoral Nerve Stretch:

Myotomes in Prone:

Resisted knee extension (L2/3)

Resisted knee flexion (L5/S1)

Gluteal contraction (S1/S2)

Reflexes:

Knee jerk (L2/3)

Ankle jerk (L5/S1)

Babinski for plantar response?

Palpation of Spinous Processes:

Any Additional Tests:

Sensation: Dermatomes, L3, L4, L5, S1, S2

CLINICAL REASONING:

DIAGNOSIS:

TREATMENT PLAN

chapter four

The Kaltenborn-Evjenth Concept

John Krauss PT, PhD, OCS, FAAOMPT

The Kaltenborn-Evjenth Concept is the culminating work of Norwegian physical therapists Freddy Kaltenborn and Olaf Evjenth. This concept uses a systematic approach to examination and intervention that is grounded in evidence-based/evidence-informed practice principles. The examination portion of the concept features symptom localization testing, which is used to link patient symptoms and movement. Interventions unique to this concept are the use of translatoric joint mobilizations and manipulations combined with therapeutic exercise. Kaltenborn (in collaboration with Evjenth and others) wrote the book entitled "Manual Mobilization of the Joints." Volume I: The Extremities and Volume II: The Spine are now in their 6th and 5th editions, respectively. Students can find more information about the approach and training opportunities by visiting http://www. oakland.edu/shs/pt/.

BACKGROUND

The Kaltenborn-Evjenth (KE) Concept was developed by Norwegian physical therapists Freddy Kaltenborn and Olaf Evjenth. Both Kaltenborn and Evjenth were trained first as physical educators and then as physical therapists. This was the required pathway to becoming a physical therapist at that time in Norway with the physical education training focusing on active exercise and athletic training, and physical therapy education focusing on passive interventions such as massage and passive motions.

Kaltenborn's path to becoming a physical therapist with a specialization in orthopedic manipulative therapy was more direct than Evjenth's. Upon completion of his physical therapy education in the late 1940s, Kaltenborn went on to study a variety of treatment approaches under Dr. James Mennel, Dr. James Cyriax, Dr. Albert Cramer, and Dr. Alan Stoddard. Kaltenborn developed a deep understanding and respect for the practice of orthopedics, osteopathy, and chiropractic based on his studies with these individuals.

In contrast, after completing his physical education training in 1954, Evjenth went on to coach track and field, gymnastics, and winter sports for the Norwegian Athletic Association. It was not until 1960 that Evjenth completed his physical therapy training and began his specialization in manual therapy under Freddy Kaltenborn. Following the completion of his manual therapy training in 1968, Evjenth then began assisting Kaltenborn on his courses and their partnership and collaboration grew.

Throughout their work together Kaltenborn and Evjenth pursued knowledge and skills that would assist in their management of patients they treated in their private practices and consulted with during their worldly travels. During these formative years of the concept, they learned, explored, and evaluated practice principles and techniques from orthopedic, osteopathic, chiropractic, and other manual therapy approaches. Examples of the techniques they explored included rotatory manipulation, dry needling, acupuncture, and neural mobilization. The overarching goal of this work was to develop a concept that would best match the practice aspirations of physical therapists throughout the world. The KE Concept made its official debut in 1973 in Gran Canary, Spain and represents a unique blending of the training, expertise, and aptitudes of its founders.

The KE Concept is a systematic examination and intervention approach consisting of orthopedic tests and measures and interventions that are selected and sequenced based upon evidence-based/evidence-informed practice principals.[1] Historically, there are three principle aspects of the concept that include the physical diagnosis, treatment, and research. The physical diagnosis is derived from a biomechanical and functionally-based examination process. Unique to the examination portion of the concept is the use of symptom localization testing, which is used to link patient symptoms and movement. Symptom localization consists of a series of examination tests that are used to identify: 1) the region of the body generating symptoms, 2) the joint(s) and soft tissue(s) generating symptoms, and 3) spinal segments generating symptoms. Each of these tests are used to either increase (provoke) or decrease (alleviate) symptoms. Another unique characteristic of the KE Concept is the emphasis of joint play testing consisting of small amplitude translatoric motions applied parallel to, or at a right angle to the "treatment plane." The treatment plane, as defined within the KE Concept, passes through the joint and lies at a right angle to a line running from the axis of rotation in the convex bony partner to the deepest aspect of the articulating concave surface.[1]

The KE Concept emphasizes that the PT diagnosis is derived from a thorough and contextually comprehensive examination process. Specifically, the examination is scaled to meet the goals of the patient and therapist, including all the necessary physical tests and measures required to derive a physical diagnosis for any given patient. The contextual nature of the examination allows the concept to adapt to various practice environments present around the world. This means that while a KE Concept examination will have similar features for each patient examination, the exact content will vary based on patient context. In addition, standard orthopedic tests and measures are typically present within a KE Concept-based examination.

The treatment portion of the concept focuses on four primary aspects: 1) to relieve pain, 2) to increase mobility, 3) to limit movement, and 4) to inform, instruct, and train. The KE Concept emphasizes that treatment used to restore function should not worsen a patient's underlying medical, pathological, and/or psychological condition. This means that the use of the KE Concept requires a foundational knowledge of anatomy, biomechanics, pathology (neuro-musculo-skeletal and medical), pathomechanics, and bio-psychosocial[2] aspects of patient management. More specifically, when pain dominates the patient's clinical presentation, the KE Concept practitioner would make every attempt to find and treat the underlying source of the patient's symptoms.

In pain-dominant cases the KE Concept practitioner would first attempt to reduce pain through the use of soft tissue techniques, including functional massage, lower grade static or oscillatory mobilizations, and low intensity hold relax-muscle stretching.[3] In cases where stiffness dominates the patient's clinical presentation, the KE Concept practitioner would use sustained end-range muscular and capsular stretching and thrust manipulations to increase mobility.[4] In the relatively rare instances when patients are unable to recognize changes in symptoms due to central nervous system processing errors[5] or due to affective and cognitive misinterpretation of sensory information, manual interventions used within the KE Concept would be conservative in nature paired with therapeutic exercise and education and coordinated with pharmacological and psychological management administered by other health professionals.

Unique intervention characteristics of the KE Concept include the emphasis on translatoric joint mobilizations and manipulations. This emphasis reflects Kaltenborn's and Evjenth's concerns that rotational motions, when used to improve mobility in stiff joints, generate compression of the articular surface (and disc joints), which may lead to or worsen cartilage and disc degeneration. Another intervention unique to the KE Concept is functional massage, which integrates soft tissue massage (in the form of manual soft tissue compressions and decompressions) and nonpainful joint motion (both angular and translatoric). The goals of functional massage are: 1) to manage musculotendinous and periarticular soft tissue pain and tension, and 2) to aid in the management of impaired segmental and/or joint motion, impaired muscle function/performance, and impaired neural dynamics caused by, or associated with musculotendinous and/or periarticular soft tissue pain and/or tension and/or gliding restrictions. Finally, the selection and sequencing of examination tests and measures and intervention strategies used within the KE Concept is dynamic and changes as new information is reported and revealed during patient care. The Kaltenborn-Evjenth Concept has evolved, and continues to evolve, into a complex and comprehensive physical therapy practice paradigm that emphasizes adaptability to the patient and practice environment.

APPLICATION OF THE KALTENBORN-EVJENTH APPROACH TO JOE LORES

Examination/Evaluation

As mentioned in the introduction, the KE Concept uses a systematic orthopedic examination along with tests and measures that are unique to the KE Concept. The first unique examination method described is symptom localization. The process of symptom localization begins during the patient interview, where symptom characteristics such as intensity, quality, location, and timing are identified and documented. Any or all of these characteristics may be used as a means of detecting the relationship between movement and symptoms. Following the patient history, these characteristics are further examined during the observation of a variety of functional movements, postural modifications, and active range of motion of the region(s) of the body that are relevant to the patient's complaint. Next, the physical examination may be directed towards more specific symptom localization testing to identify body region(s), articular, muscular, neural, vascular, or visceral structures, and spinal segment(s) that may be contributing to the patient's chief complaint.

The two primary sources of pain investigated through the use of symptom localization are: 1) pain arising in musculoskeletal tissues from stimulation of pain-sensitive (nociceptive) nerve endings by chemical and/or mechanical sources (somatic pain) and 2) pain arising from damaged or irritated nerve fibers (axons) or cell bodies (neuropathic pain). Differentiation between nociceptive and neuropathic sources of pain is initially investigated during the patient history based on patient reports of pain quality. The quality of somatic pain is usually described by the patient as "dull" or "aching" and localized, whereas neuropathic pain is usually described as "shooting," "stabbing," or "burning" and may be felt to travel along a nerve path from the spine into the arms and hands or into the buttocks, legs, or feet.[6]

Efficient use of, and interpretation of, symptom localization tests requires that tests are sequenced to implicate one region, structure, or segment at a time. When either provoking or alleviating during symptom localization, the patient is positioned so that small changes in position or load changes symptoms. When provoking symptoms, the patient is positioned at the verge of pain (VOP) where small changes in position or load will increase the patient's symptoms. When alleviating symptoms, the patient is positioned at the point of pain (POP) where small changes in position or load will decrease the patient's symptoms. When determining either the VOP or POP, several repetitions of the provoking movement or loading may be necessary for the patient to refine this position sufficiently. In practical terms the refinement of position improves the chance that the testing will provide accurate information regarding the region, structure, or segment being investigated. In our experience this is because the therapist may apply less force during symptom localization, resulting in a more controlled application of the testing load/movement.

In Joe's case, symptom localization could begin with regional localization. Typically this localization uses loading and unloading, angular and translational motions, and testing of multiregional structures (muscle, nerve, fascia) in an attempt to focus the physical examination on a specific body region. Specifically, this localization testing is a screening for regional origins of referred pain. Regional localization is most commonly performed: 1) in cases where there is no clear mechanism of injury to the local tissue (insidious onset); 2) when the location and quality of symptoms do not match the mechanism; 3) in cases where the symptoms are located at the junction of the extremities (and neck) with the trunk; 4) when symptoms are located along common nerve pathways in the extremities; and 5) when prior treatment of the local tissues has not resulted in expected improvement in physical function and/or symptoms.

To perform regional localization for pain with backward bending in standing, the patient would be positioned in standing at the verge of pain (VOP). The purpose of the test would be to determine if the buttock pain is originating from the low back, hip, or sacroiliac joint (SIJ). To implicate the hip as the source of pain the therapist posteriorly rotates the pelvis to extend the hip (Figure 4–1). This would provoke the hip and alleviate the SIJ and lumbar spine. If no pain is provoked the process is repeated; only now the apex of the sacrum is pressed ventrally to provoke the SI and alleviate the lumbar spine (Figure 4–2). If no pain is provoked then the testing would proceed to the lumbar spine. This would effectively end regional localization (since no pain was provoked in the regions adjacent to the lumbar spine) and we would begin segmental localization in the lumbar spine.

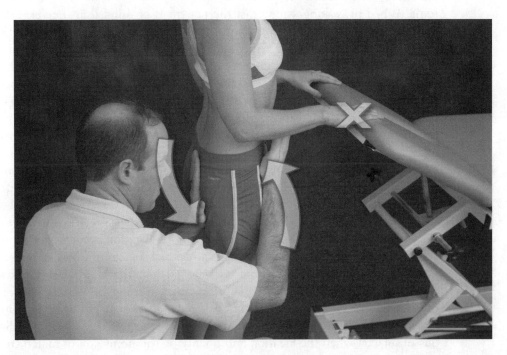

Figure 4–1 Posteriorly rotates the pelvis to extend the hip.

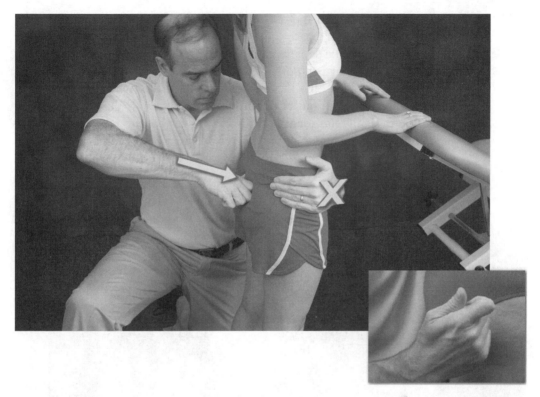

Figure 4–2 Apex of the sacrum is pressed ventrally to provoke the SI and alleviate the lumbar spine.

Segmental localization attempts to identify/diagnose individual spinal motion segments that are responsible for generating symptoms. The spinal motion segment consists of two adjacent vertebrae and all interconnecting ligamentous structures. Structures located between the vertebrae, which are potential sources of segmental pain, include the facet joints and associated ligaments, the interbody joint and associated ligaments, and intervertebral disc, spinal cord, and the spinal nerves. Because of the number and types of joints and structures that are potential sources of pain in the spinal segment, it is necessary to follow-up or precede segmental localization with structural localization when information regarding specific structural sensitivity is desired.

While it is not possible to isolate movement to only one spinal segment, it is possible to generate greater physical stress and/or motion at a tested segment through the use of either specific manual contacts, spinal locking, active and/or passive movement, or some combination thereof.[7] To perform segmental localization for extension in the lumbar spine the patient is once again positioned in standing at the VOP. Starting several spinal levels cranial to the location of symptoms the therapist presses the vertebrae in a ventral and cranial direction (Figure 4–3). If pain is provoked the therapist has identified the caudal vertebra in the painful spinal segment. In the case of Joe, we started by pressing at L2 and then progressed caudally to L3, then L4 and so forth. Pain was provoked once the base of the sacrum was pressed in a ventral slightly cranial direction, implicating the L5 spinal segment. To confirm this level was the source of symptoms Joe was positioned at the point of pain and L5 was pressed ventrally to alleviate symptoms.

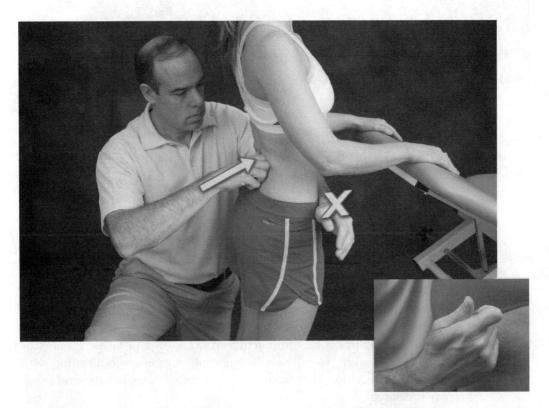

Figure 4–3 Therapist presses the vertebrae in a ventral and cranial direction.

To then differentiate the structure generating symptoms, the first step is to confirm that the pain is due to motion and not due to pressure applied to the muscle when performing the test. To accomplish this, the patient is positioned in prone and the therapist presses into the muscle adjacent to the provoked segment. If pain is elicited the therapist then supports the vertebra with an anterior to posterior pressure applied through the abdomen. If pain is present without support and absent with support then we would conclude that motion generates the pain, not just palpation alone. In the case of Joe, pain was elicited with muscular palpation with the L5 vertebra stabilized, however, it was more superficial and of lower intensity than when the vertebra was allowed to move.

To investigate other structures that could generate the symptoms with vertebral motion the therapist may perform a sciatic neural tension test.[8] This would likely be performed actively in sitting with the spine positioned on the verge of symptoms. If symptoms are reproduced then further testing of neural function (manual muscle testing, reflex testing, somatosensory testing) would be performed. In Joe's case, symptoms were not produced with neural tension testing.

To further investigate the muscular source of symptoms for pain with forward bending and left rotation the therapist may apply an active or passive muscle tendon bowstringing test. These tests combine palpation of the muscle with passive elongation or active muscle contraction (isometric, eccentric, or concentric). To perform a passive muscle tendon bowstring of the right erector spinae muscles the patient is positioned in left side lying. The therapist presses into the muscle to the VOP with his cranial hand. The therapist tilts the pelvis caudally to elongate the muscle. If pain is reproduced the palpating pressure is removed while the muscle is maintained in an elongated position. If pain increases with elongation, and is reduced with removal of the palpating pressure, the test is considered positive for a muscular impairment. To perform an active muscle tendon bowstring of the right erector spinae muscles the patient is positioned in left side lying. The therapist presses into the muscle to the VOP with his cranial hand. The therapist presses caudally on the pelvis while the patient resists the motion. If pain is reproduced the palpating pressure is removed while the muscle is maintained in a contracted state. If pain increases with contraction, and is reduced with removal of the palpating pressure, the test is considered positive for a muscular impairment. The muscle would then be palpated for quality, texture, and warmth. In the case of Joe, increased tension in the musculature was noted on the right with associated banding within the muscle. No warmth was noted.

The final piece of symptom localization information that is necessary for the management of Joe is the impact of weight-bearing on his low back pain (LBP). This is performed through the use of traction and compression testing. For compression testing the patient is positioned at the VOP in standing. The therapist then applies an axial load through the shoulder girdle and trunk (Figure 4–4). If pain is provoked the patient is then positioned at the POP and the trunk is unloaded by lifting the rib cage and thorax cranially (Figure 4–5). Care must be taken with both tests to minimize any unwanted motions other than loading and unloading during these tests. In the case of Joe, he reported increased symptoms with loading/compression and decreased symptoms with unloading/traction.

Another unique emphasis of the KE Concept-based examination is the use of passive angular and translatoric intervertebral motion testing. In the lumbar spine this testing is typically performed in side lying through either

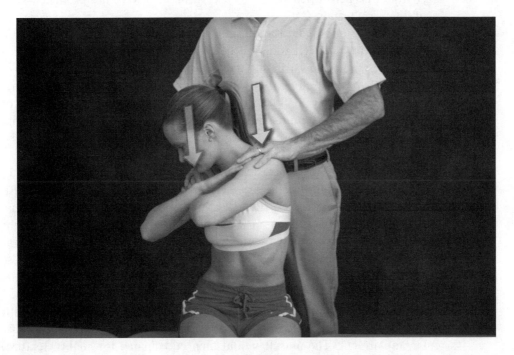

Figure 4–4 Therapist applies an axial load through the shoulder girdle and trunk.

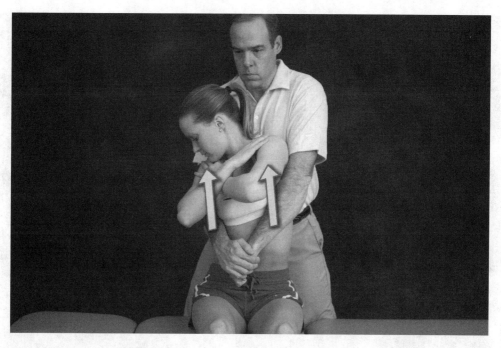

Figure 4–5 The patient is positioned at the POP and the trunk is unloaded by lifting the rib cage and thorax cranially.

femoral movement or through direct abdominal contact using a towel roll (Figures 4–6, 4–7, 4–8). These tests are performed with varying speeds, amplitudes, and stabilization. The goals of these tests are to determine if the patient presents with greater than normal (hypermobile) or less than normal (hypomobile) motion in the individual spinal segments or series of spinal segments. In addition to quantity of motion, this testing evaluates the quality of motion and end-feel. End-feel is the type of resistance felt at the end of passive motion testing and is typically described as firm (capsular), hard (boney), soft (soft tissue), empty (stopped by the patient before the end-feel is perceived), elastic (muscular), springy (meniscal), or boggy (swelling).[9] Normal end-feels vary by motion and joint. Pathologic end-feels are present when a joint demonstrates an abnormal quality or location of the end-feel (too early or too late). In the case of Joe, he presented with decreased motion at L4 and L5 with a firm end-feel. In addition he demonstrated decreased motion at the thoracolumbar junction.

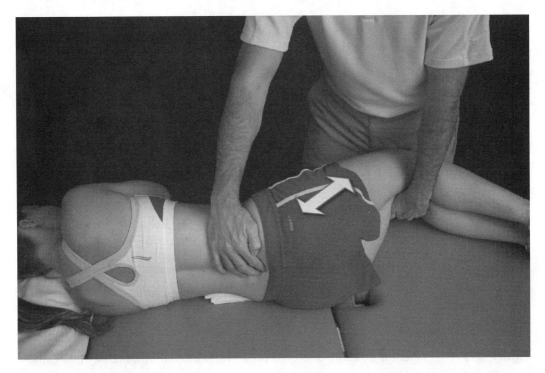

Figure 4–6 Intervertebral motion testing in side-lying through femoral movement.

Given the motion restrictions and pain present at L4 and L5, it is also important to examine the function of the lower extremity in general and the hip specifically. Upon examination, Joe demonstrates a positive right modified Thomas test.[10] This would be followed up with testing in prone to differentiate between muscle shortening (iliopsoas, or rectus femorus) and hip capsular tightness. To differentiate hip capsule versus muscle the hip would be extended in prone with the spine in neutral and then with the spine side bent to the left and right. If the hip capsule is limited then the spinal position would not affect the hip extension. If the muscle is the source of limitation then the hip extension would decrease as the spine is side bent left and would increase as the spine is side bent right. Following muscle length testing, the KE practitioner would examine hip extensor strength in prone including observing for early and/or excessive recruitment of the lumbar extensors. In Joe's case, he demonstrates early activation of the lumbar exten-

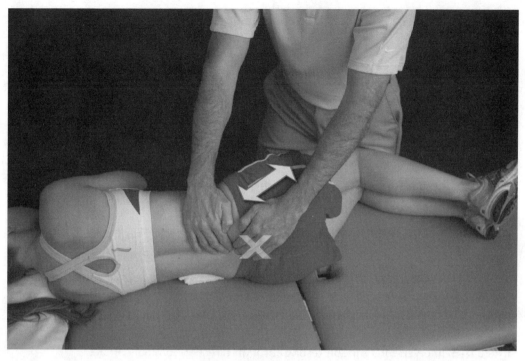

Figure 4-7 Intervertebral motion testing through femoral movement alternate position.

sors and excessive lumbar extension at L4 and L5 during hip extension. Further follow-up regarding Joe's ability to coordinate the deep extensors and transverse abdominus (TrA) revealed that he was able to perform approximately five quality contractions of TrA but that his recruitment timing was only fair.

The evaluation process used with the KE Concept uses both inductive and deductive reasoning. The process is ongoing throughout the examination and is used to determine the selection and sequencing of tests and measures and interventions used. The KE Concept also emphasizes the use of multiple tests and measures to confirm or refute a given diagnosis. The final product of the KE Concept examination is a diagnostic/differential diagnostic list. The use of the diagnostic/differential diagnostic list is an attempt within the KE Concept to limit bias due to factors such as availability of information and practitioner beliefs.

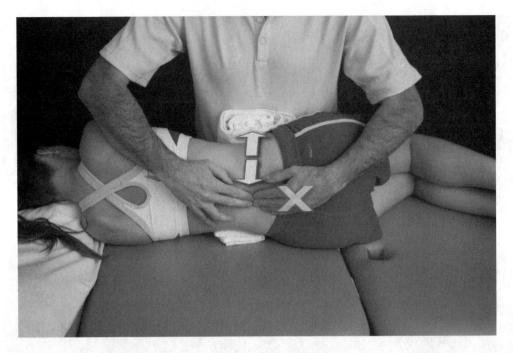

Figure 4–8 Intervertebral motion testing through direct abdominal contact.

Diagnosis

As indicated previously, the KE Concept is an integrated part of the standard physical therapy examination. As such, the differential diagnostic list for the KE Concept may contain suspected or confirmed pathological, visceral, neurological, and/or psychological diagnoses in addition to the principle physical therapy movement diagnoses. In the case of Joe, the specific movement-related diagnoses identified in the examination are hypomobile and painful L5 > L4, impaired muscle length and strength of the right lumbar paraspinal muscles, and decreased right iliopsoas muscle length.

Prognosis

In general, the physical therapy prognosis for Joe is good. His general health status is good, he reports low fear on the Fear-Avoidance Beliefs Questionnaire work subscale and physical activity subscale (this tool is described in further detail in Chapter 11),[11] and he is working full time and is well educated. The prognosis for addressing Joe's current movement impairment diagnosis is good, however it should be noted that the finding of hypomobility at L4 and L5 in a person with Joe's history is not common. While Kaltenborn and Evjenth would both treat what they diagnosed, both would suspect underlying disc changes at L4 and L5, which typically results in a hypermobility presentation. This suspicion is further strengthened by Joe's prior history of LBP. There are exceptions to this general principle (e.g., joint locking, muscle spasm) but these exceptions usually involve a change in the end-feel quality, which Joe does not present. In addition Joe presents with classic centralization phenomena[12] where repeated extension movements reduce buttock pain and increase lumbar pain and repeated flexion movements increases buttock pain. This phenomenon is also typically associated with disc changes.

When estimating a prognosis, the KE Concept relies on a foundational knowledge of anatomy, biomechanics, pathology (neuro-musculo-skeletal and medical), pathomechanics, and biopsychosocial aspects of patient management. These factors impact the development of short and long-term goals and the overall performance expectations for a given patient. For example, if Joe presented with sacroiliac joint (SIJ) hypermobility, his pain would be much more difficult to manage compared to an L4 and L5 hypomobility. This is because the SI joint relies heavily on its supporting ligaments in addition to its articular surface and joint structure for stability.[13] In order to develop muscular stability for the SIJ, extensive training is required of multiple muscles crossing between the lower extremities, pelvis, and trunk. In contrast, mobilization, manipulation, and self-mobilization of L4 and L5 may be performed in a variety of ways with relatively quick results.[14]

In addition to understanding the prognostic implications of the factors indicated in the previous paragraph, the KE Concept performs a continuous and critical appraisal of the overall therapeutic potential of the manual therapy and therapeutic exercise interventions included within the concept. This knowledge is used to refine, develop, and remove techniques that are taught within the concept as well as to assist the practitioner in the most efficient and effective selection and sequencing of interventions. To illustrate the KE Concept perspective on the selection and sequencing of intervention we can look at another example of a patient presenting with painful SI hypermobility, restricted hip joint mobility into extension, and decreased iliopsoas muscle length. In this example the KE Concept would advocate mobilization of the hip and muscle stretching of iliopsoas, while passively stabilizing the SIJ with an SI belt. Then as the SIJ became less reactive and the hip motion was improved, the muscular stabilization around the SIJ could be emphasized in the sequence of treatment.

Joe's prognosis is good based upon his initial presentation of hypomobility at L4 and L5 with concurrent paraspinal muscle shortening and weakness and concurrent hip flexor tightness on the right. However, based upon the suspected underlying disc pathology and probable hypermobility, the prognosis may change if new physical findings are identified with ongoing reexamination.

Intervention

The interventions emphasized by the KE Concept are arranged into four basic categories: 1) to relieve pain, 2) to increase mobility, 3) to limit movement, and 4) to inform, instruct, and train. As indicated in the introduction, interventions that are unique to the KE Concept include translatoric mobilizations and manipulations and functional massage.

Translatoric mobilizations and manipulation (KE intervention categories 1 and 2)

The goals of mobilization include pain relief, relaxation, and stretching. Mobilizations are performed according to three grades, which are associated with a range of translatoric motion within a joint. Grade I is described as an extremely small traction force that produces no appreciable increase in joint separation. Grade II movement takes up the slack in the tissues surrounding the joint and then tightens the tissue. Grade II is further classified into a slack zone (SZ) located at the beginning of the grade II range where there is little to no resistance to passive movement and the transition zone (TZ) where the tissues tighten and more resistance is felt. Grade III is defined as a movement applied after the slack has been taken up and all tissues become taut. Resistance within the grade III range increases rapidly.

In Joe's case, grade I-IISZ mobilizations would be used for pain relief and grade I-II mobilizations would be used for relaxation. In addition, grade III mobilization and manipulation would be used to increase mobility at L5. Finally, oscillations and vibrations may be used throughout the grades to minimize discomfort.

In the case of Joe, he appears to be a good candidate for traction manipulation of his L5 spinal segment.[15] His joint restriction is relatively small, there is a low level of reactivity to palpation, low fear of movement, the onset was only two weeks ago, and he does not present with neural compression signs. In addition, traction is particularly good given our suspicion of an underlying L5 hypermobility (i.e., the direction of traction will not stress any specific portion of the disc).

Disc traction – Thrust manipulation

To perform traction manipulation the patient is positioned in left side lying in an actual resting position as seen in Figure 4–9 (the position of maximum comfort and most free joint motion). A towel, sandbag, or other support may be used to support the resting position. The therapist stands facing the patient's pelvis and abdomen and pelvis. The therapist contacts the patient posteriorly on the sacrum with his left forearm and anteriorly on the pelvis with the left side of his torso. Slack in the lumbar spine is taken up caudally by the therapist's left arm and torso. The impulse is directed caudally through the movement of the therapist's chest and left arm.

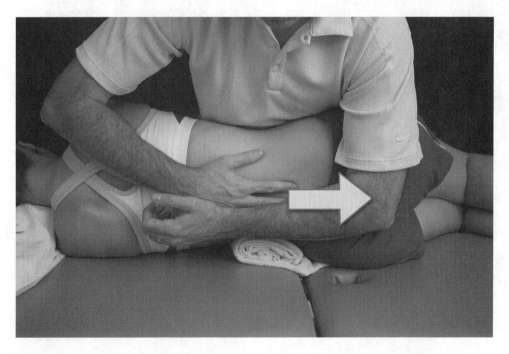

Figure 4–9 Disc traction—Thrust manipulation.

Disc traction—Mobilization

Disc traction may also be performed as a mobilization (i.e., without thrust). The technique may be performed as described for Figure 4–9, or another variation may be used with palmar contact on the sacrum. To perform this version the patient is positioned in left side lying in an actual resting position as in Figure 4–10 (the position of maximum comfort and joint motion). A towel, sandbag, or other support may be used to support the resting position. The therapist stands facing the patient's pelvis and abdomen. The therapist contacts the patient posteriorly on the sacrum with his right palm and anteriorly on the pelvis with the left side of his torso. The therapist's left hand and forearm are placed over the right to assist in supporting the right arm against the patient's sacrum. Slack in the lumbar spine is taken up caudally by the therapist's arms and torso. The mobilization is directed caudally through the movement of the therapist's chest and arms.

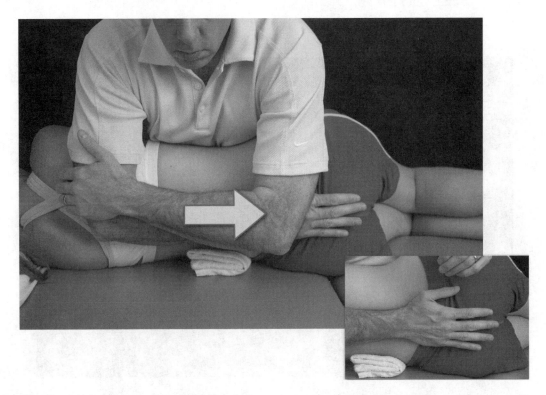

Figure 4–10 Disc traction—Mobilization.

L5 side bending mobilization (away from the side and direction of greatest restriction/symptoms)

In cases such as this one, where underlying disc pathology is suspected, but findings support facet restrictions, the KE Concept would advocate a cautious approach to restoring restricted dorsal caudal facet gliding. To explore the disc versus facet origins of symptoms and restricted motion, the KE Concept practitioner might choose to use an L5 side bending mobilization into left side bending and ventral flexion (Figure 4–11). In this technique the patient is positioned in left side lying. The lumbar spine, including L5, is positioned in ventral flexion. The patient's right hip is positioned in approximately 90° of flexion. The therapist faces the patient's pelvis and abdomen with his right thigh positioned against the abdomen (supporting lumbar ventral flexion). The therapist's right hand presses in the direction of the right side of the spinous process of L5. The therapist's left hand reinforces the position of his right wrist and hand. The therapist mobilizes L5 by leaning his body weight onto the hand contacting the spine.

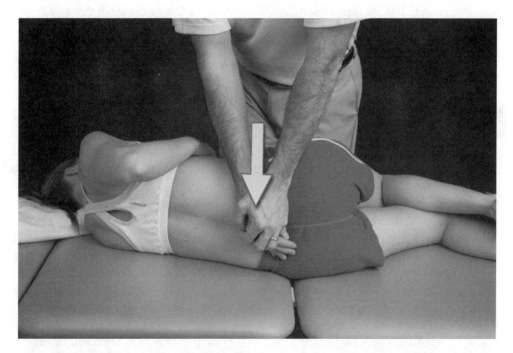

Figure 4–11 L5 side bending mobilization (away from the side and direction of greatest restriction/symptoms).

Following this mobilization the therapist would once again assess active range of motion (AROM), symptom levels/location/quality, and translatoric joint play. If AROM or symptom levels into extension, right side bending and right rotation have significantly improved, and the end-feel had changed in either quality or location then the disc or an intra-articular entrapment would be suspected as the source of the movement impairment. In such a case, treatment would continue with similar spinal movement patterns in the form of mobilization, manual muscle stretching, or functional massage. If the movement and symptoms or end-feel had not improved significantly the KE practitioner might choose to treat into the direction of restriction. In this technique the patient is positioned in right side lying. The lumbar spine including L5 is positioned in dorsal flexion and right rotation. The patient's hips are positioned in approximately 90° of flexion. The therapist faces the patient's pelvis and abdomen with his left thigh positioned against the patient's pelvis (supporting the pelvic position on the table). The therapist's left hand presses in the direction of the right side of the spinous process of L5. The therapist's right hand reinforces the position of his right wrist and hand. The therapist mobilizes L5 by leaning his body weight onto the hand contacting the spine.

Functional massage (KE intervention categories 1 and 2)

As described in the introduction, functional massage (Figure 4–12) integrates soft tissue massage (in the form of manual soft tissue compressions and decompressions) and nonpainful joint motion (both angular and translatoric). During functional massage the joint is repeatedly moved so that musculotendinous and/or periarticular soft tissues are lengthened/tensed and shortened/slackened while massage pressure is applied. Like translatoric mobilization and manipulation, functional massage is used to reduce pain and improve mobility. The integration of joint motion and massage offers several unique treatment opportunities. First, proprioceptors from both the joint and the muscle are stimulated during the massage, potentially increasing the treatment's counter-irritation effects at the spinal cord level. Second, the muscle activity during the massage may range from passive to fully active allowing for a passive intervention to be morphed into an active assistive and/or a fully active motion. Last, functional massage integrates soft tissue broadening, lengthening, and gliding of the muscles, tendons, fascia, and nerves, which occurs during normal body function. General indications for functional massage include musculoskeletal and periarticular soft tissue pain

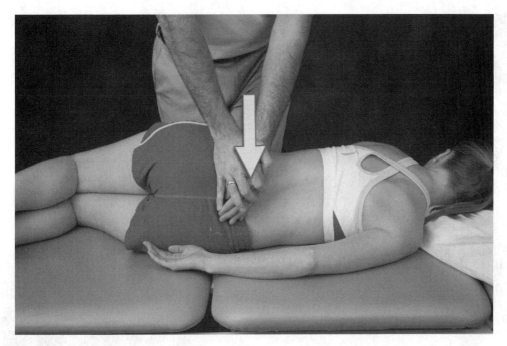

Figure 4–12 Functional massage.

and/or stiffness and resultant impairment(s) in muscle performance, joint mobility, tendon and neural mobility, and soft tissue edema/swelling. General contraindications for functional massage include severe hypomobility and injuries, medical conditions, and/or medication related conditions resulting in severe vascular or connective tissue fragility.

Functional massage into disc traction

To perform functional massage into disc traction the patient is positioned in left side lying in an actual resting position as in Figure 4–13 (the position of maximum comfort and joint motion). A towel, sandbag, or other support may be used to support the resting position. The therapist stands facing the patient's pelvis and abdomen. The therapist contacts the paraspinal muscles with the pads of his left index and middle fingers. The proximal palmar surface of the therapist's right is placed over the left to assist in pressing the fingers into the paraspinals and in generating traction. The therapist's right forearm is positioned centrally and parallel to the patient's lumbar and

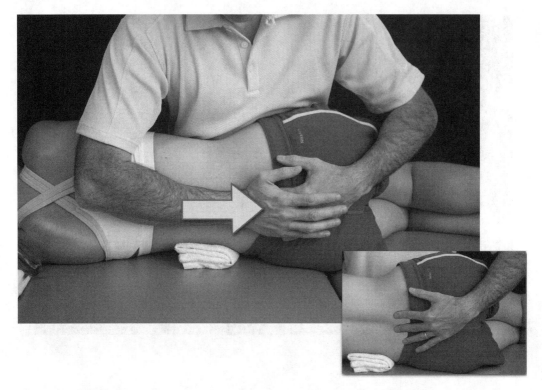

Figure 4–13 Functional massage into disc traction.

thoracic spine. The therapist massages the paraspinals by slightly flexing the left index and middle fingers and pressing his right hand into the fingers and in a caudal direction. The movement is repeated, typically at a rate of one repetition for every three seconds. The rate will vary based on the goals of the massage (e.g., relaxation, pain relief, to increase mobility), both within and between treatment sessions. Regardless of the rate, the massage should not be perceived as uncomfortable by the patient.

Functional massage into side bending

To perform functional massage into side bending the patient is positioned in left side lying as in Figure 4–14. The therapist stands facing the patient's pelvis and abdomen. The therapist contacts the paraspinal muscles with the pads of the fingers of his left and right hands. The therapist massages the paraspinals by pressing the right side of the patient's pelvis caudally and the right

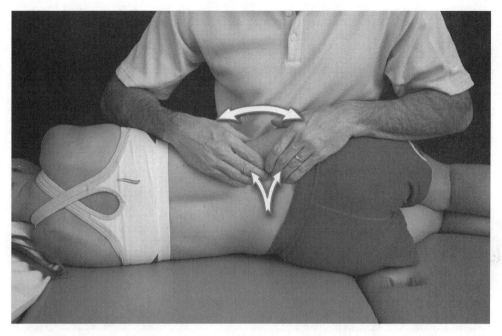

Figure 4–14 Functional massage into side bending.

side of the rib cage cranially while simultaneously pulling the paraspinals laterally and slightly cranial with the right hand and caudal with the left hand. As with massage into traction, the movement is repeated with a rate of repetition that varies based on the goals of the massage (e.g., relaxation, pain relief, to increase mobility) and the massage should not be perceived as uncomfortable by the patient.

Manual muscle stretching (KE intervention categories 1 and 2)

While manual muscle stretching is not unique to the KE Concept, its application follows the same application principles discussed previously. Specifically, manual muscle stretching should not take a joint into a restricted or painful range.[16] In addition, if underlying neural irritation is present then the muscle stretching should not move or tension the nerve in a way that provokes symptoms. Translatoric joint play testing and symptom localization are used to identify these factors within the KE Concept examination.

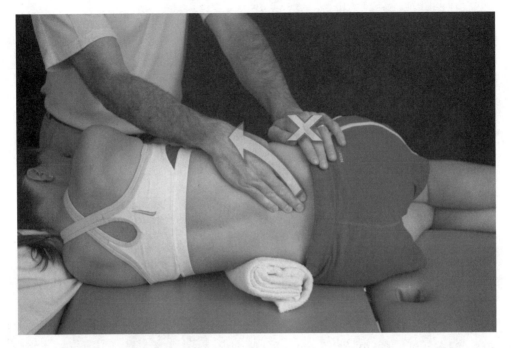

Figure 4–15 Manual muscle stretching.

In the case of Joe, examination findings support the use of a segmentally specific manual muscle stretch of the right deep extensor muscles (Figure 4–15). In this example the patient is positioned in left side lying with slight left side bending, left rotation, and flexion at L5. The therapist stands facing the patient's upper torso with his left hand contacting and stabilizing the patient's pelvis and the radial border of his right hand (index and middle fingers) contacting the patient's L5 segment. The patient is instructed to hold against a ventral and cranial force exerted by the therapist's right hand. The patient holds the contraction for 5–7 seconds and then relaxes. Slack in the muscle is taken up by further left side bending, flexing, and left rotating L5. During the stretching the therapist maintains a dialogue with the patient regarding the location, quality, and quantity of the stretch. The stretch should be maintained in a moderate to intense quantity and should fade as the stretch is maintained. The stretching procedure is repeated until the stretch intensity does not change following muscle contraction and relaxation. At this point the stretch is maintained for 30 seconds to 2 minutes or longer. Following the static stretch the patient is instructed to perform the opposing muscle action/motion to reciprocally inhibit the stretched muscles.

In addition to the segmental muscle stretching, Joe also requires manual muscle stretching of his right iliopsoas and rectus femoris muscles. This stretching (not pictured) would be performed in prone with the patient positioned at the edge of the table with his left leg off the table and positioned in flexion with the foot on the floor. A pillow would be placed under the abdomen to support the lumbar spine and a belt would be used to secure the pelvis and hip position. The right hip would then be extended to the point of moderate stretch with care taken to avoid changes in back position during hip extension. The stretching sequence would then be repeated as described in the previous paragraph. At the conclusion of the stretching the patient would be instructed to extend the hip by firing the gluteus maximus muscle. To target the rectus femoris muscle during stretching a combination of hip extension and knee flexion would be used. Care would be taken to avoid flexing the knee into any range that aggravated the prior knee surgery.

Therapeutic exercise (KE intervention categories 3 and 4)

As mentioned in the introduction to this chapter, both Kaltenborn and Evjenth were first educated as physical educators and then as physical therapists. The KE Concept places therapeutic exercise into intervention categories 3 (Immobilization) and 4 (Inform, Instruct, and Train). Specific to Joe's case, both categories would include exercises to improve the timing between the deep back extensor muscles and the transverse abdominus. In addition, both would advocate general therapeutic exercises to improve Joe's ability to perform his work without irritating his back (e.g., training of the gluteal muscles, quadriceps, and larger back and trunk muscles used during squatting, reaching, and lifting). In addition, both may use specific segmental contacts, like those illustrated in Figure 4–15 to provide direct, quick, stretch stimulus to the muscles requiring strengthening. Finally, the KE Concept advocates the continual monitoring of the patient to ensure that the therapeutic exercises they are using do not aggravate the underlying pathology/condition or movement impairment with which the patient is presenting.

Self-mobilization/Self-stretching (KE intervention category 4)

Joe's back symptoms centralized with extension during the physical examination. As indicated under the prognosis section of this chapter, this is consistent with a disc problem. While these symptoms might be treated successfully with repeated extension exercises in prone, there is still underlying concern that the hypomobility diagnosed during the examination might not be

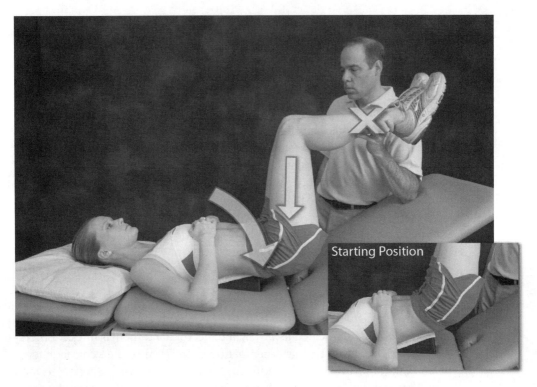

Starting Position

Figure 4–16 Self-mobilization/Self stretching.

accurate. To perform a more specific L5 extension movement, the patient would be positioned in supine as in Figure 4–16.[17] A wedge is placed with the base facing caudally and positioned under L5. The patient's hips and knees are positioned in 90° of flexion. The patient is instructed to gradually tilt the pelvis over the base of the wedge by relaxing the hamstrings. The movement is repeated 5–10 times and the motion is then reassessed by the therapist. If symptoms are reduced, movement is improved and the joint play continues to be restricted, then the patient may be instructed to perform the exercise at home taking care to monitor his symptoms prior to, during, and following the exercise. The frequency of the exercise, number of repetitions, and length of hold for each stretching movement would vary based on patient presentation.

SUMMARY

The KE Concept consists of a core set of principles with a broad scope of application. These principles thoroughly integrate into standard physical therapy practice and are intended to guide and enhance this practice. This chapter has highlighted some of the unique features and principles of the concept, however it should be noted that patient and practice context drastically impacts the content of a KE Concept-based examination and intervention. Therefore the information presented within this chapter, while comprehensive in nature, should not be considered an exhaustive representation of the concept.

REFERENCES

1. Kaltenborn FM, Evjenth O, Kaltenborn TB, Morgan D, Vollowitz E. *Manual Mobilization of the Joints Vol II: The Spine 5th ed.* Minneapolis, MN: OPTP; 2009.
2. Waddell G. 1987 Volvo award in clinical sciences. A new clinical model for the treatment of low-back pain. *Spine.* 1987;12(7):632–644.
3. Knott M, Voss DE. *Proprioceptive Neuromuscular Facilitation: Patterns and Techniques.* 2nd ed. Philadelphia: Harper & Row; 1968.
4. Maigne JY, Vautravers P. Mechanism of action of spinal manipulative therapy. *Joint, Bone, Spine.* 2003;70(5):336–341.
5. Woolf CJ. Central sensitization: uncovering the relation between pain and plasticity. *Anesthesiology.* 2007;106(4):864–867.
6. Melzack R. The McGill Pain Questionnaire: Major properties and scoring methods. *Pain.* 1975;1:277–299.
7. Huijbregts PA. Spinal motion palpation: A review of reliability studies. *J Man Manip Ther.* 2002;10(1):24–39.
8. Butler DS. *Mobilization of the Nervous System.* London: Churchill Livingstone; 1991.
9. Cyriax J. *Textbook of Orthopaedic Medicine Volume I* London: Bailliere Tindall; 1982.
10. Kendall FP, McCreary EK, Provance PG. *Muscles: Testing and Function with Posture and Pain. 5th ed.* Baltimore, MD: Lippincott Williams & Wilkins. 2005. 33–35, 57–59
11. Waddell G, Newton M, Henderson I, Somerville D, Main CJ. A Fear-Avoidance Beliefs Questionnaire (FABQ) and the role of fear-avoidance beliefs in chronic low back pain and disability. *Pain.* 1993;52(2):157–168.
12. McKenzie R. *The Lumbar Spine: Mechanical Diagnosis and Therapy.* Waikanae, New Zealand: Spinal Publications; 2003.
13. Pell JJ, Spoor CW, Pool-Goudzwaard AL, Hoek van Dijke GA, Snijders CJ. Biomechanical analysis of reducing sacroiliac shear load by optimization of pelvic muscle and ligament forces. *Ann Biomed Eng.* 2008;36(3):415–424.
14. Bronfort G, Haas M, Evans RL, Bouter LM. Efficacy of spinal manipulation and mobilization for low back pain and neck pain: a systematic review and best evidence synthesis. *Spine J.* 2004;4(3):335–356.
15. Krauss J, Evjenth O, Creighton D. *Translatoric Spinal Manipulation for Physical Therapists.* Rochester Hills, MI: Lakeview Media; 2006.
16. Evjenth O, Hamberg J. *Muscle Stretching in Manual Therapy: A Clinical Manual, Volume II.* Alfta, Sweden: Alfta Rehab Forlag; 1997.
17. Evjenth O, Hamberg J. *Auto Stretching.* Alfta, Sweden: Alfta Rehab Forlag; 1997.

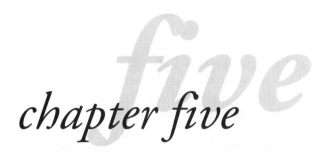

chapter five

The Maitland Concept

Kenneth E. Learman, PT, PhD, OCS, COMT, FAAOMPT
Christopher R. Showalter, PT, OCS, COMT, FAAOMPT, FABS

The Maitland Concept is named after Geoffrey D. Maitland, a physiotherapist from Australia. Students can find more information about the approach and training opportunities at the website of Maitland-Australian Physiotherapy Seminars: http://www.ozpt. com/.

The first edition of Maitland's seminal "Vertebral Manipulation" was published in 1964. His text and his work focus on clinical examination and assessment rather than focusing on technique alone. He was an advocate of "careful thought" and the relationship between clinical and critical thought to patient care. The essence of the Maitland Concept lies in the integration of examination and evaluation with intervention rendering these elements of patient care indistinguishable.

BACKGROUND

The Maitland concept is named for Geoff Maitland (1924–2010) and is underpinned by the philosophy that the patient's chief complaint (comparable sign), and its response should be the focus of the examination and treatment process.[1,2] The concept includes the examination of treatment effects in addition to the application of treatment techniques.[3] It should be further stated that the Maitland concept includes the entire clinical reasoning process around the management of a particular condition rather than focus on a specific medical diagnosis or set of manual therapy techniques alone. To this end, this chapter seeks to highlight the reasoning process used in the management of the patient Joe Lores.

The comparable sign is any combination of movement irregularity, pain, spasm, or pathomechanical abnormality (hypo vs. hypermobility) that most closely resembles the patient's interpretation of their primary subjective complaint and should not be confused with other symptoms that may not be the primary problem but are still present. These secondary complaints are referred to as joint signs[1] or a "discordant pain response."[2] This provocation model is shared with several other philosophies including the McKenzie[4] and Mulligan[5] models. It becomes self-evident when basing the clinical reasoning process on the response of the chief complaint to any and all inputs, that effective, efficient, and free flowing communication between the clinician and the patient is a must.

There are several relative advantages and disadvantages to this model, and these are outlined eloquently by Cook.[6] With the patient-focused model it is imperative that an open, honest line of communication be established between the patient and practitioner. This requires the clinician to be diligent in pursuit of valuable clinical information from the patient. Maitland referred to this diligence as "a positive personal commitment to understand what the person (patient) is enduring."[7] Maitland emphasized the practice of metacognition through the meticulous documentation of this process for future study. Any failure to adequately obtain appropriate clinical information could be considered a failure on the clinician's part and may obfuscate the appropriate plan of action. A strong advantage of using the patient-response model is in the application of evidence-based practice (EBP). Since the model is adapted to the positive response of each patient, the application of intervention should be based on the evidence of previous treatment success within the confines of each incident of care. While additional information (evidence) is applied whenever possible and applicable, this evidence does not supersede the patient's response; therefore, modeling appropriate clinical behavior on the response of individuals rather than the average behavior of groups.

Maitland employed a two compartment "brick wall" concept where any information that may apply to a given patient, be it anatomy, physiology, imaging, diagnosis, and presumed biomechanics, would be on the left side of the wall. All clinical information obtained from the patient, observation, and the physical examination would represent data on the right side of the wall.[1] The importance of this mode of thinking lies in the fact that a patient with a very specific pathoanatomical diagnosis (such as cervical spondylosis) may present with a wide variety of histories, signs, and symptoms. The infinite variation in clinical presentations certainly precludes the clinician's ability to treat them all in a uniform manner despite the same diagnosis. Variability in age, psychosocial characteristics, stage of pathology, functional limitations, and patient-directed goals will influence the treatment approach employed. Likewise, multiple patients can present with similar histories, signs, and symptoms and may be found to have differing diagnoses.[8] These findings suggest that diagnoses, theories, and any known physiologic factors may or may not clearly define the way a patient should be managed. The two-compartment mode of thinking essentially purports that each patient be treated as a case study with appropriate application of evidence as it pertains to this individual.

Using a patient-response model liberates the clinician from applying theories of biomechanics, protocols, or assessment and treatment algorithms in situations where their use may complicate the clinical reasoning process or be fundamentally flawed.[6] A patient-response model requires the clinician to alter treatment on a moment-by-moment basis in accordance with the response to the previous bout of treatment; however, as the clinical picture progresses, some components of the plan of care may remain similar as long as they are effective. A freely adaptive model does require the clinician to be willing to alter the application of a technique in some fundamental way in order to meet the needs of a patient.[1] Since potentially complicated theories of mechanics are generally avoided in the Maitland concept, the process is relatively easy to learn, often incorporates basic techniques for assessment and treatment, and can be remarkably intuitive in its application.[6] A model based on patient response tends to be impairment or functionally based, which is consistent with the *Guide to Physical Therapist Practice*[9] and is amenable to the World Health Organization's International Classification of Functioning, Disability and Health (ICF) model.[6] The choice of diagnosis tends to be impairment based as well. The Maitland model is not dependent on an absolutely correct pathoanatomical diagnosis in most cases:

> "Despite its pathology often being something of a black box, much can be done to alleviate the distress. Manipulative therapists usually approach the treatment of low back pain by observing the outputs (signs and symptoms) of the black box, then carefully and methodically applying their skills (inputs), to bring about a favourable outcome. The hypothesis of what happens inside the black box becomes less relevant except in those instances where reliable pathological data exists."[10]

Disadvantages to this model do exist. The model is potentially more time consuming in order to appropriately perform a subjective examination. Since it does not incorporate many of the tenants of other manual therapy philosophies, it is often thought to be a more "maverick" approach.[6] As previously stated, it does require the clinician to be dedicated to the concept and failure to do so can result in an inefficient process that may compromise outcomes. Since the model does not place a premium on identifying a specific diagnosis, comparative research may be lacking for other treatment models. This fact may not hinder actual outcomes since physical therapy for the treatment of LBP has gone in the direction of classification in the last 15 years;[11-13] however, the Maitland concept eschews the use of categories as well. Finally, and most importantly, to date, no manual therapy model in its entirety has been compared with other models to determine validity with respect to relative effectiveness, speed of recovery, impact on recidivism rates, or economic considerations of the process—the Maitland concept is no exception.[6]

Maitland first described and popularized the concept of irritability. Irritability is the concept of how easily a particular condition is bothered by a given degree of provocation and how long it takes for those symptoms to settle back to their baseline level.[1] It clinically represents the stability of the condition and has also been referred to as tissue reactivity.[6] The level of irritability can be viewed in two separate ways. One is to view it as a dichotomous variable and the second is to view it on a continuum that rates relative amounts of irritability. Maitland did not operationally define how to apply the concept of irritability in his writings but does give clinical guidance through case descriptions.[14] The value of the dichotomous approach is in establishing a particular level of irritability where you will make the conscious decision to alter your assessment and treatment approach in order to accommodate the likelihood of unacceptable post assessment or treatment soreness. In other words, you would not be willing to push the involved tissues past the point where symptoms are first provoked.[1] The value of the continuum approach is the obvious acknowledgement that all conditions are unique in some ways and that there are an infinite number of levels of that dimension that may be clinically present. Irritability is more about how the symptoms behave in relation to provocation rather than whether or not the symptoms are constant or severe in nature. Irritability must be estimated through the subjective examination to avoid an overly aggressive assessment during the physical examination.[10] Despite the relative lack of guidance on the application of the irritability concept, inter tester reliability has been established at a modest kappa of 0.44.[15]

Maitland promoted a teaching/learning tool referred to as movement diagrams (Figure 5–1). This tool allows the therapist to visually display the relationship between pain (or any symptom for that matter), resistance within the tissues, and the amount of force necessary to move the body segment passively through range.[16] It allows a comparison of what the clinician and patient feel and how that relates to what should be felt by the clinician and patient. If more than one diagram is created over time for the same patient, clinical progress becomes observable through diagrammatic changes much the same as one would expect through a standard documentation system.[1] The X-axis represents any range of motion for the segment. It could be the full range of motion for the joint or a subcomponent with "A" being the starting position and "B" being average normal physiologic passive movement.[16] If a clinician wants to represent full joint range, then the "AB" line can correspond to the full normal passive range of a joint. However, in a pathologic condition, it makes sense to limit the diagram to allow you to focus on the movement of interest.[16] In the case of end range pain in shoulder elevation, the last 25° may be the range that you want to study, so limiting the diagram to those last 25° makes clinical sense. The Y-axis represents the intensity of the quality under investigation.[16] Therefore, "A" would represent

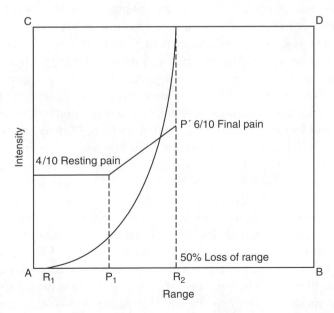

Figure 5–1 Movement diagram for lumbar flexion during the initial assessment.

the resting level of symptom and "C" being the point at which the clinician would be unwilling to push the symptoms any further. P_1 represents the point at which pain is first felt during passive oscillatory movements whereas P' refers to the intensity of pain that is experienced at the limit of range (when range is not limited by the pain). It should also be pointed out that the maximum symptom one would be willing to provoke is dependent upon the concept of irritability previously discussed, the nature of the symptoms, and the experience and confidence of the clinician in similar situations. If a particular movement causes symptoms of back pain to spread into the buttock and down the leg (not that uncommon in dealing with spinal pain as we are in this case), the clinician has to make the determination at what point in assessment this peripheralization becomes unacceptable and discontinues the assessment through range.

One could also view the "AC" line as the force required to move the segment through range. When the primary limiting factor is resistance, the "AC" line represents the limit of the clinician's willingness to push into that resistance.[7] R1 is the point at which any resistance to movement is first appreciated. One might say that this occurs when the toe region has been taken up and we enter the elastic range, but R1 could also be a neurophysiologic response (guarding) to movement. While the exact mechanism of first resistance may be unclear in any given scenario, R1 is the point when that subtle resistance to movement, by any mechanism, is appreciated. The joint movement typically ends in R2 when pain is not a limiting concern; however, there are scenarios when the therapist may be unwilling to push firmly into R2 and limit the motion voluntarily at a point short of the joint's true range. In the case of a patient with knees or elbows that hyperextend easily, the therapist can push into end range without a noticeable bony block occurring. Since the end-feel never seems to become very firm, R2 may be established not on true end range but on the perception that pushing more forcefully into range could result in further joint damage. The slope of the line used to represent the intensity vs. range behavior of the condition can further refine the complex relationship between the variables in question.[1]

There are several ways in which movement diagrams can be used as a teaching/learning tool. The student can be provided with a blank movement diagram and the mentor could request them to fill it out with some basic instruction on what representation pain and restriction may have on the diagram.[16] Since there is not necessarily an absolute value for either P2 or R2, a student and mentor can compare the values they would obtain and the difference between them could suggest that the student is either too forceful or not forceful enough in their assessment.[1] The mentor can also use the movement diagram to emphasize the interrelationship between the various joint signs, pain, stiffness, and spasm that may be present during a joint assessment as well as diagrammatically represent the range and excursion of a particular passive treatment technique. This complexity of application can also be used to show progression of a condition over time through the course of treatment. The judicious use of movement diagrams forces the clinician to engage metacognition, evaluate their own strengths and weaknesses, and enhance their own clinical reasoning abilities.

Movement diagrams can also be used to define the oscillatory grades of manipulative treatment. Maitland's description of oscillatory grades can be defined by where they end in range with relationship to barriers. These barriers can either be provocation of pain (additional pain where constant) or the appreciation of resistance or spasm. In essence, the only difference between a grade III and IV is the size of the oscillation; grade III being larger, but where they are in range remains constant; approximately halfway into resistance where the end feel is soft or at the end of range when the end-feel is hard.[1] Further delineation of where in resistance the oscillation occurs can be made by the use of pluses and minuses, with pluses nearing the end of the resistance barrier and minuses nearing the onset of the barrier.[1] See Figure 5–2 for oscillatory grades superimposed on a movement diagram.

APPLICATION OF THE MAITLAND CONCEPT TO JOE LORES

Examination

Since the Maitland concept is dependent on a carefully performed subjective examination, a thorough history must be taken. While using a subjective examination is not unique to the Maitland concept, there are some specific categories of inquiry that are felt to be exceedingly important to uncover factors that may guide the clinician in the physical examination to follow by narrowing down the vast array of potential tests and measures that could be selected in the physical examination. There is evidence that history taking contributes to the diagnostic process[17] even though this relationship to the selection of treatment techniques has not been well established.[18] Free-flowing communication is essential to allow the patient to present the narrative of their condition in their own words. The clinician must remain active, vigilant, and flexible in their subjective examination and data collection. The clinician must remain vigilant that they do not cut off the patient

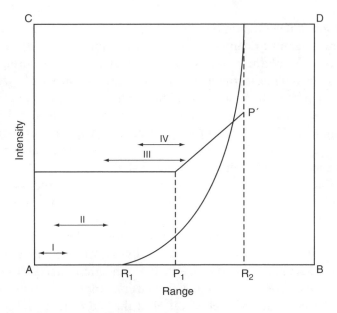

Figure 5–2 Grades of passive oscillatory movement.

mid-narrative and thus prematurely block a fruitful, perhaps essential line of enquiry. Flexibility is required for the therapist to allow the subjective exam to take its own natural course, and yet return to relevant components to gather important clinical data. The subjective exam is an active process akin to solving a puzzle by collecting data and proposing, modifying, and rejecting hypotheses. This process makes it unnecessary to have a "Maitland specific" data collection sheet. The following is a narrative obtained during an initial examination with the patient Joe.

Nature and kind of disorder

Joe reported that his main concern is right-sided low back pain (LBP) that radiates into his right buttock. The primary problem is pain; he does report that some stiffness is present as well, but denies the sense of weakness or giving way. The pain is described as aching and deep, and has spread since the initial onset from LBP to include buttock pain. The pain is constant and variable ranging from 2–6 on a 0–10 scale and is currently a 4/10. Joe's chief complaint is pain in the low back and buttock so this is the cluster of symptoms important to him.

Behavior of symptoms

The pain is activity dependent and demonstrates the following 24-hour behavioral pattern. Joe has level 2/10 pain upon waking and whenever he is lying down. His symptoms increase to 3/10 upon rising from lying down. Sitting for 10 minutes increases the pain to 6/10 and the pain continues to rate 6/10 upon rising from the chair. The fact that Joe's symptoms are constant requires clarification to determine that they are truly constant, so he was questioned whether those symptoms ever go away at any point in time during the day, even if only for a while, and he reported that they do not. Bending forward and sitting aggravates the symptoms and nothing takes the symptoms away but lying down and medications reduce the intensity. Since typical movements like bending twisting, sitting, and lifting all increase symptoms from level 2–4/10 to level 6 within 5–10 minutes of activity and he is unable to determine exactly how long it takes to settle back down but they ultimately do settle, irritability level cannot be definitively determine; however, it does not appear that the problem is irritable enough to substantially alter a typical examination pattern. He will be monitored as to how he responds to testing in case further examination requires modification of tactics to accommodate irritability. Joe would rather stand than sit, but even though he does tend to work in a standing position at times, the work is compromised because he does have to bend forward, twist, and lift, as well as maneuver himself into tight places when doing private jobs at home.

The symptoms began 2 weeks ago in a forward bent and rotated position under a kitchen sink connecting the plumbing during installation. No other unusual activities were performed that day. He has not sought any medical treatment besides going to his physician who prescribed a radiograph (negative), relative rest, and medication (he was prescribed Flexeril and was already on Lotensin for hypertension). The symptoms improved during the first week but reached a plateau since that time. In addition to the Flexeril, Joe is taking 220 mg of Aleve at night or as needed throughout the day. The Aleve does seem to help with symptoms.

Past history

Joe had one previous episode of LBP back in 2002 while helping a friend move a couch. This is the only episode of LBP, he did not seek medical attention, and it fully resolved with over-the-counter medication. He has no history of neck problems but does note that his knees sometimes feel stiff and achy. This lack of progressive history may imply that the condition is not degenerative in nature; however, a previous history of back pain has been linked to frequency and severity of future back and neck pathology[19] and delayed recovery,[20] but not necessarily the development of disabling back pain.[21]

Special questions: There is no change with bowel and bladder function or body weight. With his young age (38) and the short duration of symptoms so far (2 weeks), and the apparent mechanical mechanism of injury and behavior of symptoms, there is little concern for contribution from sinister pathology.[22] It is, however, always a good idea to monitor for that possibility since approximately 3% of LBP is from nonmechanical sources[23] and since a small percentage of general practice physicians routinely screen for red flags upon examination.[24]

Additional factors obtained from the examination included an Oswestry Disability Index (ODI)[25] score of 42% (on a 0–100% scale) and a Fear-Avoidance Belief Questionnaire (FABQ)[26] score of 34 total, with 16 and 18 on the work and physical activity subscales, respectively. Joe was asked "During the past month, have you been bothered by feelings of being down depressed or hopeless?" and "During the past month, have you been bothered by little pleasure in doing things?"[27] These questions are a quick screen for depression with diagnostic accuracy values of 96–97% for sensitivity and 57–67% for specificity.[28,29] Both questions were negative for Joe.

Observation

Maitland refers to the observation examination as part of the physical examination, recognizing the fact that observation generally begins upon first meeting the patient and continues throughout the entire clinical process. It is common to all major orthopedic philosophies to perform some form of postural assessment, even a perfunctory one even though postural asymmetry does not predict spinal[30] or pelvic[31] pathology. It is generally accepted that these asymmetries are noteworthy despite their lack of predictive validity.

Joe's resting symptoms were established before beginning the examination (4/10). Since forward flexion was identified as a provocative movement that is required for his work, we began the exam with this comparable movement. He was willing to bend forward and moved through 50% range of motion without hesitation or aberrant movement patterns. Extension was equally limited and the movement pattern was also good. Both sagittal plane movements increased his symptoms slightly. Side flexion to the right was limited to 75% normal range and side flexion left was full and did not alter symptoms; however, overpressure mildly increased pain. Maitland routinely used passive overpressures to fully assess and clear a movement pattern that was not provocative during active range of motion. The overpressure increases the sensitivity of the test since it allows assessment to the extent of the passive range unobtainable by active movement alone. Rotations were mildly limited at 80% of range and did not alter symptoms. Repeated movements into flexion made his symptoms worse and repeated movements into extension reduced his symptoms in buttock area and reduced the overall intensity of his symptoms. Passive physiologic flexion was full in range and increased his symptoms and passive physiologic extension was mildly limited and increased his symptoms. Passive accessory intervertebral movements (PAIVMS) are used to identify painful segments that may have altered mobility. The PA glide has variable reliability depending on whether or not it is being used to identify painful or stiff segments, with painful response being more reliable[19,32,33] but is likely better at identifying a specific segmental level to treat rather than identifying a specific degree of stiffness.[6] In this case PAIVMs reveal that L4 and L5 were provocative and hypomobile. Unilateral PAIVMS were stiff and painful on the right at L4-5 but were less stiff and pain free on the left. As unilateral PA glides were performed repeatedly on the right, both the symptoms and stiffness reduced. Transverse PAIVMS on the spinous process were stiff and painful directed toward the right at L4-5 and were less stiff and pain free toward the left (Figure 5–3).

Evaluation

Initially it was established that LBP that radiates into the right buttock was his chief complaint and therefore comparable symptoms. It was established in the subjective history and confirmed during the physical examination that forward flexion, prolonged sitting, twisting, and lifting all increase his symptoms within minutes of initiation of activity, making them all comparable active movements. The passive physiological examination further confirmed that both flexion and extension increase symptoms and are limited. The passive accessory examination revealed limitation of movement and painful response to

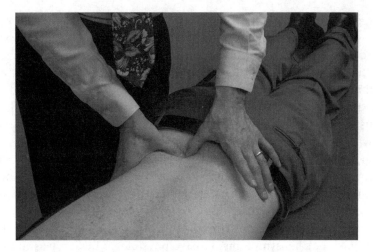

Figure 5–3 Lumbar unilateral PA glide.

both central and right unilateral vertebral pressures (PAIVMs) at both L4 and L5, with the right L4–L5 articular pillar being the most provocative movement. These findings suggest that multiple comparable signs were available for reassessment and treatment so a decision needed to be made as to which movement to base treatment on. Since he did not respond to the assessment in an irritable fashion, the clinician could proceed with the use of the most comparable sign. In this circumstance, the most comparable sign for treatment, because it produced the most provocation of symptoms earliest in range and with the least amount of force, was the unilateral PA glide on L4–L5. Active forward flexion is the most comparable sign that Joe would appreciate as a problematic functional movement pattern so it was selected as the most comparable sign for reassessment. A thorough assessment identified these multiple comparable signs and graded them in order to determine which sign was the most comparable for his condition. This simply could not be determined without adequate communication with active input from the patient.

Diagnosis

The Maitland concept does not use a particular nomenclature for arriving at a diagnosis nor does it find it necessary to assign specific pathoanatomic causation to a condition in order to treat. Grieve stated that signs and symptoms have a greater relationship to treatment selection than the identification of a particular diagnosis.[34] The condition can be defined by assessment of specific impairments identified in the clinical examination[33] and the patient response to inputs from the clinician.[1,20] In our case, it can be stated that Joe has mechanical LBP that is exacerbated by the comparable movements of flexion, extension, and right sidebending. Maitland found that the final pathomechanical diagnosis was difficult to make, especially when based on the initial patient encounter alone.[35] One may surmise that it is discogenic in origin but that cannot be guaranteed at this point as there is no prima facie evidence for a discogenic disorder at this point.

Prognosis

Joe's condition demonstrates a very good prognosis to achieve full resolution of symptoms over the next 3 weeks with a return to full activity secondary to his fairly young age, an absence of significant comorbidities known to prolong this type of condition, no known psychosocial factors that are known to protract care, the fact that this is only his second episode of LBP, and, most importantly, the fact that within-session changes were noted during the examination. Centralization with repeated extension has been shown to predict good short term outcomes,[36] even though recent evidence would suggest that long term prognostic value is less compelling.[37] This centralization was confirmed through the use of unilateral PA glides on L4–L5. Maitland believed that accurate prognosis can be a difficult task and a level of uncertainty is always present, making prognosis an estimation of probabilities rather than certainties, perhaps more of an art than science.[1]

Intervention

There were several treatment options available for Joe and all would likely show progress over time. The condition responded favorably to movements that mechanically close down the right side of the involved segment though; therefore, any treatment or position that closed the L4–L5 segment was available to reduce his symptoms. There may be some dissention regarding exactly what happens at a given facet joint. We may agree that there could be a different affect when we consider three alternative points of contact during a unilateral PA glide depending on whether we are on the superior articular process, the joint line, or the inferior articular process.

The Maitland concept prompts us to explore these different inputs at all three points and determine which one reproduces the comparable sign with the least amount of force. (It should be acknowledged that a clinician's ability to discriminate these different points is limited.) If treatment is chosen to be based exclusively off the movements used in the assessment, and unless the clinical reasoning would prompt the clinician to select a technique otherwise (more on this later), a unilateral PA glide on the right side of L4–L5 would work well. The assessment already found that performing a trial bout relieved his comparable sign and this technique is easy to guide a more localized, focused treatment. Placing thumbs across the right articular pillar and performing a bout of oscillation that engages resistance to the point of a mild increase in pain was warranted. The direction of the force would be straight toward the floor, regardless of facet orientation since there is no compelling evidence that performing techniques in specific planes yields superior outcomes,[21] even though variation in angle may alter the clinician's perception of stiffness[32] or the comparable sign. A bout of mobilization could last anywhere from 30 seconds to a couple of minutes depending on irritability. With Joe having constant pain, a slightly shorter treatment time of around 45 seconds could be recommended, then reassess the response to the treatment before continuing. Multiple bouts (3 to 4) would be a good place to start. The grade of the mobilization can be variable, but since resistance has been engaged we know that it is either a grade III or IV depending on the size of the oscillation. The smaller grade IV oscillations may be preferable to treat constant pain.

An equally valid treatment approach would have been to select an alternative treatment option that may not necessarily be the most provocative movement pattern but shows promise for reducing the condition. In this case, a lumbar rotation, performed in sidelying on the painful side would enhance closure of the involved segment. On the surface, this choice would not appear to necessarily be a valid technique based on the tenants of the concept, yet there are circumstances in which a clinician may recognize specific patterns that allow them to employ their expertise from previous experiences. One could begin by bringing Joe's legs up into a little flexion until the beginning of movement was felt in the L4–L5 segment, then rotating the trunk up toward the ceiling (left rotation) until movement was felt at the same segment. Then the therapist could direct rotation to the involved segment by oscillating the subject with force on the anterior shoulder and posterior hip. This sidelying position theoretically closes down the involved segment by placing it in right side flexion and left rotation. Again, multiple bouts of mobilization, either grade III or IV, would be appropriate, a grade

IV in this case might be the best recommendation since it could be used to reduce the comparable sign while enhancing movement.

In general, Maitland did not use spinal manipulation as his first treatment option for most conditions. Maitland believed that the majority of conditions responded favorably to mobilization without the risks of increased post-treatment soreness. This is particularly true when the clinician is not certain how stable the symptoms may be. Once the patient has been treated with gentler techniques and the response to more aggressive treatment could be more accurately predicted, a manipulation may become a viable treatment option.[1] In this case, I would not elect to manipulate Joe's spine initially, despite the fact that the initial examination revealed satisfaction of a clinical prediction rule for short-term treatment success with four out five known factors and patient characteristics that meet the inclusion criteria for the rule.[38,39] If progress plateaus and the condition became less severe in nature with intermittent symptoms, the case could be made to perform a manipulation for this patient. Initially, mobilization is less likely to result in unacceptably high levels of post-treatment soreness, making it the more conservative treatment.

Since lumbar extension repeatedly reduced Joe's symptoms, a logical home exercise program would include repeated lumbar extension. It can easily be performed standing by having Joe place his hands on his posterior hips for stability and extending backward as far as he can without exacerbating his

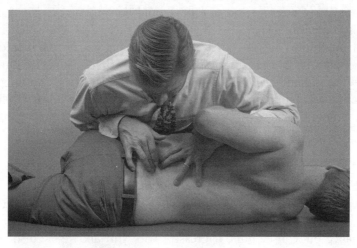

Figure 5–4 Lumbar rotation mobilization.

symptoms unacceptably. This can be done for up to 10 repetitions several times per day, particularly after just standing up from sitting. One recommendation would be that Joe avoid too much sitting and forward bending for a few days until his symptoms become more manageable (stable). Alternative or additional home exercises could include lying on his right side and rotate back to his left and hold this posture (or gently oscillate it) for several minutes 3–4 times per day since this treatment option reduces pain, Joe could also stand straight up and while keeping his knees straight he could reach back with his right hand to his right popliteal fossa, creating a stronger closure of the right side of his spine with a functional quadrant (tri-planar) position. Over the course of treatment we will progress treatment by increasing the duration of mobilization, increase the number of bouts and/or intensity of the grade to IV+ or even IV++ in an effort to move the pain curve off the movement diagram and to change the resistance curve to reflect an increase in range of motion and to normalize the relationship between the R1 and R2 points.

Ideally, an intrasession improvement of approximately 30–50% is desirable. Often the patient loses some of the progress between sessions but it should not return to pretreatment levels, especially if an appropriate home exercise program is implemented to address notable impairments or functional movement losses. As the patient progresses through treatment, the improvements get larger and progress is maintained. Anywhere from 3–8 sessions, depending on many variables in and out of the therapist's control, over a 2–4 week period of time should be sufficient to satisfactorily reduce his comparable sign initiate his home exercise program that is designed to maintain the progress noted while enhancing strength. It would be advisable to start with 2–3 sessions in the first week with declining treatment frequency as the patient becomes able to control their own symptoms to stimulate active self-management of their condition to ensure full rehabilitation.

SUMMARY

The Maitland concept is a free flowing, dynamic clinical reasoning process that focuses on continual reassessment of the comparable sign and its response to treatment techniques employed by the physical therapist. The concept is just as gentle as needed to accommodate irritability and pain dominance but can be quite aggressive with stiff and stable disorders. The concept is not rooted in the fallacious dogma that pervades unfounded biomechanical theories yet is flexible and adaptable to these theories when clinically warranted. The concept also can accommodate treatment techniques that may be ascribed to other philosophies while maintaining the basic tenets of Maitland. Even though there is a growing body of evidence to validate components of the concept, it is still, like all other assessment and treatment philosophies, understudied at an overarching conceptual level.

REFERENCES

1. Maitland GD, Hengeveld E, Banks K, English K. *Maitland's Vertebral Manipulation*. 6th ed. London: Elsevier Health Sciences; 2001.
2. Laslett M, Young SB, Aprill CN, McDonald B. Diagnosing painful sacroiliac joints: A validity study of a mckenzie evaluation and sacroiliac provocation tests. *Aust J Physiother*. 2003; 49:89–97.
3. Maitland GD. *Neuro/Musculo-Skeletal Examination and Recording Guide*. 5th ed. Glen Osmond, South Australia: Lauderdale Press; 1992.
4. McKenzie R. *The lumbar spine: Mechanical diagnosis and therapy*. Wellington, NZ: Spinal Publications Limited; 1981.
5. Mulligan BR. *Manual therapy "NAGs", "SNAGs", "MWMs" etc*. 3rd ed. Wellington, NZ: Plane View Services LTD; 1995.
6. Cook CE. *Orthopedic Manual Therapy: An Evidenced-based Approach*. 2nd ed. Upper Saddle River, NJ: Pearson Prentice Hall; 2012.
7. Maitland GD. *Peripheral Manipulation*. 3rd ed. Oxford: Bitterworth-Heinemann; 1991.
8. Macnab I. Negative disc exploration. An analysis of the causes of nerve-root involvement in sixty-eight patients. *J Bone Joint Surg Am*. 1971;53:891–903.
9. American Physical Therapy Association. Guide to physical therapy practice. *Phys Ther*. 2001;81:S1–S738.
10. Maitland GD. Examination of the lumbar spine. *Aust J Physiother*. 1971;17:5–11.
11. Fritz JM, Cleland JA, Childs JD. Subgrouping patients with low back pain: Evolution of a classification approach to physical therapy. *J Orthop Sports Phys Ther*. 2007;37:290–302.
12. Kent P, Keating JL, Leboeuf-Yde C. Research methods for subgrouping low back pain. *BMC Med Res Methodol*. 2010;10:62.
13. Kamper SJ, Maher CG, Hancock MJ, Koes BW, Croft PR, Hay E. Treatment-based subgroups of low back pain: A guide to appraisal of research studies and a summary of current evidence. *Best Pract Res Clin Rheumatol*. 2010;24:181–191.
14. Barakatt ET, Romano PS, Riddle DL, Beckett LA, Kravitz R. An exploration of maitland's concept of pain irritability in patients with low back pain. *J Man Manip Ther*. 2009;17:196–205.
15. Barakatt ET, Romano PS, Riddle DL, Beckett LA. The reliability of maitland's irritability judgments in patients with low back pain. *J Man Manip Ther*. 2009;17:135–140.
16. Hickling J, Maitland GD. Abnormalities in passive movement: Diagrammatic representation. *Physiotherapy*. 1970;56:105–114.
17. McGregor AH, Dore CJ, McCarthy ID, Hughes SP. Are subjective clinical findings and objective clinical tests related to the motion characteristics of low back pain subjects? *J Orthop Sports Phys Ther*. 1998;28:370–377.
18. Woolf AD. How to assess musculoskeletal conditions. History and physical examination. *Best Pract Res Clin Rheumatol*. 2003;17:381–402.
19. Van Nieuwenhuyse A, Crombez G, Burdorf A, Verbeke G, Masschelein R, Moens G, Mairiaux P. Physical characteristics of the back are not predictive of low back pain in healthy workers: A prospective study. *BMC Musculoskelet Disord*. 2009;10:2.

20. McKenzie R. Mechanical diagnosis and therapy for disorders of the low back. In: Twomey L, Taylor J, eds. *Physical therapy of the low back*. New York: Churchill Livingstone; 2000.
21. Chiradejnant A, Maher CG, Latimer J, Stepkovitch N. Efficacy of "therapist-selected" versus "randomly selected" mobilisation techniques for the treatment of low back pain: A randomised controlled trial. *Aust J Physiother*. 2003;49:233–241.
22. Deyo RA. Diagnostic evaluation of lbp: Reaching a specific diagnosis is often impossible. *Arch Intern Med*. 2002;162:1444–1447; discussion 1447–1448.
23. Deyo RA, Weinstein JN. Low back pain. *N Engl J Med*. 2001;344:363–370.
24. Bishop PB, Wing PC. Knowledge transfer in family physicians managing patients with acute low back pain: A prospective randomized control trial. *Spine J*. 2006;6:282–288.
25. Fairbank JC, Couper J, Davies JB, O'Brien JP. The Oswestry Low Back Pain Disability Questionnaire. *Physiotherapy*. 1980;66:271–273.
26. Waddell G, Newton M, Henderson I, Somerville D, Main CJ. A fear-avoidance beliefs questionnaire (FABQ) and the role of fear-avoidance beliefs in chronic low back pain and disability. *Pain*. 1993;52:157–168.
27. Spitzer RL, Williams JB, Kroenke K, et al. Utility of a new procedure for diagnosing mental disorders in primary care. The prime-md 1000 study. *Jama*. 1994;272:1749–1756.
28. Whooley MA, Avins AL, Miranda J, Browner WS. Case-finding instruments for depression. Two questions are as good as many. *J Gen Intern Med*. 1997;12:439–445.
29. Arroll B, Khin N, Kerse N. Screening for depression in primary care with two verbally asked questions: Cross sectional study. *BMJ*. 2003;327:1144–1146.
30. Fann AV. The prevalence of postural asymmetry in people with and without chronic low back pain. *Arch Phys Med Rehabil*. 2002;83:1736–1738.
31. Levangie PK. The association between static pelvic asymmetry and low back pain. *Spine*. 1999;24:1234–1242.
32. Caling B, Lee M. Effect of direction of applied mobilization force on the posteroanterior response in the lumbar spine. *J Manipulative Physiol Ther*. 2001;24:71–78.
33. Spitzer W. Diagnosis of the problem (the problem with diagnosis). In: Scientific approach to the assessment and management of activity-related spinal disorders. A monograph for clinicians. Report of the quebec task force on spinal disorders. *Spine* 1987;12:S1–59.
34. Grieve G. *Common vertebral joint problems*. 2nd ed. Edinburgh: Churchill Livingstone; 1988.
35. Maitland GD. General session. *IFOMPT International Congress*. Vail, CO.1992.
36. Werneke M, Hart DL, Cook D. A descriptive study of the centralization phenomenon. A prospective analysis. *Spine*. 1999;24:676–683.
37. Christiansen D, Larsen K, Jensen OK, Nielsen CV. Pain response classification does not predict long-term outcome in sick-listed low back pain patients. *J Orthop Sports Phys Ther*. 2010.
38. Flynn T, Fritz J, Whitman J, et al. A clinical prediction rule for classifying patients with low back pain who demonstrate short-term improvement with spinal manipulation. *Spine*. 2002;27:2835–2843.
39. Childs JD, Fritz JM, Flynn TW, et al. A clinical prediction rule to identify patients with low back pain most likely to benefit from spinal manipulation: A validation study. *Ann Intern Med*. 2004;141:920–928.

chapter six

McKenzie Approach: Mechanical Diagnosis and Therapy

Helen Clare, PhD, FACP, Dip Phy, Dip MDT

The McKenzie approach is named after Robin McKenzie, a physiotherapist from New Zealand. Practitioners refer to this approach as mechanical diagnosis and therapy (MDT). Students can find more information about the approach and training opportunities at the website for the McKenzie Institute: http://www.mckenziemdt.org/.

In 1956, while treating a patient with acute low back and leg pain, Robin McKenzie noted that when the patient was lying in end range lumbar extension his symptoms improved. This patient's experience led McKenzie on a career long path exploring the effect of position and specific directional movement on pain. In 1981 he published his first book, The Lumbar Spine: Mechanical Diagnosis and Therapy, *a text that shifted many therapists away from the prevailing paradigm of flexion-based exercises.*

BACKGROUND

The McKenzie approach, more commonly known as "mechanical diagnosis and therapy" (MDT), classifies patients into subgroups or "syndromes" that are based on a patient's symptom response to repeated movements and sustained postures. In general, symptom response procedures have better levels of reliability than procedures using palpation or observation.[1] Using this model, the therapist ascertains two key patient-based components during examination: 1) centralization and 2) directional preference (see box).

> *Centralization occurs when distal pain is abolished in response to repeated movements or sustained postures and remains better. Centralization also occurs when remaining spinal pain is abolished in response to repeated movements.*
>
> *Directional preference refers to the direction in which pain is centralized or reduced in response to repeated movements. Directional preference may also be the direction in which a patient's range of motion increases in response to repeated movements.*

The ability to identify centralization and directional preference has proven to yield good patient outcomes, lending to the prognostic validity of this approach.[2–5]

Mechanical Syndrome Classifications

There are four nonspecific mechanical syndromes unique to the MDT approach that are used in classifying patients. Classification into each syndrome is based on the patient's response to sustained mechanical loading and repeated movements of the spine.

1. Reducible Derangement
   In this syndrome, patients experience centralization in response to therapeutic loading strategies. In other words, the pain moves from a distal to more proximal direction. If the patient is experiencing back pain only, the pain moves from a widespread to a more central location. In patients with reducible derangements, pain is reduced and then abolished during the application of therapeutic loading strategies, such as repeated movements. The changes in pain location, or reduction or abolition of pain remain better, and are usually accompanied or preceded by improvements in the mechanical presentation (range of movement and/or deformity).

2. Irreducible Derangement
   In this syndrome patients experience peripheralization of symptoms (i.e., increase or worsening of distal symptoms in response to therapeutic loading strategies). In addition, there is no reduction, abolition, or centralization of pain.

3. Articular Dysfunction/Adherent Nerve Root
   Patients with Articular Dysfunction experience intermittent spinal pain only. At least one movement is restricted, and the restricted movement consistently produces concordant pain at end-range. In addition, there is

no rapid reduction or abolition of symptoms, and no lasting production of distal symptoms. Patients with adherent nerve root have a history of sciatica or surgery in the last few months that has improved, but is now unchanging. Symptoms are intermittent and are experienced in the thigh and/or calf. Movements such as flexion in standing, long sitting, and straight leg raise are clearly restricted and consistently produce concordant pain or tightness at end range. There is no rapid reduction or abolition of symptoms, and no lasting production of distal symptoms.

4. Posture

Patients with postural syndrome experience spinal pain only, which is brought on by static loading. There is no pain during movement, no loss of range of movement, and no pain with repeated motion testing. Symptoms are abolished with postural correction.

Evidence suggests that the majority of patients with back pain classified by MDT-experienced clinicians are classified into one of the mechanical syndromes, of which the majority were classified with derangement syndrome.[1,4] Derangement syndrome has been identified in about 70–80% of patients with spinal problems.[1,4,6] In a systematic review, centralization, which only occurs in the derangement syndrome, was identified in 70% of 731 patients with sub-acute and 52% of 325 patients with chronic low back pain (LBP).[2] In a randomized controlled trial, directional preference, again only occurring in the derangement syndrome, was identified at the initial mechanical evaluation in 230 of 312 (74%) acute to chronic patients with LBP.[4]

Tests and Measures Unique to the MDT Approach

An MDT examination uses a standardized MDT assessment sheet (Appendix 6–1 and Appendix 6–2) that promotes a hypothesis-generating process to determine the possible presence of one of the mechanical syndromes. The presence of the MDT syndromes can be suspected or ruled out from items in the history-taking, such as the nature and history of the episode, aggravating and relieving factors, and, in particular, whether a directional preference might be present. The history also includes standard red-flag questions to rule out the presence of serious spinal pathology. In addition to excluding serious spinal pathology, the history may also alert the clinician to the presence of "yellow flags," which are psychosocial barriers to recovery that can impact negatively on treatment.

The physical examination considers the patient's posture, the response to posture correction, takes a baseline range of movement assessment, and then uses repeated movements to monitor symptom and mechanical responses. Where appropriate, a neurological examination is performed before the repeated movements. Not all the repeated movements on the assessment form (Appendix 6–1) are performed; the selection is related to the clinical reasoning process of the clinician. The clinical reasoning process may be diagramed in the format of a classification algorithm (Figure 6–2). In the physical examination, the standard algorithmic thought is to consider sagittal plane movements before frontal plane movements, except in the presence of a lateral shift. If sagittal plane movements exacerbate or peripheralize symptoms, frontal plane movements are explored.

APPLICATION OF MCKENZIE MODEL TO JOE LORES

Tests and Measures

Figure 6–1 contains the completed examination form with Joe's data. Joe was taken through both repeated flexion and extension. He was not tested in the frontal plane, as centralization and directional preference were determined through sagittal plane testing.

Evaluation

Joe gave a history of injuring himself while he was installing a sink, which suggests that flexion forces created the injury. The initial mechanical loading may have been sufficient to cause tissue damage and to initiate an inflammatory response. The chemical exudate that formed with the inflammatory response, secondary to tissue damage, activated the nociceptive receptor system and resulted in a constant pain, while the level of chemical activation was above the threshold for stimulation.[7,8] This response would account for the constant pain Joe was reporting in his low back. However, the injury occurred 2 weeks ago, which suggests that any chemically mediated pain should have subsided by this time.[7] Chemically mediated pain does not usually reduce with changes of position, unloading, or exercise, and in Joe's case, his pain did.[9,10] The behavior of his symptoms is not typical of chemically mediated pain but is more suggestive of mechanical pain.

THE McKENZIE INSTITUTE
LUMBAR SPINE ASSESSMENT

Date   05/04/2010

Name   Joseph Lores   Sex M / F

Address

Telephone

Date of Birth   Age

Referral: *GP / Orth / Self / Other*

Work: Mechanical Stresses   Self-employed Plumber- Bending.
    lifting, working in awkward positions

Leisure: Mechanical Stresses   Reading, TV, home projects

Functional Disability from present episode   Limited lifting

Functional Disability score   Modified Oswestry 42%

VAS Score (0-10)   Range 2-6 depending on activity

SYMPTOMS

HISTORY

Present Symptoms   Right low back pain, extending into right buttock

Present since   2 weeks   *Improving / Unchanging / Worsening*

Commenced as a result of   Performing a sink installation   *Or no apparent reason*

Symptoms at onset: *back / thigh / leg*

Constant symptoms: *back / thigh / leg*   Buttock intermittent   Intermittent symptoms: *back / thigh / leg*

Worse   *bending*   *Sitting / rising*   *standing*   *walking*   *lying*

    am / as the day progresses / pm   *when still / on the move*

    other

Better   *bending*   *sitting*   *standing*   *walking*   Variable   *lying* back either side

    am / as the day progresses / pm   *when still / on the move*

    other

Disturbed Sleep   *Yes / No*   Sleeping postures: *prone / sup / side R / L*   Surface: *firm / soft / sag*

Previous Episodes   0   1-5   6-10   11+   Year of first episode   2002

Previous History   Low back pain in 2002 related to lifting - resolved after one

Previous Treatments   Rest, Analgesic medication- Tylenol

SPECIFIC QUESTIONS

Cough / Sneeze / Strain / +ve / -ve   Bladder: *normal / abnormal*   Gait: *normal / abnormal*

Medications: *Nil / NSAIDS / Analg / Steroids / Anticoag / Other*   Advil/Aleve, Lotensin, Flexeril

General Health: *Good / Fair / Poor*

Imaging: *Yes / No*   Negative report from X-ray

Recent or major surgery: *Yes / No*   Night Pain: *Yes / No*

Accidents: *Yes / No*   Unexplained weight loss: *Yes / No*

Other:

Figure 6–1 Joe Lores assessment form. © The McKenzie Institute International.

EXAMINATION

POSTURE

Sitting: Good / *Fair* / Poor   Standing: Good / *Fair* / Poor   Lordosis: *Red* / Acc / Normal   Lateral Shift: Right / Left / *Nil*

Correction of Posture: Better / Worse / *No effect* _____   Relevant: Yes / No

Other Observations: _____

NEUROLOGICAL

Motor Deficit	L4	Reflexes	L4
Sensory Deficit	Negative	Dural Signs	SLR Lpos

MOVEMENT LOSS

	Maj	Mod	Min	Nil	Pain
Flexion		X			X
Extension		X			X
Side Gliding R				X	
Side Gliding L			X		

TEST MOVEMENTS   **Describe effect on present pain – During:** produces, abolishes, increases, decreases, no effect, centralising, peripheralising. **After:** better, worse, no better, no worse, no effect, centralised, peripheralised.

	Symptoms During Testing	Symptoms After Testing	↑Rom	↓ Rom	No Effect
Pretest symptoms standing:	Right low back and buttock 4/10				
FIS	Increased right buttock				
Rep FIS	Increased right buttock	Worse 6/10	X		
EIS	Increased right low back				
Rep EIS	Decreased right buttock	Better 3/10	X		
Pretest symptoms lying:					
FIL	Increased right buttock				
Rep FIL	Increased right buttock	No worse			X
EIL	Increased right buttock				
Rep EIL	Decreased right buttock and right low back	Better- only right back	X		
If required pretest symptoms:					
SGIS – R	Not tested				
Rep SGIS - R	Not tested				
SGIS - L	Not tested				
Rep SGIS- L	Not tested				

STATIC TESTS

Sitting slouched	Increases symptoms, Worse	Sitting erect	Decreases symptoms. No Better
Standing slouched	Increases symptoms, Worse	Standing erect	Unable to do due to loss of lordosis
Lying prone in extension	Better	Long sitting	Not tested

OTHER TESTS

_____

_____

PROVISIONAL CLASSIFICATION

Derangement   Dysfunction   Posture   Other

Derangement: Pain location   Central/symmetrical _____

PRINCIPLE OF MANAGEMENT

Education   Posture correction sitting, avoidance of flexion   Equipment Provided   Lumbar roll for sitting

Mechanical Therapy: Yes / No _____

Extension Principle: Extension in standing. Extension in lying   Lateral Principle: _____

Flexion Principle: _____   Other: _____

Treatment Goals: Centralise the pain, restore range of flexion and extension, improve function

Figure 6–1 Joe Lores assessment form (continued).

Joe reported that his symptoms were worse with flexion forces, both dynamic (bending) and sitting (sustained), and better with movement in and out of extension (walking). This suggests that Joe had a directional preference to extension. He reported that his symptoms were better when he unloaded his lumbar spine (lying). This pattern of aggravating and relieving factors is highly indicative of the mechanical pattern of pain seen in the MDT derangement syndrome.

Joe gave a negative response to the standard red-flag questions, so there was no suggestion of the presence of serious spinal pathology. He continued to remain at work, was not taking excessive amounts of medication, demonstrating fear-avoidance behaviors, or passive coping strategies. Therefore, it is unlikely that he had significant psychosocial barriers that would impede his recovery. Joe scored 42% on his modified Oswestry questionnaire and gave a pain rating of 2–6 out of 10 on a pain rating scale, which is indicative of a moderate level of disability.

The physical examination was used to confirm or disconfirm the hypothesis of derangement determined from the history. On physical examination, Joe demonstrated a loss of lumbar lordosis in both sitting and standing, and reported pain in these positions. Sitting erect was possible and Joe reported that his symptoms were reduced in this position, which provides initial support from the physical examination for a directional preference for extension.

Joe had a movement loss into both flexion and extension, and both movements reproduced pain, which suggested that investigation of repeated movements in the sagittal plane was appropriate. Repeated spinal movement testing demonstrated a directional preference for extension with repeated lumbar flexion in standing worsening his most distal pain (the right buttock symptoms). Repeated lumbar extension decreased his buttock pain when performed both in standing and in lying, and his pain remained better after testing. Movements in the frontal plane were not tested because his symptoms had been altered with sagittal movements.

Diagnosis

An algorithmic reasoning (Figure 6–2) is used in MDT to identify mechanical responders with mechanical syndrome classification, to rule out red flags, and to identify nonresponders who might fit one of a number of specific categories, and who may benefit from alternative interventions, including medical ones.

At the end of the physical examination the provisional classification was derangement with a directional preference to extension. This supported the

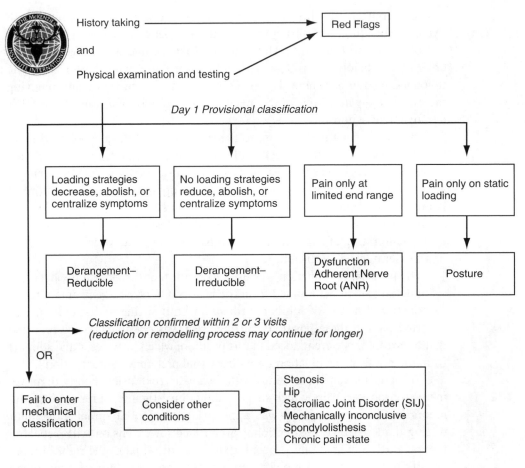

Figure 6–2 Classification algorithm.

hypothesis established from the history. In a clinical setting, the therapist would provide management for this provisional classification and the classification confirmed or reconsidered at follow-up.

Prognosis

Numerous factors are associated with the failure of recovery from an acute episode of LBP. These typically relate to three different aspects of the patient's presentation: clinical, biomechanical, and psychological/social factors.

Clinical prognostic factors

- History of previous back pain is a considered a prognostic factor for prolonged symptoms.[11,12]
  Joe reported one previous episode.
- Reported leg pain at onset is associated with poor outcomes.[13]
  Joe did not report the presence of leg symptoms.
- Centralization of leg pain predictor of good outcome.[14-16]
  Joe did not report leg pain but he did demonstrate signs of centralization.
- Inability to centralize the pain found to be the strongest predictor of chronicity compared with a range of psychological, clinical, and demographic factors.[17]
  Joe was able to centralize his pain.
- Higher level of reported pain and disability.[18,19]
  Joe had a VAS score range 2–6 and a modified Oswestry score of 42%, which are not regarded as high scores.
- Disc herniation/structural specific diagnosis.
  It is reported that Joe has a negative X-ray report, which suggests that there was no specific structural pathology present. However, as he has not had a CT scan or MRI, it is not possible to exclude a disc herniation.

Biomechanical prognostic factors

Occupational physical factors are strongly associated with the occurrence of back pain but there is uncertainty regarding their role in prognosis—i.e., ability to return to work and persisting symptoms.[20]

- Heavy or frequent lifting.
  Joe's occupation requires this.
- Whole body vibration (e.g., as when driving).
  Not applicable for Joe.
- Prolonged or frequent bending or twisting.
  Joe's occupation requires this.
- Postural stresses (high spinal load or awkward postures).
  Joe's occupation requires this.

Psychosocial prognostic factors

Psychosocial factors are now clearly linked to the transition from acute to chronic LBP and disability, and these variables generally have more impact than biomechanical factors on disability.[21]

The following psychological factors have been shown to influence prognosis:

- fear-avoidance behavior
- depression
- anxiety about pain
- passive coping strategies
- catastrophizing
- low self-efficacy belief
- external health locus
- poor general health
- higher levels of reported pain and disability

Although specific evaluation of these psychological factors was not performed, Joe did not appear to be displaying these characteristics. He continued to try and work, was not using excessive amounts of medication, and his reported pain scores and his score from his modified Oswestry questionnaire suggested that he was continuing to function at a reasonable level.

Social prognostic factors

- lower education level
- lower income
- heavy manual labor
- sitting occupation
- lack of alternative work duties to perform
- low job satisfaction
- over-protective spouse

These specific social factors were not screened for in the initial assessment so it is difficult to comment on how they may influence his prognosis.

In summary, factors that cause acute pain to become chronic are complex, multiple, and specific to the individual. It is likely that a combination of clinical and psychosocial factors influence prognosis. There is evidence that the patient-clinician relationship has a role to play in the patient's recovery, with inappropriate advice or management preventing or prolonging recovery.[22]

The MDT therapist would anticipate the prognosis for Joe to be good. He has symptoms of recent onset—the recovery of which will be assisted by natural history. His symptoms are local to the lumbar spine and buttock, are not radiating into the leg, and his symptoms change with variations in mechanical loading. On examination, his symptoms and his spinal mechanics change quickly with repeated spinal movements and remain better after the movement has ceased. Joe is able to reduce his symptoms with his own mechanical forces, which implies that he can "treat" his symptoms regularly throughout the day. His symptoms displayed the initial signs of centralization with repeated spinal movements and this has been associated with good outcomes. At the initial assessment, Joe did not display significant psychosocial factors that would play a role in hindering his prognosis.

His job does involve some heavy labor and working in sustained awkward positions, which he may need to try and modify. To avoid future recurrences and the possibility of persisting symptoms, Joe will need to be educated about the ways of managing these mechanical loading situations. The MDT approach to the management of LBP focuses on patient involvement, education, self exercise, and encouraging activity, all of which are recommended in many of the guidelines for the treatment of acute LBP and may assist in influencing prognosis.

Intervention

As mentioned earlier in this chapter, the principle of management using MDT is classification into one of the identified subgroups, determination of the patient's directional preference, the achievement of centralization of symptoms, patient self care, independence through exercise and education, and, where necessary, the progression of forces.[23] Generally stated, treatment for each subgroup is outlined as follows:

- Patients classified with derangement are treated using movements and forces that centralize and abolish the symptoms. Correction of static postures is emphasized as a technique for maintaining derangement reduction and symptom control.
- Patients with irreducible derangement may be referred for medical care, taught a program of stabilization exercise, and reexamined after a prolonged period of time to ascertain if their symptoms have changed and their response to testing results in reclassification.
- Patients who have an articular dysfunction are treated by techniques aimed at restoring normal range of motion to the joints. The adherent nerve root classification is a special case of dysfunction in which the

restriction is soft tissue and related to nerve length. The techniques for treating adherent nerve root are directed to restoring normal range and function of the shortened nervous system tissue.

- For patients classified in the posture subgroup the treatment is postural correction. Typically this revolves around reducing the impact of performing activities of daily function (e.g., sitting) for prolonged periods of time at the end of the normal tissues' range of motion. Correction may include modification of seating and workstation through ergonomic consultation. The patient is educated about the relationship of posture to LBP and the importance of back pain prevention.

In MDT the progression of forces typically follows a path from patient-generated forces, patient-generated forces with self-overpressure, clinician-generated mobilization, and clinical generated manipulation. The management of Joe will follow these principles.

On examination, Joe's symptoms displayed a directional preference toward extension. Use of directional preference has been shown to be associated with better outcomes[4] and will therefore guide treatment. The European guidelines for the management of acute nonspecific LBP recommend involving the patient in the treatment, education, and encouragement of self-management,[24] and these principles form key components to the management with MDT.

During the physical examination Joe was able to decrease both his buttock and back pain and improve his range of motion with repeated extension exercises in standing and lying. This is evidence that the mechanical forces he can generate with his own exercises are sufficient to have the desired effect on his symptoms.

"If a patient can change their symptoms with their own mechanical forces it is our responsibility to educate them about how to do so."[25] Hence, the MDT therapist would initially manage Joe with a routine of extension in standing and extension in lying exercises (Figures 6–3 and 6–4). The frequency of performing the exercises and the number of repetitions required would be influenced by the symptom response, but a typical guide is doing 10–20 repetitions every 2 hours. It is essential, however, that Joe understands that the exercises are aimed at symptom relief so he can perform them as often as is required to achieve this. The therapist would ensure that Joe understands the desired effect of the exercise, which is to decrease, centralize, and abolish the symptoms. Joe would also be advised to cease the exercises if the opposite occurs—symptoms are produced or peripheralize. Joe would also be advised

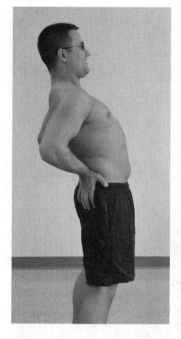

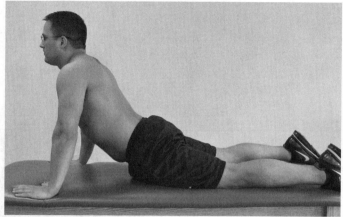

Figure 6–3 Extension in standing.

Figure 6–4 Extension in lying.

about the possibility of the onset of "new" pains in other spinal regions in response to different postural and mobility demands. He would be advised that these are common and should normally only last for one or two days as the body adapts to the new mechanical forces being applied.

In both the history and the physical examination it was determined that flexion of the lumbar spine, be it as a movement in standing or as a sustained position in sitting, worsened his symptoms. Joe would therefore be advised to limit flexion activities such as bending, and to use a lumbar support when sitting to keep his lumbar spine in a lordotic position (Figure 6–5). This advice will reduce the flexion forces being applied to his lumbar spine and thus reduce the degree of continued mechanical stimulation of the nociceptors.

Subsequent consultations: Joe would be reassessed in 1–2 days and his symptomatic and functional response to the exercises provided would be determined. Of particular interest is the location of his symptoms, as the desired response to the management provided is centralization of his pain. With Joe, this would equate to abolishment of his right buttock pain and an

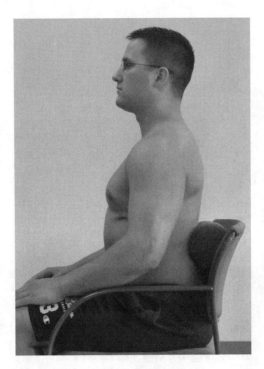

Figure 6–5 Posture correction.

initial increase in the intensity of his central back pain. Associated with a change in the location of his pain, an improvement in his range of spinal movement would be anticipated. If there is both a symptomatic and a mechanical improvement, the management would not be altered. The way he has been performing the exercises would be checked and Joe would be encouraged to try and move to the very end of his extension range by breathing out and "sagging" at end range (patient-generated overpressure). His posture correction would be checked and the advice about the temporary avoidance of flexion reinforced.

While Joe's symptoms are continuing to centralize and abolish, the management plan would not be altered. Once his central pain is abolished, his range of spinal motion fully restored, his functional restrictions recovered, and he reports only intermittent pain at the end range of flexion, recovery of function would be implemented. Recovery of function involves the introduction of what had previously been provocative movements, which in Joe's case was flexion. The symptomatic and mechanical response to flexion would be tested by Joe performing repeated flexion in lying exercise (Figure 6–6). The desired symptomatic response to this movement is to produce a stretch in the lumbar spine at the end of the flexion movement that abolishes on the return to the neutral position and the symptoms do not increase when the flexion is repeated. The range of lumbar extension would be assessed before performing the flexion exercises and after to determine if the range reduces as a result of the repeated flexion. If the range does reduce and the symptoms increase with the flexion exercise it would be regarded as "unsafe" to introduce flexion. Joe would then continue managing his symptoms with his extension-focused management and the response to flexion would be reassessed in a few days. When the flexion in lying exercises can be performed without resulting in a worsening of his symptoms or a loss of extension range, Joe would be advised to perform these 2 or 3 times per day until his flexion range was full and pain free. The flexion exercises would always be followed by a set of extension in lying exercises as a safety measure.

Once Joe reports resolution of his symptoms and on examination he has recovered his normal range of spinal mobility, he would be discharged. He would be encouraged to continue to be diligent about maintaining a lordotic posture while sitting, which is best achieved by the use of a lumbar support and to balance periods of sustained flexion by performing extension movements. There is evidence to suggest that the daily performance of a set of

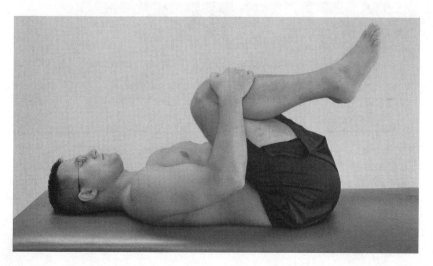

Figure 6–6 Flexion in lying.

extension in lying exercises and the regular performance of extension in standing after bending and sitting reduced the incidences of acute LBP,[26] so this advice would be given to Joe.

If at any time Joe's symptoms plateau (i.e., they do not fully centralize or improve with his current exercise but do not remain better and he is reporting no further functional improvement), an assessment of the symptomatic and mechanical response to the application of stronger extension forces would be investigated. The first progression of force would be the application of clinician overpressure while Joe performs extension in lying. (Figure 6–7) Again, the desired response to this procedure would be centralization/ abolishing of his residual symptoms and an increase in his extension range. Once this is achieved the use of the clinician overpressure would cease and Joe would continue with his own exercises and management would continue as described previously.

If the introduction of the clinician overpressure fails to achieve the centralization and abolishment of his symptoms, a second progression of extension mobilization (Figure 6–8) would be applied. Both the symptomatic and mechanical response would be evaluated. The mobilization would be applied over the spinal segment that achieved the desired response of centralization/ abolish. If required, a further progression can be achieved by performing the mobilization with the patient in an end-range extended position. Again, once

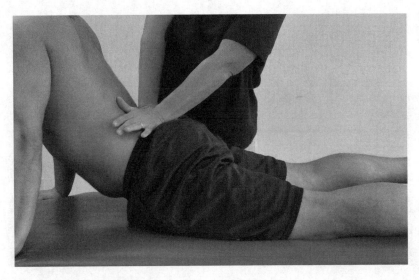

Figure 6–7 Extension in lying with clinician overpressure.

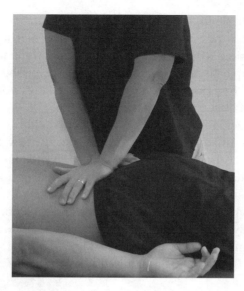

Figure 6–8 Extension mobilization.

the desired response is achieved, the use of the mobilization is ceased and Joe self manages.

If at any time Joe's symptoms fail to centralize with the extension procedures, the effect of adding lateral forces should be explored. On the initial assessment Joe presented with no loss of right side glide and a minimum loss of left side glide, which suggests that lateral forces are unlikely to be required. However, if the symptoms do not fully respond to the movements in the sagittal plane, the effect of performing the extension movements with Joe in a position of right side glide (hips moved to the left while in the prone position) should be assessed. He would then be instructed to perform the extension in lying exercise with his hips shifted to the left. The aim of this procedure is to apply more force to the right side of the spine and the desired response is for the symptoms to shift to a more central location. If the addition of this force has no effect it should be discontinued. If it does result in more central symptoms it should be continued until the symptoms are centrally located, and then discontinued. This is usually for a period of 2–3 days.

Occasionally, patients are able to fully abolish their symptoms, but have difficulty keeping their symptoms resolved. Clinically, the most common reason for this is the inability of the patient to either avoid sufficient flexion activities or they do not pay sufficient attention to their sitting posture. If patients are able to achieve centralization of their symptoms with their own exercises, it is not necessary to progress the mechanical forces, although more attention would need to be paid to avoidance of any aggravating postures. Typically this is only necessary for a period of 1–2 weeks, then as recovery of function is introduced, the patient would not need to be as diligent at avoiding flexion forces.

It is anticipated that Joe's symptoms should resolve in a period of 3–4 weeks. This timeframe will be influenced by how quickly the symptoms centralize and abolish and how well Joe is able to maintain the centralization by the avoidance of flexion and control of his sitting postural stresses. In the initial stages of treatment Joe will have to avoid/limit his flexion activities, which will be difficult because of his work as a plumber. If not able to fully avoid flexion, he will need to interrupt the flexion with extension movements. Restrictive tape applied to his lumbar spine to restrict his flexion may be required if he continues to reaggravate because of his work.

Long-term management for Joe would include regular performance of his extension in standing exercises to interrupt the flexed postures he is required to work in. He would be advised to continue the use of the extension in lying exercise morning and evening as a preventative strategy and encouraged to also perform them as soon as he recognizes the onset of any back pain or stiffness. Joe would also be advised to continue to be aware of maintaining a good sitting posture, especially at the end of a work day when his spinal structures have been mechanically loaded and are at a greater risk of being overloaded by sustained flexed postures. He would be encouraged to self manage and to seek further assistance if his own management strategies were not being effective in abolishing his symptoms.

SUMMARY

The McKenzie approach is characterized by a classification system for diagnosis and an algorithm that is used in examination. The uniqueness of this approach is its incorporation of repeated movement and its application of the principles of centralization, peripheralization, and directional preference. All of these elements were demonstrated through the case of Joe, both in developing a conclusion about the nature of his LBP problem and in planning for intervention.

REFERENCES

1. May S. Classification by McKenzie mechanical syndromes: A survey of McKenzie-trained faculty. *J Manipulative Physiol Ther.* 2006;29(8):637–642.
2. Aina A, May S, Clare H. The centralization phenomenon of spinal symptoms—A systematic review. *Man Ther.* 2004;9(3):134–143.
3. Chorti AG, Chortis AG, Strimpakos N, McCarthy CJ, Lamb SE. The prognostic value of symptom responses in the conservative management of spinal pain: A systematic review. *Spine.* 2009;34(24):2686–2699.
4. Long A, Donelson R, Fung T. Does it matter which exercise? A randomized control trial of exercise for low back pain. *Spine.* 2004;29(23):2593–2602.
5. Long A, May S, Fung T. Specific directional exercises for patients with low back pain: A case series. *Physiother Can.* 2008;60(4):307–317.
6. Hefford C. McKenzie classification of mechanical spinal pain: Profile of syndromes and directions of preference. *Man Ther.* 2008;13(1):75–81.
7. Enwemeka CS. Inflammation, cellularity, and fibrillogenesis in regenerating tendon: Implications for tendon rehabilitation. *Phys Ther.* 1989;69(10):816–825.
8. Evans P. The healing process at cellular level: A review. *Physiotherapy.* 1980;66(8):256–259.
9. McKenzie RA. *The Lumbar Spine: Mechanical Diagnosis and Therapy.* Waikanae, New Zealand: Spinal Publications Limited; 1981.
10. McKenzie RA. *The Cervical and Thoracic Spine: Mechanical Diagnosis and Therapy.* Waikanae, New Zealand: Spinal Publications Limited; 1990.
11. Frank JW, Kerr MS, Brooker AS, et al. Disability resulting from occupational low back pain. Part I: What do we know about primary prevention? A review of the scientific evidence on prevention before disability begins. *Spine.* 1996;21(24):2908–2917.
12. Ferguson SA, Marras WS. A literature review of low back disorder surveillance measures and risk factors. *Clin Biomech.* 1997;12(4):211–226.
13. Carey TS, Garrett JM, Jackman AM. Beyond the good prognosis. Examination of an inception cohort of patients with chronic low back pain. *Spine.* 2000;25(1):115–120.
14. Donelson R, Silva G, Murphy K. Centralization phenomenon. Its usefulness in evaluating and treating referred pain. *Spine.* 1990;15(3):211–213.
15. Long AL. The centralization phenomenon. Its usefulness as a predictor or outcome in conservative treatment of chronic law back pain (a pilot study). *Spine.* 1995;20(23):2513–2520.
16. Werneke M, Hart DL, Cook D. A descriptive study of the centralization phenomenon. A prospective analysis. *Spine.* 1999;24(7):676–683.
17. Werneke M, Hart DL. Centralization phenomenon as a prognostic factor for chronic low back pain and disability. *Spine.* 2001;26(7):758–764.
18. Potter RG, Jones JM, Boardman AP. A prospective study of primary care patients with musculoskeletal pain: The identification of predictive factors for chronicity. *Br J Gen Pract.* 2000;50(452):225–227.
19. Henschke N, Maher CG, Refshauge KM, Herbert RD, Cumming RG, Bleasel J, York J, Das A, McAuley JH. Prognosis in patients with recent onset low back pain in Australian primary care: inception cohort study. *BMJ.* 2008;337.
20. Burdorf A, Sorock G. Positive and negative evidence of risk factors for back disorders. *Scand J Work Environ Health.* 1997;23(4):243–256.
21. Linton SJ. A review of psychological risk factors in back and neck pain. *Spine.* 2000;25(9):1148–1156.
22. Weiser S, Cedraschi C. Psychosocial issues in the prevention of chronic low back pain–A literature review. *Baillieres Clin Rheumatol.* 1992;6(3):657–684.

23. McKenzie RA, May S. *The Lumbar Spine-Mechanical Diagnosis and Therapy.* 2nd ed. Waikanae, New Zealand: Spinal Publications Limited; 2003.

24. van Tulder M, Becker A, Bekkering T, et al. Chapter 3. European guidelines for the management of acute nonspecific low back pain in primary care. *Eur Spine J.* 2006; 15:S169–191.

25. McKenzie RA, May S. *The Human Extremities Mechanical Diagnosis and Therapy.* Waikanae, New Zealand: Spinal Publications Limited; 2000.

26. Larsen K, Weidick F, Leboeuf-Yde C. Can passive prone extensions of the back prevent back problems? A randomized, controlled intervention trial of 314 military conscripts. *Spine.* 2002;27(24):2747–2752.

appendix one

The McKenzie Institute Lumbar Spine Assessment

THE McKENZIE INSTITUTE
LUMBAR SPINE ASSESSMENT

Date _____

Name _____ Sex M / F _____

Address _____

Telephone _____

Date of Birth _____ Age _____

Referral: *GP / Orth / Self / Other* _____

Work: Mechanical Stresses _____

_____

Leisure: Mechanical Stresses _____

Functional Disability from Present Episode _____

Functional Disability Score _____

VAS Score (0–10) _____

SYMPTOMS

HISTORY

Present Symptoms _____

Present Since _____ *Improving / Unchanging / Worsening*

Commenced as a Result of _____ *Or no apparent reason*

Symptoms at Onset: *back / thigh / leg* _____

Constant Symptoms: *back / thigh / leg* _____ Intermittent Symptoms: *back / thigh / leg*

Worse	*bending*	*sitting / rising*	*standing*	*walking*	*lying*
	am / as the day progresses / pm			*when still / on the move*	
	other _____				

Better	*bending*	*sitting*	*standing*	*walking*	*lying*
	am / as the day progresses / pm			*when still / on the move*	
	other _____				

Disturbed Sleep   *Yes / No*   Sleeping Postures: *prone / sup / side R / L*   Surface: *firm / soft / sag*

Previous Episodes   0   1-5   6-10   11+   Year of First Episode _____

Previous History _____

_____

Previous Treatments _____

_____

SPECIFIC QUESTIONS

Cough / Sneeze / Strain / +ve / -ve   Bladder: *normal / abnormal*   Gait: *normal / abnormal*

Medications: *Nil / NSAIDS / Analg / Steroids / Anticoag / Other* _____

General Health: *Good / Fair / Poor* _____

Imaging: *Yes / No* _____

Recent or Major Surgery: *Yes / No* _____   Night Pain: *Yes / No* _____

Accidents: *Yes / No* _____   Unexplained Weight Loss: *Yes / No*

Other: _____

EXAMINATION

POSTURE

Sitting: *Good / Fair / Poor*   Standing: *Good / Fair / Poor*   Lordosis: *Red / Acc / Normal*   Lateral Shift: *Right / Left / Nil*

Correction of Posture: *Better / Worse / No effect* _____ Relevant: *Yes / No*

Other Observations: _____

NEUROLOGICAL

Motor Deficit _____ Reflexes _____

Sensory Deficit _____ Dural Signs _____

MOVEMENT LOSS

	Maj	Mod	Min	Nil	Pain
Flexion					
Extension					
Side Gliding R					
Side Gliding L					

TEST MOVEMENTS   **Describe effect on present pain – During:** produces, abolishes, increases, decreases, no effect, centralizing, peripheralizing. **After:** better, worse, no better, no worse, no effect, centralized, peripheralized.

	Symptoms During Testing	Symptoms After Testing	Mechanical Response		
			↑Rom	↓ Rom	No Effect
Pretest symptoms standing:					
FIS					
Rep FIS					
EIS					
Rep EIS					
Pretest symptoms lying:					
FIL					
Rep FIL					
EIL					
Rep EIL					
If required pretest symptoms:					
SGIS – R					
Rep SGIS - R					
SGIS - L					
Rep SGIS- L					

STATIC TESTS

Sitting Slouched _____ Sitting Erect _____

Standing Slouched _____ Standing Erect _____

Lying Prone in Extension _____ Long Sitting _____

OTHER TESTS _____

_____

PROVISIONAL CLASSIFICATION

Derangement   Dysfunction   Posture   Other

Derangement: Pain location _____

PRINCIPLE OF MANAGEMENT

Education _____ Equipment Provided _____

Mechanical Therapy: *Yes / No* _____

Extension Principle: _____ Lateral Principle: _____

Flexion Principle: _____ Other: _____

Treatment Goals: _____

appendix two

Guidelines for Completion
of Assessment Forms

McKenzie Institute Assessment Forms

Guidelines for the Completion of the Assessment Forms

History: Page One *Patient responses are recorded but supplemented by the clinician as appropriate*	
Referral:	Circle the appropriate, may record date of follow-up appointment.
Postures / Stresses:	**Work: Mechanical stresses:** Record work activities and indicate frequency of activity (e.g., 50% sitting, 50% standing). **Leisure: Mechanical stresses:** Record leisure or hobby activities and indicate frequency of activity (e.g., 75% sitting, 25% bending, or could say walking 3x week 40 mins, gardening 3 hours/week).
Functional Disability from Present Episode:	Ask patient-specific activities that they are unable to perform or have difficulty performing because of current symptoms.
Functional Disability Score:	Note the test being used, and the score.
VAS Score:	Tend to scale the intensity of the pain, must include most distal pain. Can use to define pain range, not just its upper limit.
Body Chart:	Used to record "all symptoms this episode" (i.e., all the symptoms the patient is complaining of, not signs). All symptoms may not still be present.
Present Symptoms:	Record here the location/type of symptoms that are still concerning the patient. May differ from the body chart as not all may still be present.
Present Since:	Usually given in weeks or days. Can write a specific date if known or if needed for legal reasons.
Improving / Unchanging / Worsening:	Circle as appropriate, and ask patient how, or in what way, if they say they are improving or worsening.
Commenced as a Result of:	If appropriate describe mechanism of injury (e.g., lifting and twisting) Or circle no apparent reason.
Symptoms at Onset:	Circle give time frame of onset of distal pain (e.g., circle back then comment 2 days later in the leg).
Constant / Intermittent:	Circle as appropriate. Back = to gluteal fold, Thigh = above knee, Leg = below knee.
Better / Worse Section:	Recording *Circle* for always – if not clarified this means immediate pain response. If relates to time need to clarify outside the circle with e.g. 10 minutes, prolonged. *Line under* – sometimes. *Oblique line through* – no effect. Put a ? above activity if patient still unsure even after further questions, rather than leave blank. If two unrelated areas of pain, may need to indicate if dealing with back or leg pain for each activity.
Disturbed Sleep:	If always, circle Yes, sometimes, underline Yes. Not affected, circle No. If was previously, circle Yes but write "previously".
Sleeping Postures:	Circle usual, indicate if unable to use this because of current pain and indicate present position – best and worse.
Sleeping Surface:	Circle as appropriate.

History: Page One	
Patient responses are recorded but supplemented by the clinician as appropriate	
Previous Episodes:	Circle 0, between 1-5 episodes, 6-10 episodes or 11+, indicate year of first episode
Previous History:	Write if episodic, which areas affected before and what was it like between episodes (e.g., 100% between episodes)
Previous Treatment:	Write what treatments they have had for this episode and, if appropriate what treatments/interventions they have had for previous episodes. May indicate what has helped if appropriate.
Specific Questions:	Circle appropriate answers and write any clarifications on the lines provided.

Physical Examination: Page Two	
It is not essential to perform all components of the physical examination with every patient. If any section is not performed an oblique line is drawn through it.	
Posture:	Circle appropriate response.
Correction of Posture:	Circle response and indicate which pain changes, if appropriate.
Other Observations:	Record any significant musculo-skeletal differences (e.g., wasting, swelling redness etc.)
Neurological Examination:	Qualify which deficit in each section, recorded if abnormal (e.g., decreased S1 reflex). Can add Babinski / Clonus to reflexes if required. Record as NAD if testing was normal. Oblique line through if not applicable
Movement Loss:	The boxes Maj/Mod/Min/Nil can be used as a line (i.e., more as a continuum). Can also record as a tick in the "pain" box, if patient is reporting pain, indicate location of the pain.
Test Movements:	Indicate the order performed by numbering if order is different to standard. Useful also to record the number of repetitions performed to gain theresponse. **Symptomatic response**—Use standard terms only. Monitor and describe effect on most distal symptoms predominantly. **Mechanical response**—Tick appropriate box. Can indicate which movement has been effected by the change if it is different to the one being tested.
Static Tests:	Record with standard "After" words.
Other Tests:	State which and the response achieved.
Provisional Classification:	Circle the classification, record the pain location for Derangement, indicate the direction of Dysfunction, or clarify the type of Other.
Principle of Management:	**Education Circle**—Record specifics (e.g., posture correction, avoidance of flexion). **Mechanical Therapy** - Circle Yes or No and write the specific exercises on the line for Extension Principle, Flexion Principle or Lateral Principle. **Treatment Goals**—Indicate what you expect to change by next visit and things you wish to reassess on Day 2. Short and Longterm goals can be recorded also.

chapter seven

The Mulligan Concept

Donald K. Reordan PT, MS, OCS, MCTA

*The Mulligan Concept is named after Brian Mulligan, a physiotherapist from New Zealand. This concept is based on the premise that joint mobilization can restore the normal articular relationship of a joint that has altered positional alignment. A key feature of the examination is the use of a trial intervention, which ultimately guides further treatments. Mulligan developed unique treatments that combine mobilization with active or passive movements. The first edition of Mulligan's book entitled, *Manual Therapy: NAGs, SNAGs, MWMs, etc.*, was published in 1989. Students can find more information about the approach and training opportunities at www.bmulligan.com and www.na-mcta.com.*

BACKGROUND

The famous scientist, Louis Pasteur observed, "Chance only favors the prepared mind." Such mental preparation combined with the practical experience of physiotherapist Brian R. Mulligan from Wellington, New Zealand resulted in development of the Mulligan Concept approach to manual physical therapy.

Brian Mulligan qualified as a physiotherapist in 1954 and achieved his diploma in manipulative therapy in 1974. Along with continually working in clinical practice in Wellington, New Zealand, he has been teaching manual therapy in New Zealand since 1970, and internationally since 1972. The first edition of Mulligan's book entitled, *Manual Therapy: NAGs, SNAGs, MWMs, etc.* was published in 1989, and currently is in its sixth edition, printed in 2010.[1]

Mulligan's interest in the analytical development of manual therapy and in the collection of reliable evidence in support of its practice has influenced him to continue to teach and further refine his approach. In order to meet the increasing international demand from therapists wishing to learn the Mulligan Concept and to ensure high standards of instruction, Mulligan established the Mulligan Concept Teachers Association (MCTA) in 1993. Currently there are over 40 physical therapists worldwide who are accredited instructors of this approach. In addition to instruction, the MCTA is dedicated to generate funding and promote research related to the validity of these concepts and the clinical efficacy of these techniques. MCTA instructors as well as published references are accessible at www.bmulligan.com and www.na-mcta.com.

The development of the Mulligan Concept was born from Mulligan's desire to more efficiently achieve optimal mechanical and functional results in the management of musculoskeletal disorders of the spine and extremities. The manual therapy techniques adopted within this approach incorporate the use of active, passive physiological, passive accessory, and functional movements. From his experience at his busy practice, Mulligan identified the importance of immediately evaluating the effectiveness of his manual interventions. He also often observed that patients receiving traditional orthopedic manual therapy procedures did not make significant or lasting improvement. His intolerance for the use of techniques that lacked timely results led Mulligan toward the investigation of new paradigms.

When treating one such patient who presented with chronic (several months) index finger pain and movement restriction in the proximal interphalangeal (PIP) joint, Mulligan had exhausted his traditional manual therapy, exercise, and modality options. Frustration at the lack of improvement by the second visit gave way to inspiration when he attempted a technique that he had not been taught nor had he consciously performed previously. He changed the direction of joint mobilization from a traditional sagittal plane posterior-to-anterior (PA) glide of the concave joint surface (proximal end of middle phalanx) to a passive accessory mobilization in the frontal plane. The first attempt, a medial glide, produced pain prior to the commencement of movement. Though initially inclined to discontinue this pursuit, Mulligan was compelled to persevere with his experiment. To his and the patient's interest, upon the application of a lateral glide the patient reported not only no pain but actual elimination of symptoms. Intrigued, Mulligan asked the patient if she could now flex her finger, which she did painlessly. He observed that the previously restricted and pain-provoking joint motion was immedi-

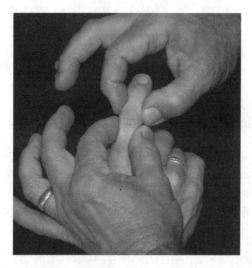

Figure 7–1 PIP mobilization in the frontal plane.

ately restored to normal range without pain in response to sustaining a manual repositioning of the articular surfaces

This unexpected experience led to further experimentation with the use of similar mobilizations in other joints of both the spine and extremities. Mulligan consistently found that, when indicated, the combination of accessory joint mobilization with concurrent physiological movement provided immediate, significant, and lasting changes in the patient's condition. The improvements that Mulligan observed in response to these new techniques occurred so quickly and were of such magnitude that they could not be explained by the gradual nature of the typical healing process.

Theoretical Framework for the Mulligan Concept

Through empirical evidence gained by frequent and consistent trials using the strategy of combining accessory mobilization with physiologic movement, Mulligan further developed the theory that a joint may assume a faulty position that might restrict motion and produce pain. Such a positional fault may be the result of trauma, aging, muscle imbalance, or poor posture and may not be detectable through conventional diagnostic imaging procedures.

What has become known as the *positional fault theory* suggests that joints having less than optimal positional relationships will adopt faulty movement patterns that lead to reduced function and/or pain. Mobilization is performed for the purpose of restoring the normal articular relationships. This theory is in contrast to previously established approaches that often utilize joint mobilization for the purpose of stretching, breaking, or gating pain associated with capsular restrictions of the joint. When operating under this more traditional theoretical construct, immediate changes in motion and symptoms in response to mobilization cannot be expected. The amount of time that is anticipated for joint mobilization techniques that are designed to stretch or break adhesions to have their desired effect is greater than that demonstrated through Mulligan's clinical experiences. There is growing evidence in the literature in support of immediate changes in pressure-pain threshold[2] and sympathoexcitatory response[3] resulting from application of Mulligan's "mobilization with movement" (MWM).

The positional fault theory is neither new nor unique to this approach. The concept that articular malalignment leads to altered kinematics and eventual dysfunction is a fundamental principle among several other orthopedic manual therapy approaches as well. The osteopathic approach to orthopedic manual therapy, for example, is based on the theory that joint malalignment, particularly in the spine, leads to dysfunction. This approach is based on the identification and reduction of positional faults for the purpose of improving joint kinematics. Other approaches have attempted to apply these principles to the joints of the extremities as well. McConnell[4] discusses the concept of "tracking problems" in the management of patellofemoral syndrome and Sahrmann[5] describes the "displaced path of the instantaneous center of rotation" in patients with alignment and movement impairments.

To test the positional fault theory, the manual therapist need only to reposition the joint and have the patient undertake the previously restricted, or symptom-provocative movement, while taking note of any obvious changes in the patient's range of motion or symptoms. Theories that support the pathogenesis and sequealae of adaptive shortening and capsular adhesions suggest that such restrictions may *only* be addressed after stresses are applied repeatedly over a period of time. However, the immediate results often experienced in response to MWM techniques seem to provide face validity in support of the positional fault theory. Perhaps nonresponders are those individuals who are truly experiencing issues with adaptive shortening and capsular adhesions. When applied as one component of the physical examination, this process of clinical exploration may assist in determining the differential functional diagnosis and guiding subsequent therapeutic intervention.

Principles of Examination

As with other approaches, the Mulligan Concept advocates a thorough examination, which includes a detailed history as well as measurement of joint motion and an appreciation of joint kinematics. Standard examination procedures including measurement of active range of motion (ROM), passive ROM, strength testing, neurologic testing, and palpation are performed as indicated. The exam seeks to comprehensively identify the nature and origin of the patient's presenting dysfunction. Additional examination procedures are performed to provide information concerning diagnosis, prognosis, the need for additional nonmanual interventions, and appropriateness for manual interventions. These procedures, however, do not serve as the primary indicators for the specific type and manner of manual therapy intervention that is warranted.

The primary examination procedure that is used to make clinical decisions and guide subsequent manual therapy intervention lies in the concept of the trial treatment, or trial intervention. First popularized by Kaltenborn[6] (see Chapter 4) the trial treatment approach involves the initiation of a low dosage intervention that is employed for the primary purpose of evaluating the immediate and delayed effects of such an intervention on the patient's primary presenting impairment. Within this approach, the specific procedure chosen for this trial intervention is based primarily on the location of symptoms and the posture and specific movement that provokes or increases the patient's chief complaint.

One of the primary advantages of the Mulligan Concept is the simplicity with which these techniques may be tested for effect. The immediate effect of each trial manual intervention on the patient's chief impairment becomes the primary indicator for intervention. As the trial mobilization is performed, the therapist notes the patient's symptom response, and the quantity and quality of the movement during and immediately after the mobilization has been performed. In order to ascertain the effect of each chosen technique on the patient's chief impairment, the process must involve examination, trial intervention, then followed immediately by reexamination.

The expectation is that the patient's pain will be immediately abolished and that motion will significantly improve in response to the trial intervention.

If such a response is not realized, the therapist should make slight alterations in the location, direction, and/or the amplitude of mobilization force. If the patient continues to fail to respond, the technique may be abandoned altogether in favor of another. Common errors in technique performance include failure to apply force in the ideal direction of the joint treatment plane, alteration of the mobilizing force during the physiologic movement, application of force over the wrong segment or joint, or mobilization with either too little or too much force. Therefore, when considering the principle features of the examination that serve to guide the use of these techniques, the concept of the trial intervention is paramount. Most assuredly, the other components of a thorough examination are performed, but to determine the efficacy of this approach, a trial of low load mobilization is advocated with close observation of the patient's response. No time is wasted, as the value of these techniques will be immediately apparent.

Principles of Intervention

The transition from examination to intervention is immediate and lends to the overall efficiency of this approach. The specific trial procedure that was proven to be effective in altering symptoms and enhancing range during the examination becomes the intervention. Using this approach for a variety of impairments over the course of 50 years of physical therapy practice, Mulligan has chronicled a collection of techniques that have proven to be effective for a myriad of disorders. These techniques have collectively become known as mobilizations with movement (MWM) based on the fact that active or passive physiologic movement occurs simultaneous with passive accessory mobilization. Although modifications have been made depending on the anatomic region in question, these techniques have in common the basic tenets of MWM that were previously articulated.

The use of joint mobilization and active or passive movement are common tools in the arsenal of the manual physical therapist. It is the combination of these two interventions, however, that makes this approach unique. Although specific manual contacts may differ, the application of articular accessory glides utilized during MWM follows the mobilization principles espoused by Kaltenborn (see Chapter 4). In particular, two fundamental principles of his Nordic approach are strictly followed when performing MWM. First, the manual therapist must be sure to gain contact and apply force as close to the joint as possible. Secondly, the mobilizing force must be applied parallel to the treatment plane, which is defined by the line that extends across the concave articular surface of the joint.

Mobilization with Movement (MWM) Clinical Practice Guidelines

There are several important clinical practice guidelines that make the performance of MWM unique. First and foremost, mobilizations must be applied in the direction in which pain is eliminated. If pain is produced then either the technique is not indicated or the technique is being performed incorrectly. With the onset of pain, the manual therapist must modify or discontinue the technique immediately. When applying MWM the manual therapist must be sure to use the minimum amount of force necessary to achieve pain-free mobilization. The mobilizing force is typically applied directly to the region from which symptoms are emanating. The manual therapist's hand contacts must enable the application of an accessory glide parallel to the treatment plane and not restrict normal physiologic movement. Lastly, many MWM techniques are performed in weight bearing. Most other orthopedic manual therapy approaches implement techniques that are performed in non weight-bearing positions. An advantage to weight bearing mobilization is that motion gains that are accomplished in functional positions are more likely to be retained. Furthermore, utilizing the weight-bearing position may be more functional. It is the posture in which active range is often examined and, in many cases, the posture in which pain is produced. Some individuals may also have difficulty assuming a lying position that may be required for implementation of non weight-bearing manual procedures. Once MWM efficacy has been established, sufficient repetitions (usually 5–10 repetitions) for effective training are performed in order to sustain the corrected articular position after the accessory glide is released.

Another difference between MWM and those techniques described by others like Kaltenborn and Maitland[7] is their nonoscillatory nature. MWM techniques typically use patient-assisted overpressure at end range as opposed to the use of oscillations. Furthermore, the primary objective in using MWM is to reduce joint malalignments and eliminate positional faults through the application of light, sustained pressure as opposed to stretching a restricted capsule. Therefore, unlike traditional joint mobilization, the guiding indication for the degree of mobilizing force is not the joint's end-feel, but rather the onset of the patient's symptoms and functional restrictions.

An advantage to the use of MWM is the manner in which its immediate efficacy is established. Efficacy is determined by repositioning the joint using the appropriate amount of force, then repeating the previously restricted and/or provocative motion and noting any changes in movement or symptoms. If the range of movement and/or symptoms significantly improves, MWM is indicated in the management of the patient, and the presence of a positional fault is suspected. If the provocative and/or restricted joint motion is improved but not cleared in response to mobilization, the manual therapist may slightly modify the direction, force, or location of the mobilization in attempt to improve the response. The manual therapist must make every attempt to persist with minor modifications until, ideally, symptoms are eliminated and full motion has been restored.

Mobilization with Movement (MWM) of the Spine in the Management of Low Back Pain

The use of MWM in the management of spinal conditions has become widely practiced among the orthopedic manual therapy community due to repeated claims of their clinical efficacy. Some advocate their use based on the expediency of results as compared to other manual and nonmanual interventions. A survey[8] of 3,295 physical therapists in Britain was conducted for the purpose of investigating the current use of MWM for the management of low back pain (LBP). Forty-one percent of the respondents, 1,136 therapists, reported being involved in the management of LBP, with greater than 50% of these using MWM on at least a weekly basis. Over 62% were using MWM predominantly for treatment of mechanical LBP. An increase in range of motion was reported by 54.4% as the most common immediate finding in response to MWM and 27.5% reported an immediate relief in pain. The lower lumbar levels were the most commonly treated region and, on average, two spinal levels were mobilized. The majority of therapists utilized other interventions in combination with MWM in the management of LBP.

The following techniques for the spine were developed by Mulligan, and later modified by both he and his colleagues through years of clinical practice. These techniques have been well described in Mulligan's text. Within this chapter, Mulligan's techniques will be described for the purpose of providing the reader with the clinical application of the principles previously discussed as they relate to LBP. The reader is encouraged to read Mulligan's text as well as the references cited at www.bmulligan.com for additional information on the philosophy and practice of this approach, and to take lab courses offered by the Mulligan Concept Teachers Association (www.na-mcta.com) to assist with motor skill and clinical reasoning development.

Sustained Natural Apophyseal Glides (SNAGs)

SNAGs are nonoscillatory mobilizations that are useful throughout the entire spine. These techniques were among the first procedures described by Mulligan that fully demonstrated the major tenets for use of MWM. As their name implies (i.e., sustained natural apophyseal glides), the mobilizing force is applied in accordance with the anatomic features of the joint along the plane of the concave joint surface. This force is applied as the pain-producing physiologic motion is superimposed either actively or passively. It is important that the manual therapist sustain the mobilizing force throughout the entire range of physiologic movement until the joint returns from the provocative range. Pain often ensues if the therapist fails to maintain the mobilizing force throughout the movement. Once the end of available range of motion is engaged, passive overpressure is applied. The patient may provide overpressure at end range. SNAGs for the lumbar spine are indicated for patients with painful or restricted lumbar motion.

The patient should be treated in their provocative posture. If the patient presents with pain or restriction of lumbar motion in standing, then they should be treated in standing. If symptomatic in sitting, they should be treated in sitting. If the patient is symptomatic in sitting *and* standing, treat in sitting; if SNAGs are indicated, the retest will typically be clear in both positions.

To perform lumbar SNAGs in sitting, the therapist stands behind the seated patient with a belt around the therapist's hips and the patient's lower abdomen, just inferior to the ASIS level. The belt is used to offer counterforce to the anterior pressure of the mobilizing hand. The therapist's mobilizing hand contacts the patient with the hypothenar border of the hand just distal to the pisiform, with the fifth metacarpal "horizontal" to the "vertical" spine. The contact target is the spinous process or transverse process of the superior vertebra of the segment to be mobilized. The mobilizing hand is supinated to hook on to the soft tissue and the mobilizing force applied in a cranial direction to match the treatment plane of the apophyseal joints. If SNAGs are indicated, an accessory glide will result in full, painless motion of the patient's lumbar spine through the previously provocative range. Repetitions and overpressure (the weight of the body is usually sufficient) precede the retest. The lumbar SNAG technique described previously is for the L1–L4 levels, as the PSIS bilaterally prevent contacting L5 in this fashion.

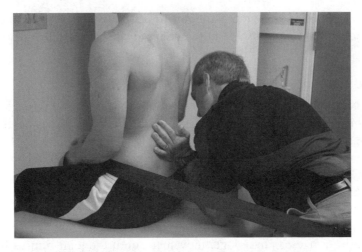

Figure 7–2A Right L4 SNAG during seated flexion.

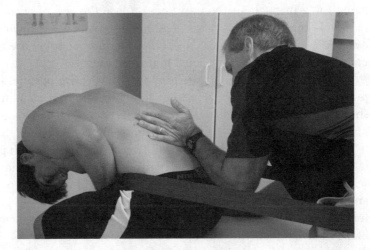

Figure 7–2B Right L4 SNAG during seated flexion.

L5 SNAGs

The L5 SNAG requires mobilization using both thumbs: the ipsilateral thumb is placed between L5 and the sacrum with the thumbnail vertical for contacting the articular pillar of L5 on the side of symptoms or restricted movement, the other thumb underneath providing a cranially directed mobi-

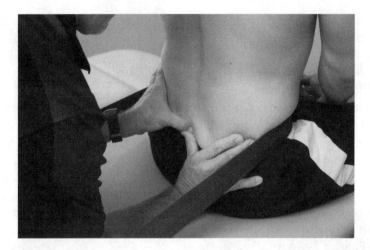

Figure 7–3 L5 SNAG.

lization force through the lateral border of the contact thumb. L5 SNAGs follow all the principles of MWM previously discussed.

APPLICATION OF THE MULLIGAN CONCEPT TO JOE LORES

Examination

It is during the subjective and physical exam process previously noted that the indications for use of Mulligan Concept techniques would be initially determined. As stated, standard examination procedures including measurement of active ROM, passive ROM, strength testing, neurologic testing, and palpation are performed as indicated. In the particular case of Joe, the patient indicates sudden onset right sided low back and buttock pain of two weeks duration. The subjective indicators of interest include aggravating factors of sitting, getting up from sitting, bending, and lifting. Symptoms are eased by lying and rest. No paresthesia is noted.

Objectively, standing flexion and extension provoke the patient's pain at 50% of expected normal ROM. Other movements are symptomatic and restricted but not to the extent of flexion and extension, which are therefore the initial focus to the practitioner of Mulligan Concept techniques. If the patient has pain in standing, active movement tests would next be performed in sitting. In this case, sitting ROM is similarly provocative with flexion producing more pain than extension. Of note, the neurologic exam, hip, SI and SLR tests are negative.

Evaluation and Diagnosis

The initial clinical reasoning process indicates primary lumbar involvement. The next question to answer is if the Mulligan approach is indicated. In Joe's case, sitting and standing flexion and extension are equally restricted, but flexion is more painful than extension. It is also noted that spring testing (posterior to anterior pressure) over L4–L5 and L5–S1 are positive, with greater pain reproduction on the right than in the center. Therefore the indicated *mobilization* is a right L4 SNAG concurrent *with* the seated flexion *movement,* and is chosen for initial trial intervention (Figures 7–2A and 7–2B).

Before Mulligan techniques are used to assist differential functional diagnosis during the physical exam, it is important to educate the patient. He is told that if this manual therapy technique is to be useful it must eliminate his pain. If *any* pain is felt during the MWM the therapist must be told immediately—this guides the treatment. Mulligan achieves better patient understanding and involvement by showing them the anatomy of a plastic lumbar spine model and describing that a stiff (hypomobile) facet joint or segment can result in unacceptable pressure on the disc during movement. SNAGs treat both the facet joints and the disc simultaneously. This is easily demonstrated to the patient on a spine model by lifting L3 cranially off of L4. They can also be taught that pain would likely result if the clinician SNAGs L4 when they were intending to SNAG L3, as this would close/compress the segment intended for opening/decompression.

Prognosis

Typically, a patient like Joe would be expected to improve quickly with resolution within approximately 2 weeks, about 6 visits, in the absence of poor compliance with home program, exacerbating factors, or reinjury. Manual therapy would be indicated at subsequent visits only if symptoms or restrictions returned and could not be resolved with positioning, therapeutic exercise, or repetitive movements. The usual therapeutic exercises, posture, and body mechanics instructions for prevention of reinjury would be discussed. The expected outcome is full, pain-free lumbar ROM.

Intervention

If this trial manual therapy intervention eliminates the pain and restores normal flexion ROM, 4–6 repetitions of these mobilizations with movement are performed. The overpressure advocated by the Mulligan Concept is provided by the patient's body weight with gravity assist. The manual intervention is immediately followed by retesting active ROM: seated lumbar flexion. If the patient is now pain-free with full lumbar flexion ROM, extension is tested. If in likewise manner seated extension is also full and painless, the movements are retested in standing.

Complete resolution/Assessment

If it is the ideal case and full pain-free lumbar ROM has been achieved by an L4 SNAG then the assessment is dysfunction of the L4–L5 segment. The manual part of the first treatment is over and the patient is educated in improved sitting posture (knees below hips is primary), as sitting is one of his described provocative positions. If deemed important from the subjective data, the low back may be taped with an "X" across the neutral lumbar area to give a proprioceptive reminder to stay away from end-range stress.

Incomplete resolution

If a right L4 SNAG for seated lumbar flexion resulted in partial improvement of pain-free movement, for example increasing first pain with flexion from 50–75%, the clinical indication is to either:

a) perform more repetitions of a right L4 SNAG if full pain-free range is achieved; if not,
b) modify the L4 SNAG by changing the mobilization contact hand placement (location), direction or force, or
c) perform a right L5 SNAG if repetitions or a modified L4 SNAG do not resolve the problem.

If partial resolution was achieved with L4 SNAGs, and complete resolution after L5 SNAGs, the assessment would be changed to dysfunction of L4–L5 and L5–S1. If symptoms were eliminated during SNAGs but are not fully resolved upon retest of lumbar flexion, the patient may be shown how to perform self-SNAGs with either his fist or a belt.

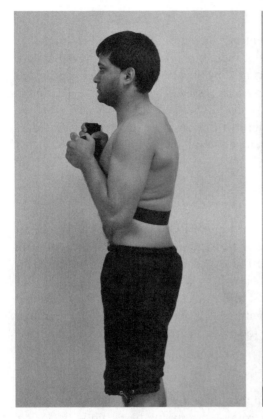 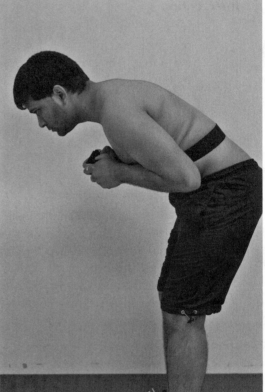

Figure 7–4A Self SNAG in flexion.   **Figure 7–4B** Self SNAG in flexion.

Once again, Mulligan Concept techniques are described with the acronym "PILL," reminding the clinician that when indicated they are (P) Pain-free when applied, produce an (I) Immediate change in the patient's condition, and have a (LL) Long Lasting benefit. Manual therapy sessions are typically 2 or 3 days per week, seldom daily. The majority of improvement achieved should be retained at subsequent visits.

If symptoms and movement restrictions return between visits, Joe would be advised to avoid or minimize positions or activities involving lumbar flexion, especially interrupting prolonged positions of flexion and repetitive flexion tasks. Careful consideration of disc-type symptom behavior is important and underscored by the findings in the examination that repetitive flexion in standing (RFIS) increased symptoms and extension (REIS) decreased them.

The Mulligan Concept recognizes the contributions of the McKenzie approach in the diagnosis and treatment of LBP. If full resolution of the patient's symptoms and movement restrictions occur with repetitive lumbar extension, there would be no need to apply Mulligan techniques. Mulligan's sitting advice would still be instructed, and perhaps taping applied if considered useful. If, however, extension exercises in standing were not completely pain-free, SNAGs may be applied or self-SNAGs taught so his home exercise program would be pain-free instead of merely centralizing the pain.

SUMMARY

The Mulligan Concept is rooted in the framework of the positional fault theory, which suggests that malalignment of a joint leads to pain and dysfunction. The model utilizes a clinical reasoning process that is based on the patient's response to a manual therapy trial intervention that is designed to restore normal articular relationships through the entire range of movement. The immediate effect of each trial manual intervention on the patient's chief impairment becomes the primary indicator for intervention. Accessory mobilizations combined with physiologic movements are the hallmark techniques of the Mulligan approach.

REFERENCES

1. Mulligan, BR. *Manual Therapy: NAGs, SNAGs, MWMs, etc.* 6th Edition. New Zealand: Plane View Services Ltd.; 2010.
2. Teys P, Bisset L, Vicenzino B. The initial effects of a Mulligan's mobilization with movement technique on range of movement and pressure pain threshold in pain-limited shoulders. *Manual Therapy.* 2008;13(1):37–42.
3. Paungmali A. Hypoalgesic and sympathoexcitatory effects of mobilization with movement for lateral epicondylalgia. *Physical Therapy.* 2003;83(4):374–383.
4. McConnell J. The management of chondromalacia patellae: a long term solution. *The Australian Journal of Physiotherapy.* 1986;32(4):215–223.
5. Sahrmann S. *Diagnosis and Treatment of Movement Impairment Syndromes.* St. Louis, MO: Mosby; 1992.
6. Kaltenborn FM. *Manual Mobilization of the Extremity Joints: Basic Examination and Treatment Techniques.* Minneapolis, MN: Orthopedic Physical Therapy Products; 1989.
7. Maitland GD. *Peripheral Manipulation.* 4th ed. Oxford, UK: Butterworth-Heinemann. 2006.
8. Konstantinou K. The use and reported effects of mobilization with movement techniques in low back pain management; a cross-sectional descriptive survey of physiotherapists. *Manual Therapy.* 2002;7(4):206–214.

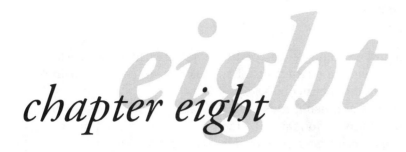

chapter eight

The Paris Approach

Jeffrey A. Rot, PT, DHSc, OCS, MTC, FAAOMPT
James A. Viti, PT, MSc, DPT, OCS, MTC, FAAOMPT

Stanley V. Paris is a physical therapist who trained in England under the mentorship of James Cyriax MD, Alan Stoddard DO, and Freddy Kaltenborn PT. During this time, he recognized each practitioner's significant contributions as well as their similarities and differences. These observations formed the underlying foundation of his approach, which draws from many schools of thought.

Dr. Paris teaches that joint dysfunction is treated with specific spinal manipulation or muscular stabilization for restoring normal movement needed for return of function. He has written extensively about spinal hypermobility and hypomobility and how each can contribute to joint dysfunction. He published his first book in 1965, which was titled The Spinal Lesion. *Currently, Dr. Paris is the founding and acting president of the University of St. Augustine for Health Sciences, Institute of Physical Therapy (www.usa.edu).*

BACKGROUND

"Whenever a body of knowledge that defines a discipline is greater than the individual's ability to remember and interpret it, there develops a need for a philosophy of management that can serve as a guide to practice within that discipline."[1] Over the years, the Institute of Physical Therapy, founded by Dr. Stanley V. Paris, has developed its own philosophy for the practice of orthopaedic physical therapy. The philosophy is based on the following principles[1]:

1. Joint injury, including such conditions referred to as osteoarthrosis, instability, and the after-effects of sprains and strains are impairments (dysfunctions) rather than diseases.

2. Impairments are manifest as either increases or decreases of motion from the expected normal or by the presence of aberrant movements. Thus, impairments are represented by abnormal movement.

3. Where the impairment is detected as limited motion (hypomobility), the treatment of choice is manipulation to joint structures, stretching to muscles and fascia, and the promotion of activities that encourage a full range of movement.

4. When the impairment is manifested as increased movement (hypermobility), laxity, or instability, the treatment of the joint in question is NOT manipulation, but stabilization by instruction of correct posture, stabilization exercises, and the correction of any limitations of movement in neighboring joints that may be contributing to the hypermobility.

5. The primary cause of degenerative joint disease is from long-standing joint impairments (dysfunctions). Therefore the presence of debilitating clinical joint disease is from the failure to provide timely physical therapy interventions that reverse the degenerative process thus negating the need for surgery.

6. The physical therapist's primary role is in the examination, evaluation, and treatment of impairments (dysfunctions), whereas that of the physician is the diagnosis and treatment of disease. These are two separate but complimentary roles in health care.

7. Since impairments are the cause of pain, the primary goal of physical therapy should be to correct the impairments rather than the pain. When, however, the nature of the pain interferes with correcting the impairments, the pain will need to be addressed as part of the intervention.

8. The key to understanding impairments, and thus being able to examine and treat them, is to understand anatomy and biomechanics. It therefore behooves us in physical therapy to develop our knowledge and skills in these areas, so that we may safely assume leadership in the nonoperative management of neuromusculoskeletal disorders.

9. It is the patient's responsibility to restore, maintain, and enhance their health. In this context, the role of the physical therapist is to serve as an educator, to be an example to the patient and to reinforce a healthy and productive lifestyle.

10. Autonomous practice is paramount because our body of knowledge is sufficiently unique and is of sufficient volume that to depend on referral

for patients is no longer morally defensible. Today's doctorally prepared physical therapists have the competencies to detect serious pathology, recognize neural compromise, and be able to identify psychosocial stress and to make appropriate referrals.

The Paris Approach is classified as a pathoanatomical (impairment-based) model with the clinical understanding that pain is a direct result of pathomechanics and tissue-specific impairments. Treating just the symptoms without addressing the causative and contributing impairment would produce only short-term outcomes. Usually multiple impairments exist before the level of noxious stimuli reaches the patient's awareness for pain. The goal of this approach is to identify, measure, and treat the impairments, whether they are the source (e.g., facet, disc, ligament, muscles) of the symptoms or merely contribute to the source of symptoms (e.g., tight hip flexors, weak abdominals, poor posture/body mechanics). Identifying impairments requires a thorough manual physical therapy examination. The examination process identifies historical, subjective, and objective findings that help to establish the physical therapy diagnosis. The intervention strategy addresses the impairments as well as the contributing factors rather than the pain. Syndrome identification may greatly assist the management of each particular patient. A syndrome is a consistent set of signs and symptoms that corresponds to a particular physical therapy diagnosis.[2] When the patient is effectively treated with impairment-based interventions, using syndromes as a guide, they should become pain-free without functional limitations. The principle syndromes of the lumbar spine and pelvis that can produce low back and leg pain follow in order of greatest to least observed clinical frequency.

The Paris Classification System Syndromes[2]

1. Myofascial states
2. Facet dysfunction
3. Sacroiliac dysfunction
4. Ligamentous weakness
5. Instability
6. Disc dysfunction
7. Spondylolisthesis
8. Lumbar spine stenosis (central spine stenosis, and lateral foraminal stenosis)
9. The lesion complex

10. Lumbar spine: Kissing spines (Baastrap's disease)
11. Thoracolumbar syndrome

The Paris examination process follows a systematic framework that is designed to identify relevant joint and soft tissue impairments. The examination consists of the following 14-Step process:[2]

1. Pain assessment
2. Initial observation
3. History and interview
4. Structural inspection
5. Active movements
6. Neurovascular assessment
7. Palpation for condition
8. Palpation for position
9. Palpation for mobility
10. Upper and/or lower quarter assessment
11. Radiologic, other tests, and medical data
12. Summary of findings
13. Intervention/treatment plan
14. Explanation and prognosis

APPLICATION OF THE PARIS APPROACH TO JOE LORES

Examination

Steps 1–11 of the 14-step process will be presented in this section. Joe was asked to fill out the following examination intake forms: Medical History Questionnaire, Modified Oswestry Low Back Disability Questionnaire, McGill Pain Questionnaire, and a Body Chart Pain Drawing. Figure 8–1 contains a completed examination form for Joe. A blank Paris examination form can also be found at the end of this chapter.

1. Pain assessment, 2. Initial observation, 3. History and interview

The initial observation began in the reception area when the physical therapist introduced himself/herself to the patient and walked to the examination/treatment room with the patient. Mr. Lores' transition from sitting to standing was guarded. He exhibited normal gait. He reported that his back pain was

PARIS APPROACH   UNIVERSITY OF ST. AUGUSTINE
                                            FOR HEALTH SCIENCES

SPINE EVALUATION   Date: ____ / ____ /20____

Mr/Mrs/Miss/Ms: JOSEPH LORES

Age: 40 yo.   Dr.: _____

Diagnosis: LBP

Medical Orders: — P.T. EVAL +RX

· **SUBJECTIVE/Complaint:** LBP + BUTTOCKS PAIN
  ON (R)

How sustained: STARTED – WHEN INSTALLING A SINK. (PLUMBER)

HE WAS FLEXED + ROTATED – IN A TIGHT SPOT   Date of Onset ___ / ___ / 20___, n.a. ____

Occupation/Activities: FULL TIME – SELF EMPLOYED, PLUMBER   (Photocopy I.D.)

Medical History: not significant ✓ , _____

Medical Tests and Results: n.a. ____ , X-RAYS – RADIOGRAPHS (–)

·**OBJECTIVE/Findings:**

Structure,	not significant____,	see page 3 ✓ ·
Active Mvts. (ROM)	not significant____,	see page 3 ✓ ·
Neurovascular	not significant ✓ ,	see page 3 & 4 ·
U. and L. Quarter	not significant____,	see page 4 ✓ LE ·
Palpation Findings	not significant____,	see page 5 ✓ ·

EVALUATION/IMPAIRMENTS   **INTERVENTIONS**
  STG = Short Term Goals   LTG = Long Term Goals

1. STRUCTURE – POSTURE | LUMBAR EXT PROG.
   STG: ⊕ ↑ LUMBAR LORDOSIS | LTG: NORMAL LORDOSIS
2. ↓ AROM & ↓ PIVM | MANIPULATION & THEN EX
   STG: ↑ AROM | LTG: AROM + PIVM = (N)
3. MYOFASCIAL HYPERTONICITY & TENDERNESS | MYOFASCIAL MANIPULATION
   STG: ↓ TONE & ↓ TENDERNESS | LTG: TONE + TENDERNESS (N) WNL
4. ↓ ↓ HIP AROM – PROM + TIGHT HAMSTRINGS | PASSIVE STRETCHING MANUALLY + HOME PROGRAM
   STG: ↑ HIP ROM | LTG: HIP ROM WNL & WNL HAMSTRINGS.
5. ↓ STRENGTH + MM CONTROL | STRENGTHEN, STABILIZE AGE + MM CONTROL EX.
   STG: ↑ STRENGTH & MM CONTROL ABDOMINAL MUSCLES | LTG: STRENGTH + MM CONTROL = WNL
6. OSWESTRY = SEVERE DISABILITY 42% | EDUCATION, FUNCTIONAL TRAIN, BACK-SCHOOL
   STG: 20% | LTG: OSWESTRY < 10

Education to Receive: Back School ✓ , Neck School ____ , Other_____

Present Stage: Immediate ____, Acute ____, Sub Acute ✓ , Settled ____, Chronic ____,

Other _____

Impression: Facet ✓ , Muscle ✓ , Ligament ____ , Disc ____ , Stenosis ____ , Spondylogenic____,
Neurogenic____, Other: _____

Frequency: _____   Duration: _____

PROGNOSIS: GOOD _____   **PHYSICAL THERAPIST SIG.:** _____

Page 1

Figure 8–1 Completed examination form for Joe Lores. *Source:* Reprinted with permission from Stanley V. Paris.

1. **PAIN QUESTIONNAIRE and BODY CHART:** completed _✓_ , n.a. _____
2. **INITIAL OBSERVATION:** ambulatory _✓_ bedridden _____
   Gait: normal _✓_ , guarded _____ , leg problem _____
   Comments: _GUARDED MOVT = TRANSITIONING FROM CHAIR TO STANDING_
   Resting position: sitting chair _✓_ , stool _____ , table _____ , other _____
   Behavior, if any: acute facet _✓_ , acute disc _____ , ligamentous _____ , other _SUB ACUTE_

3. **HISTORY and INTERVIEW**
   Present History
   1. Where precisely did the pain start (draw it in with an "X")
   2. Where did it spread to (draw it in): _✓_
   3. Where is it now / currently / today: _(R) LB + BUTTOCKS_
   _____
   4. What makes it hurt worse: _SITTING > STANDING,_
   FLEXION — BENDING FORWARD
   _____

   5. Does it hurt at night: yes _____ , no _✓_ ,
      5b. If yes, can the pain be affected by a change in position or
      activity of any kind: yes _____ , no _____
   6. What its like first thing in the morning: better___, stiff _✓_ , sore ___,
   7. What its like by mid-day: same _____ , better _✓_ , worse _____ ,
   8. What its like by late afternoon: same ___, better _____ , worse _✓_ ,
   9. What its like in the evening: same _____ , better _____ , worse _✓_ ,
   10. Pain Level 0–10: at best _2_ , worst _6_ , present _3_
   11. What have you learned that makes your back better: _____
       REST , MEDS , LYING DOWN

   Neurological
   12. Do you have any tingling, numbness or loss of skin sensation: no _✓_ , yes _____ , if yes, where _____
   13. Do you have any altered sensation, pain / numbness in the S4 region: no _✓_ , yes ____ , explain _____
   14. Do you experience any dizziness with change in neck positions? _NO_ _____
   15. What treatments have you had: none ___ , or _MEDS_ _____
       Did they help: yes _✓_ , no____ , other _A LITTLE_ _____
   16. Presently, are you getting better____ , worse____ , or staying much the same _✓_ ,
   Previous History
   17. Have you had anything similar before: yes _✓_ , no____ , if yes, describe _BACK PAIN - WENT AWAY_
       AFTER 2 WKS
       If yes, are they increasing in **frequency**: yes___ , no _✓_ , **severity**: yes___ , no _✓_ ,
   Miscellaneous
   18. Are you taking any medications: yes _✓_ , no____ , if yes, describe _ADVIL + FLEXERIL_
   19. When do you see your physician next: _____
   Behavioral
   20. What concerns you most: your pain _✓_ , or restriction of activities _✓_ , both _____ , n.a.____ ,
   21. What are your goals in coming to me: n.a.____ , (define some goals starting with functional goals) n.a.____ ,
       WORK - PAIN FREE - GET INTO TIGHT PLACES + BENDING W/ NO PAIN
   22. Now, is there anything else you would like to tell me before I examine your back / neck: no____
   _____

Figure 8–1 Completed examination form for Joe Lores (continued).

STRUCTURAL EXAMINATION n.a. ____, bed ridden ____, other _____

Patient is Typically   Comments: _____

  endomorph ____   ↓ LUMBAR LORDOSIS

  mesomorph ✓

  intermediate ____

  ectomorph ____

Pelvis

  neutral ____

  Ant. tilt ____

  Post. tilt ____

  R side down ____

  L side down ____

Head Position and Bearing: good ____, forward head ____, suspect S/C fault _____

5. ACTIVE MOVEMENTS n.a. ____, too acute ____, other ® LUMB.
        PAIN ® LUMB. & BUTTOCKS ®

Key	Range of motion	I
	Location of block	II
	Limited by pain	X

Area _____ LUMBAR _____

Comments: PAIN REPORTED and IN ® LB & BUTTOCKS DURING FB & ® SB

6. NEUROVASCULAR ASSESSMENT unnecessary ____, other _____

Key
0 = no contraction
1 = trace
2 = poor
3 = fair
4 = good
5 = normal

Lower Quarter

Muscle	Left	Right
L1, 2 Psoas	5/5	5/5
L3 Quads		
L4 Tib Ant		
L5 E.H.L.		
S1 F.H.L.		
S2 Hams	↓	↓

Upper Quarter

C1-2 apr chin in
C1-2 ppr chin up
C3 lat. nk. press
C4 upper trapezius
C5 biceps
C6 wrist ext.
C7 triceps
C8 thumb extensors
T1 intrinsics

	Left	Right

Reflexes
0 = absent
1+ = diminished
2+ = normal
3+ = increased
4+ = clonus

Reflexes	Left	Right
Knee Jerk	2+	2+
S1 Ankle Jerk	2+	2+
Babinski	Ⓘ	Ⓘ
Clonus	Ⓘ	Ⓘ

Reflexes
0=absent
1+=diminished
2+=normal
3+=increased
4+=clonus

	Left	Right
C5-6 biceps		
C5-6 brachio-radialis		
C7 triceps		

Sensation   not tested ____, area tested *LE's*, findings WNL / INTACT THROUGHOUT

Page 3

Figure 8–1 Completed examination form for Joe Lores (continued).

Lumbar - additional tests performed _____,

SLR tested_____, L _____ R _____

cm_____ _____

Passive Kernig: tested_____, normal ✓, limited_____, _____

Compression/distraction and quadrant: tested_____, normal_____, positive_____, _____

_____

Cervical - additional tests performed _____,

Compression/distraction and quadrant: tested_____, normal_____, positive_____, _____

_____

7. UPPER AND/OR LOWER QUARTER ASSESSMENT n.a. _____,

Upper Quarter, performed _____, normal _____, n.a._____, _____

Shoulder

Left: limited_____, painful_____, capsular_____, non-capsular_____, _____

Right: limited_____, painful_____, capsular_____, non-capsular_____, _____

Craniomandibular

Left: limited_____, painful_____, capsular_____, non-capsular_____, _____

Right: limited_____, painful_____, capsular_____, non-capsular_____, _____

Thoracic outlet findings: none_____, comments, _____

_____

Lower Quarter: performed_____, normal_____, n.a._____,

Hip (*Faber, Thomas, Hip Joint Distraction*)

Left: limited_____, painful_____, capsular_____, non-capsular_____, $IR = 40°$ $EXT = 10°$

Right: limited ✓, painful_____, capsular_____, non-capsular_____, $IR = 30°$ $EXT = 5°$

Sacroiliac: examined ✓, nothing significant ✓, n.a._____,

Test: ASIS compression,   positive left_____, right_____, comments_____ WNL ✓

ASIS gap,   positive left_____, right_____, comments_____

Anterior torsion,   positive left_____, right_____, comments_____

Post torsion   positive left_____, right_____, comments_____

Post. Gap/Shear painful positive left_____, right_____, comments_____

Post. Gap/Shear limited positive left_____, right_____, comments_____

Faber Test,   positive left_____, right_____, explain:_____

Supine to Sit Test,   positive _____, negative _____

Other sacroiliac tests/comments: _____

_____

_____

_____

_____

_____

_____

_____

Figure 8–1 Completed examination form for Joe Lores (continued).

PALPATION:

CONDITION   n.a._____.   9. POSITION   n.a._____.   10. MOBILITY   n.a._____.

Key:
X   Tender
⊗   Center Pain
≢   Spasm
//// Guarding
↕   Reflex Contr.

Key:
0 – Ankylosed
1 – Considerable Restriction
2 – Slight Restriction
3 – Normal
4 – Slight Increase
5 – Considerable Increase
6 – Unstable

Segment	FB	SBL	SBR	RL	RR	Other
L1-2	2			2	2	
L2-3	2			2	2	
L3-4	2			2	2	
L4-5	2			2	2	
L5-S1	2			2	2	

11. RADIOLOGIC AND OTHER MEDICAL DATA
Radiographs have been taken ✓ , reports are to hand_____,
Findings to relate _____

Other medical data: _____

PROGRESS, REASSESSMENT AND TREATMENT NOTES:

Page 5

Figure 8–1 Completed examination form for Joe Lores (continued).

NAME: _____

Where is your pain?
Please mark on the drawings below the areas where you feel your pain.

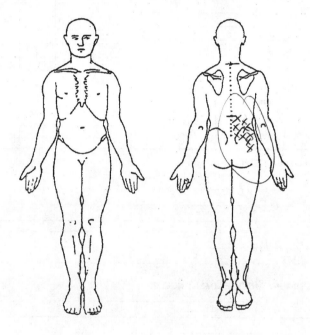

Figure 8–1 Completed examination form for Joe Lores (continued).

Body Chart and the McGill Pain Questionnaire

This we have already presented under Neuroanatomy, Pain and Pain Management in the FCO seminar.

Here are many words that describe pain. Some of these are grouped below. Check (✓) any words that describe the pain you have these days.

1.	2.	3.	4.
Flickering	Jumping	Pricking	Sharp
Quivering	Flashing	Boring	Cutting
Pulsing	Shooting	Drilling	Lacerating
Throbbing		Stabbing	
Beating			
Pounding			

5.	6.	7.	8.
Pinching	Tugging	Hot	Tingling
Pressing	Pulling	Burning	Itchy
Gnawing	Wrenching	Scalding	Smarting
Cramping		Searing	Stinging
Crushing			

9.	10.	11.	12.
Dull	(Tender)	Tiring	Sickening
(Sore)	Taut	Exhausting	Suffocating
Hurting	Rasping		
(Aching)	Splitting		
Heavy			

13.	14.	15.	16.
Fearful	Punishing	Wretched	(Annoying)
Frightful	Gruelling	Blinding	Troublesome
Terrifying	Cruel		Miserable
	Vicious		Intense
	Killing		Unbearable

17.	18.	19.	20.
Spreading	Tight	Cool	Nagging
Radiating	Numb	Cold	Nauseating
Penetrating	Drawing	Freezing	Agonizing
Piercing	Squeezing		Dreadful
	Tearing		Torturing

Page 7

Figure 8–1 Completed examination form for Joe Lores (continued).

reproduced when he moved from sitting to standing. He also stated that his pain was worse in sitting when compared to standing. The history and interview session is a key element for identifying a working hypothesis related to a particular clinical syndrome, which then assists with patient management.

Joe is a 38-year-old Hispanic male who was self-employed as a plumber where his occupational tasks involved lifting and working in tight places. His past medical history was positive for high blood pressure, a fracture to his clavicle (15 years prior), and arthroscopic knee surgery (14 years prior). He stated that he had low back pain (LBP) of 1-week duration in 2002 when he was helping a friend move a couch. He reported that his current low back and buttock pain began two weeks ago while installing a sink. He was working in a tight area, which required him to flex and rotate his trunk when he experienced immediate LBP.

The specific pain assessment consists of four features; the location, intensity, nature, and behavior. The location of pain was assessed using the pain drawing on the body chart. The pain drawing has been shown to have high test-retest reliability in patients with LBP.[3] Joe illustrated his pain to be on the right side of his back and buttock (see Appendix). He reported that his pain started in his right low back and had spread to his right buttock region. He denied pain or paraesthesias in either leg. The verbal analogue scale (0 = no pain, 10 = emergency room pain) was used to quantify the intensity of his pain. In a study by Williamson et al. the verbal analogue scale was compared to the visual analogue scale and both were found to have good and comparable reliability and validity.[4] Joe reported his pain to be constant with variable intensity ranging from 2–6/10 where the least amount of pain occurred when he awakened in the morning and the worst amount was when he sat for longer than 10 minutes and transitioned from sitting to standing.

Functional tasks such as sitting, bending, work activities, lifting, and transitioning from sitting to standing made his pain worse. Lying down, resting, and taking medication made his pain better. He reported that the pain did not wake him from sleeping. The McGill Pain Questionnaire was used to identify the nature (type) of Joe's pain. He described his pain as being sore, hurting, aching (category 9), tender (category 10), annoying (category 16). Melzack described the sensitivity of this questionnaire to changes in pain after various treatments and cited this as evidence for the validity of this assessment.[5] The pain descriptors used by Joe indicated that the nature of his pain represented that of a musculoskeletal condition. Pain behavior appeared to be related to movement and position and no systemic signs or red flags were noted.

In addition, Joe completed the Modified Oswestry Back Pain Questionnaire, which measures the patient's function in relation to their complaints of pain. He scored a 42%, which represented a severe disability with the goal being a disability score less than 10%.[9] The questionnaire has high test-retest reliability and is a valid indicator of functional improvement.[6]

Joe reported that he was currently taking the prescribed medication of Lotensin for his high blood pressure and Flexeril for his current low back and buttock pain. He also took over-the-counter anti-inflammatory medication as needed to decrease his symptoms. Joe's primary goal was to work pain-free in his full-time job.

4. Structural inspection

Structural inspection began with visually observing the patient in standing. The patient was observed from the front, the back, and the side, which revealed a slightly reduced lumbar lordosis. The patient's body type was mesomorphic. This means that he had a stocky muscular build. Body types may indicate natural abilities that should be considered in job and sport selection.

In the posterior view, hypertonic muscle guarding was observed more on the right when compared to the left from L3 to S1. Hypertonic muscle guarding is a state of increased tension in the muscle that may manifest as a protective response. Palpation of the iliac crests, posterior superior iliac spines (PSIS), greater trochanters, and anterior superior iliac spines (ASIS) revealed relatively symmetrical landmarks. Palpation of the spinous processes revealed that no step deformity was present. A step deformity may indicate the presence of a spondylolisthesis.[7] This diagnosis requires radiographic confirmation.[7]

5. Active movements

Lumbar active range of motion was examined using visual estimates. Forward bending was limited 50% with minimal reversal of his lumbar lordosis. The patient reported pain in the right low back and buttock. The lumbar lordosis should "reverse" during normal forward bending. Backward bending was also limited 50% with reproduction of similar symptoms on the right. Right side bending increased the patient's symptoms and was limited 20% compared to left side bending, which was normal. Rotation was limited 20% bilaterally. Repeated backward bending relieved the patient's symptoms in the buttock.

6. Neurovascular exam

A neurovascular assessment was performed due to the patient's reported distal pain in the right buttock. The dermatomes, myotomes, reflexes, and straight leg raise/ neural tension tests were all found to be negative.

7. Palpation for condition

In the prone position, the patient's skin was examined for superficial findings such as temperature change, moisture/dryness findings, moles, scars, ulcers, and skin mobility. There were no significant findings. The condition of the subcutaneous tissue was examined next. Tissue features such as edema, subcutaneous nodules, tenderness, and fascial plane mobility were all examined. The right gluteus medius, gluteus maximus, piriformis, quadratus lumborum, and multifidus were found to be tender and hypertonic.

8. Palpation for position

Palpation for position was unremarkable.

9. Palpation for mobility

Mobility testing was performed for the thoracic and lumbar spinal segments (Figure 8–2). The Paris' Passive Intervertebral Mobility (PIVM) rating scale (Figure 8–3) was used to measure the spinal intervertebral mobility.[8,9] All lumbar segments were measured as a 2/6, which was described as a slight restriction of the spinal segments. While mobility testing has been found to have fair intratester reliability and poor intertester reliability[8-10] it has been found to have good clinical utility or usefulness for determining intervention strategies for patients with LBP.[11] According to the PIVM data, Joe presents with a generalized stiff lumbar spine.

10. Lower quarter assessment

Hip passive range of motion in prone was positive for decreased internal rotation (35°) on the right when compared to the left (40°). Hip extension was limited to 5° on the right and 10° on the left. The hamstrings were tight bilaterally. Sacroiliac provocation tests were found to be negative. Selected provocation tests for the sacroiliac joint have been found to be reliable and/ or valid.[12–14] The patient was asked to draw in his abdominals and maintain this position in order to test the motor control and endurance of the trans-

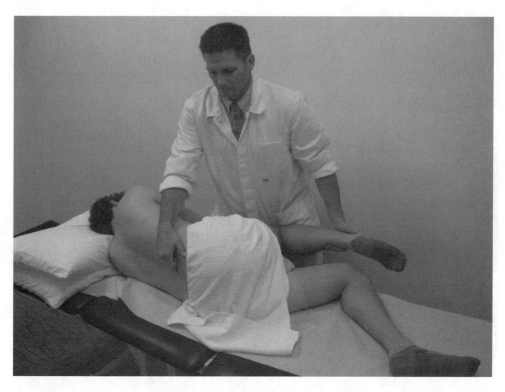

Figure 8–2 PIVM testing. *Source:* Reprinted with permission from Jeffrey A. Rot.

Table 8–1 PIVM Rating Scale[1]

Grade	Description	Criteria
0	Ankylosed	No detectable movement
1	Considerable hypomobity	Significant decrease in expected range and significant resistance to movement
2	Slight hypormobility	Slight decrease in mobility and resistance to movement
3	Normal	Normal expected movement
4	Slight hypermobility	Slight increase in expected mobility and less than normal resistance to movement
5	Considerable hypermobility	Significant increase in expected mobility, eventually restricted by periaricular structures
6	Unstable	Increase in expected mobility without restraint of periarticular structures

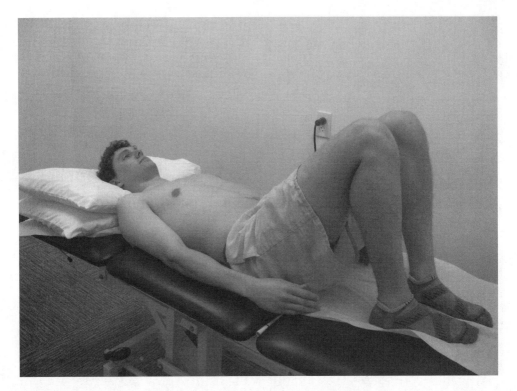

Figure 8–3 Transversus abdominus contractions. *Source:* Reprinted with permission from Jeffrey A. Rot.

versus abdominus muscle.[15,16] (Figure 8–3) Joe demonstrated difficulty performing isolated contraction of this muscle. His abdominal muscle strength was tested using the double leg lowering test (DLLT) described by Kendall.[17] This test was found to have excellent intratester reliability.[18] Abdominal strength was found to be fair (3/5).

11. Radiologic, other tests, and medical data

Imaging studies were negative.

12. Summary of examination findings

Summarizing examination findings is the 12th step in Paris' 14-step examination process. Examination findings were categorized into the impairments that were during the physical examination process. Refer to Table 8–2 for the list of identified impairments.

Table 8–2 Summary of Impairments

	Impairments
1.	Structural/posture = Decreased lumbar lordosis
2.	Decreased AROM = Forward bending limited 50% with pain Backward bending limited 50% with pain Right side bending limited 20% with pain Bilateral rotation limited 20%
3.	Muscle hypertonicity and tenderness: Right gluteus medius, right gluteus maximus, right quadratus lumborum, right piriformis, and right multifidus
4.	Hypomobility (stiffness) of the lumbar spine L1-2–L5-S1
5.	Right hip internal rotation limitation of 35° Right hip extension limitation 5°
6.	Hamstrings were tight bilaterally
7.	Muscle control deficit of transversus abdominus
8.	Abdominal weakness = Fair grade (Double leg lowering test)
9.	Oswestry Low Back Pain Questionnaire = 42% = Severe disability
10.	Poor body mechanics

Evaluation and Diagnosis

As mentioned previously, the Paris classification system categorizes patients into specific pathoanatomical syndromes determined from the impairments measured throughout the examination process. Within each syndrome there are several subcategories.[19] Based on the historical, subjective, and objective findings, a model-specific diagnosis of facet synovitis/restriction with hypertonic muscle guarding was developed. There are five subcategories for the facet syndrome in the Paris system. They include: 1) Facet synovitis/ hemarthrosis (acute sprain), 2) Facet stiffness/restrictions, 3) Facet painful entrapment, 4) Facet mechanical block, and 5) Chronic facet dysfunction. Joe initially experienced an acute facet sprain (facet hemarthrosis/synovitis), which had (2 weeks post injury) developed into facet restrictions that is limiting active range of motion in conjunction with hypertonic muscle guarding. The facet joints have been identified as a source of pain in a number of studies [20–24] and can refer to the buttock region.[20]

Acute synovitis or hemarthrosis is perhaps the most common source of acute LBP.[25,26] The signs and symptoms in the low back will be localized lumbar pain with minimal referred pain, perhaps to the iliac crest and buttock.[20] Changes in the myofascia will invariably accompany LBP, regardless of its origin.[19] Not all myofascial changes, particularly those relating to tone, require treatment, but always require consideration.[19] Actively loading the facet as in backward bending and bending to the same side may be painful at this stage, but may reduce with repetitive movements due to firing of mechanoreceptors located in the facet joint capsules.[27,28] Stimulation of mechanoreceptors may gate pain and inhibit muscle guarding of the surrounding musculature.[27,28] Repeated movements may also improve range of motion by stretching facet restrictions if present.

The negative sacroiliac provocation tests ruled out sacroiliac dysfunction.[13] In addition Laslett[14] found that no peripheralization or centralization of pain with repeated extension combined with three or more positive sacroiliac provocation tests was highly predictive of sacroiliac dysfunction. This was not the case with this patient. The lack of positive neural-tension and neurological signs ruled out disc dysfunction.

Prognosis

Joe's prognosis is good based on his age, stage of condition, level of tissue reactivity, multiple musculoskeletal impairments, and that he is a very motivated self-employed hard worker. Based on the examination, evaluation, and intervention strategy, Joe would be seen for a total of 10 physical therapy visits over a 6-week period of time. He would be seen three times a week for one week, two times a week for two weeks, one time a week for two weeks, and one follow up visit two weeks after the last visit. Patient outcome will be measured with the same assessment tools that were used to assess and measure the identified musculoskeletal impairments listed in Figure 8–3. Joe should achieve normal pain-free work functions within this six-week period of physical therapy. He would need to continue with a home exercise program that addressed his weak spinal musculature to decrease the likelihood of recurrent LBP.[29]

Intervention

The impairments and appropriate interventions are listed in Table 8–3.

The intervention strategy is to address all the impairments that were identified in the physical examination process. In Joe's case, the main interventions included myofascial manipulation and stretching, spinal manipulation, exercise, and education.[30-33] Treating the impairments is critical for achieving the most effective and efficient outcomes. The rationale for a particular intervention is based on the patient's stage of condition and the level

Table 8–3 Summary of Impairments and Associated Interventions

Impairments		Interventions
1.	Structural/postural findings: Decreased lumbar lordosis	Therapeutic exercise: Lumbar extension program
2.	Decreased AROM: Forward bending limited 50% with pain Backward bending limited 50% with pain Right side bending limited 20% with pain Bilateral rotation limited 20%	Manipulation to: Restore facet joint mobility and decrease pain Therapeutic exercise to restore restricted motions
3.	Muscle hypertonicity and tenderness: Right gluteus medius Right gluteus maximus Right quadratus lumborum Right piriformis Right multifidus	Myofascial manipulation to: Reduce tone and tenderness
4.	Hypomobility (stiffness) of the lumbar spine L1/2–L5/S1	Manipulation to restore facet mobility and segmental motion
5.	Right hip internal rotation Limitation of 30° Right hip extension limitation 0–5 degrees	Passive stretching to: Restore normal passive pain-free motion at the hip joint
6.	Tight hamstrings bilaterally	Myofascial stretching to restore normal length
7.	Muscle control deficit of: Transversus abdominus	Therapeutic exercise and stabilization Exercises to improve muscle control
8.	Abdominal weakness: Fair grade (Double leg lowering test)	Strengthening and stabilization exercises
9.	Oswestry Low Back Pain Questionnaire 42%: Severe disability	Education, functional training, and back school All the above interventions
10.	Poor body mechanics	Education, back school, and work hardening

of reactivity. These two factors will determine the dosage and duration of interventions. Joe was in the subacute (2 weeks post-injury) stage of condition and had moderate reactivity (pain with restriction), which allowed treatment to be focused on the source of pain (facet joints) and the associated sources of pain (myofascial). Myofascial impairments will be addressed with myofascial manipulation and stretching in order to decrease tone, tenderness, guarding, and pain. Specific myofascial manipulative techniques would include quadratus lumborum myofascial manipulation (Figure 8–4) and multifidus lamina release myofascial manipulation (Figure 8–5).

Spinal manipulation would be utilized to increase range of motion and decrease symptoms in the lumbar spine.[34] The specific grades of manipulation typically begin with mid-range movements and then progress to end-range movements stretching within the patient's tolerance (Figure 8–6). Range of motion loss is addressed with manipulation (spinal and myofascial) combined with exercise to maintain the manipulation effects and restore normal motion in the directions that were limited (extension, side bending, rotation, and flexion).

As range of motion and muscle length is restored the patient is gradually progressed on a stabilization program to restore muscle control and strength to the abdominals and lumbar multifidus (Figures 8–7, 8–8, 8–9, 8–10). The multifidus is targeted based on the evidence that it will atrophy in patients

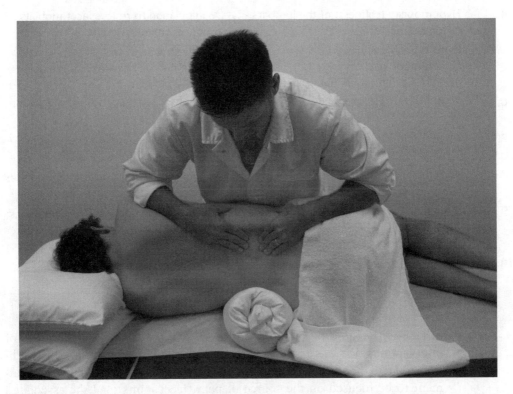

Figure 8–4 Quadratus lumborum myofascial manipulation. *Source:* Reprinted with permission from Jeffrey A. Rot.

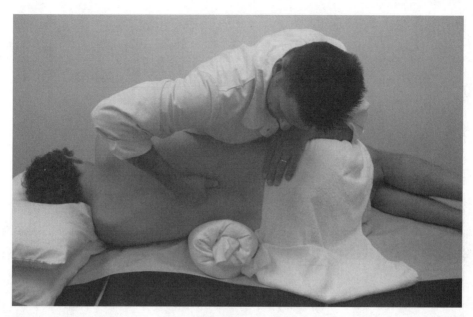

Figure 8–5 Multifidus lamina release myofascial manipulation. *Source:* Reprinted with permission from Jeffrey A. Rot.

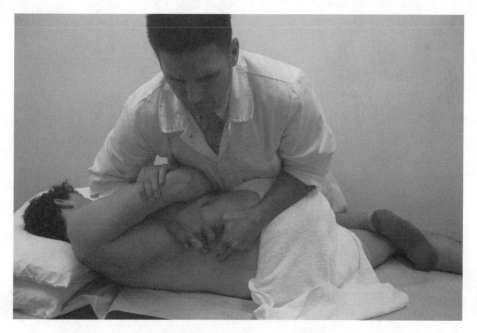

Figure 8–6 Lumbar end range manipulation. *Source:* Reprinted with permission from Jeffrey A. Rot.

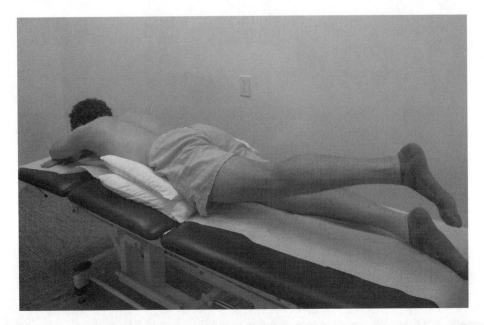

Figure 8–7 Multifidus exercise in prone. *Source:* Reprinted with permission from Jeffrey A. Rot.

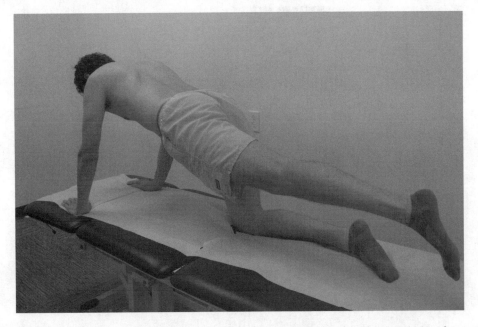

Figure 8–8 Multifidus exercise in quadruped. *Source:* Reprinted with permission from Jeffrey A. Rot.

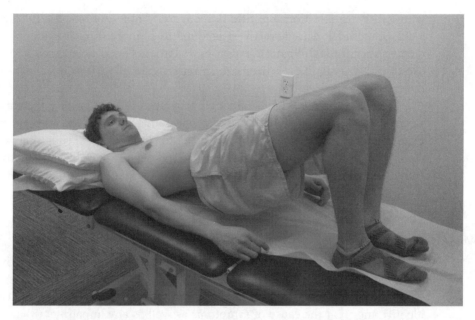

Figure 8–9 Bridging for back and hip extensors. *Source:* Reprinted with permission from Jeffrey A. Rot.

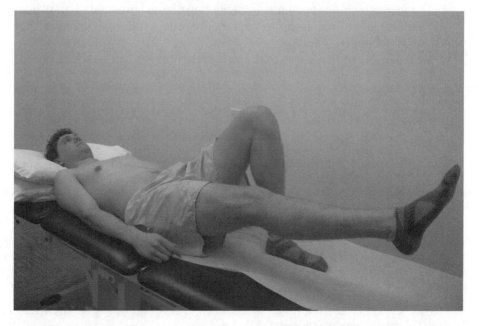

Figure 8–10 Single leg abdominal exercise. *Source:* Reprinted with permission from Jeffrey A. Rot.

with LBP.[35] In addition, multifidus recovery is not spontaneous following resolution of LBP. Muscle recovery is found to be more rapid in patients who receive specific stabilization exercises.[29] Patients who performed specific exercise had a significant decrease in recurrence of LBP at one, two, and three years follow-up.[29]

The final phase of the rehabilitation program would be to have the patient perform the functional activities that replicate his specific job requirements. Examples of the job-specific activities would include repeated squatting while maintaining neutral spine, lifting objects from the floor to a table, and reaching activities that replicate plumbing work. When the patient had demonstrated competence and safety with all work activities he would be discharged.

SUMMARY

The Paris approach is guided by 10 philosophical principles, with the over-arching belief that pain is a direct result of pathomechanics and tissue-specific impairments. As such, the goal of the approach is to systematically identify and treat the cause of symptoms as well as any impairment that may contribute to the symptoms. The approach utilizes a classification scheme that categorizes patients into specific pathoanatomical syndromes. Treatment strategies include spinal manipulation, myofascial manipulation, patient education, functional training and therapeutic exercise to restore mobility, strength and stability.

REFERENCES

1. Paris SV, Loubert PV. *Foundations of Clinical Orthopaedics.* 3rd ed. St. Augustine, FL, Institute Press; 1999.
2. Paris SV. *Introduction to Spinal Evaluation and Manipulation, Seminar Manual.* St. Augustine, FL: University of St. Augustine; 1999.
3. Ohnmeiss DD. Repeatability of pain drawings in a low back pain population. *Spine.* 2000; 25(8):980–988.
4. Williamson A, Hoggart B. Pain: A review of three commonly used pain rating scales. *Journal of Clinical Nursing.* 2005;14:798–804.
5. Melzack R. The McGill Pain Questionnaire: Major properties and scoring methods. *Pain.* 1975;1:277–299.
6. Fritz JM, Irrgang JJ. A comparison of a modified Oswestry Low Back Pain Disabilty Questionnaire and the Quebec Back Pain Disability Scale. *Physical Therapy.* 2001;81(2):776–778.
7. Pitkanen M, Manninen HZ, Linderen KA, et.al. Limited usefulness of traction-compression films in the radiographic diagnosis of lumbar spinal instability: Comparison with flexion-extension Films. *Spine.* 1997;22(2):193–197.
8. Gonella C, Paris SV, Kutner M. Reliability in evaluating passive intervertebral motion. *Physical Therapy.* 1982;62(4):436–444.

9. Insco EL, Witt PL, Gross MT, Mitchell RU. Reliability in evaluating intervertebral motion of the lumbar spine. *JMMT*. 1995;3:135–143.

10. Peter A. Huijbregts. Spinal motion palpation: A review of reliability studies. *The Journal of Manual & Manipulative Therapy*. 2002;10(1):24–39.

11. Fritz JM, Whitman JM, Childs JD. Lumbar spine segmental mobility assessment: An examination of the validity for determining intervention strategies in patients with low back pain. *Archives of Physical Medicine and Rehabilitation*. 2005;86(9):1745–1752.

12. Broadhurst NA, Bond MJ. Pain provocation tests for the assessment of sacroiliac dysfunction. *Journal of Spinal Disorders*. 1998;11:341–345.

13. Freberger JA, Riddle DA. Using published evidence to guide the examination of the sacroiliac joint region. *Physical Therapy*. 2001;81(5):1135–1143.

14. Laslett M, Williams M. The reliability of selected pain provocation tests for SI pathology. *Spine*. 1994;19(11):1243–1249.

15. Richardson CA, Jull GA. Muscle control-pain control. What exercises would you prescribe? *Manual Therapy*. 1995;1:2–10.

16. Richardson CA, Snijders CJ, Hides JA, Damen L, Pas MS, Storm J. The relation between the transversus abdominis muscles, sacroiliac joint mechanics, and low back pain. *Spine*. 2002;27:399–405.

17. Krause DA, Youdas JW, Hollman JH, Smith J. Abdominal muscle performance as measured by the double leg lowering test. *Arch Phys Med Rehabil*. 2005;86:1345–1348.

18. Youdas JW, Garrett TR, Egan KS, Therneau TM. Lumbar lordosis and pelvic inclination in adults with chronic low back pain. *Physical Therapy*. 2000; 80(3):261–275.

19. Paris SV, Viti J. Differential diagnosis. In: Vleming A, Mooney V, Stoeckart. Churchill Livingstone, eds. *Movement, Stability, and Lumbo Pelvic Pain: Integration of Research and Therapy*. 2nd ed. New York: Elsevier; 2007:381–390.

20. Mooney V, Robertson J. The Facet syndrome. *Clin. Orthop*. 1976; 115:149–156.

21. Datta S, Lee M, Falco F, Bryce D. Systemic assessment of diagnostic accuracy and therapeutic utility of lumbar facet joint interventions. *Pain Physician*. 2009;12:437–460.

22. Cohen SP, Raja SN. Pathogenesis, diagnosis, and treatment of lumbar zygapophysial (facet) joint pain. *Anesthesiology*. 2007;106:591–614.

23. Binder DS, Nampiaparampil DE. The provocative lumbar facet joint. *Curr Rev Musculoskeletal Med*. 2009;2(1):15–24.

24. Rihn JA, Lee JY, Khan M, et al. Does lumbar facet fluid detected on magnetic resonance imaging correlate with radiographic instability in patients with degenerative lumbar disease? *Spine*. 2007;32(14):1555–1560.

25. Manchikanti L, Boswell MV, Singh V, Pampati V, Damron KS, Beyer CD. Prevalence of facet joint pain in chronic spinal pain of cervical, thoracic, and lumbar regions. *BMC Musculoskeletal Disorder*. 2004;5:15.

26. Manchikanti R, Pampati V, Manchikanti L. Facet joint pain in chronic spinal pain: an evaluation of prevalence and false-positive rate of diagnostic blocks. *J Spinal Disord Tech*. 2007;20:539–545.

27. Wyke B. The neurology of joints: a review of general principles. *Clinics in Rheumatic Diseases*. 1981;7(1):223–239.

28. Wyke B. Articular neurology—a review. *Physiotherapy*. 1972;58:94–99.

29. Hides JA, Jull GA, Richardson CA. Long term effects of specific stabilizing exercise for first-episode low back pain. *Spine*. 2001;26(11):E243–248.

30. Agency for Health Care Policy and Research (AHCPR). *Clinical Practice Guideline: Number 14, Acute Low Back Problems in Adults*. Washington D.C.: U.S. Department of Health and Human Services Public Health Service; 1994:95–0642.

31. Engers AJ, Jellema P, Wensing M, van der Windt DAWM, Grol R, van Tulder MW. Individual patient education for low back pain. *Cochrane Database Syst Rev*. 2008;(1).

32. Treweek SP, Glenton C, Oxman AD, Penrose A. Computer-generated patient education materials: Do they affect professional practice? A systematic review. *J Am Med Inform.* 2002;9:346–358.

33. Ullrich PF, Vaccaro AR. Patient education on the Internet: opportunities and pitfalls. *Spine.* 2002;27:E185–E188.

34. Bronfort G, Haas M, Evans RL, Boulter LM. Efficacy of spinal manipulation and mobilization for low back pain and neck pain: A systematic review and best evidence synthesis. *The Spine Journal.* 2004;4:335–356.

35. Hides JA, Richardson CA, Jull GA. Multifidus muscle recovery is not automatic after resolution of acute, first episode low back pain. *Spine.* 1996;21(23):2763–2769.

Blank Paris Assessment

Source: Reprinted with permission from Stanley V. Paris.

SPINE EVALUATION Date: _____/ _____/20 ____

Mr/Mrs/Miss/Ms: _____

Age: _____ Dr.: _____

Diagnosis: _____

Medical Orders: _____

_____

• **SUBJECTIVE/Complaint:** _____

_____

_____

How sustained: _____   (Photocopy I.D.)

_____ Date of Onset ____/ ____/ 20___, n.a. _____

Occupation/Activities: _____

Medical History: not significant _____, _____

Medical Tests and Results: n.a. _____, _____

• **OBJECTIVE/Findings:**

Structure,	not significant____,	see page 3 _____	•
Active Mvts. (ROM)	not significant____,	see page 3 _____	•
Neurovascular	not significant____,	see page 3 & 4 _____	•
U. and L. Quarter	not significant____,	see page 4 _____	•
Palpation Findings	not significant____,	see page 5 _____	•

EVALUATION/IMPAIRMENTS   **INTERVENTIONS**

  STG = Short Term Goals   LTG = Long Term Goals

1. _____ /   _____
   STG: _____ /   LTG: _____
2. _____ /   _____
   STG: _____ /   LTG: _____
3. _____ /   _____
   STG: _____ /   LTG: _____
4. _____ /   _____
   STG: _____ /   LTG: _____
5. _____ /   _____
   STG: _____ /   LTG: _____
6. _____ /   _____
   STG: _____ /   LTG: _____

Education to Receive: Back School ____, Neck School _____, Other _____

Present Stage: Immediate ____, Acute ____, Sub Acute ____, Settled _____, Chronic _____,

Other _____

Impression: Facet ____, Muscle ____, Ligament ____, Disc ____, Stenosis ____, Spondylogenic____,
Neurogenic____, Other: _____

Frequency: _____ Duration: _____

PROGNOSIS: _____ **PHYSICAL THERAPIST SIG.:** _____

1. **PAIN QUESTIONNAIRE and BODY CHART**: completed _____, n.a. _____
2. **INITIAL OBSERVATION**: ambulatory _____ bedridden _____
   Gait: normal _____, guarded _____, leg problem _____
   Comments: _____
   Resting position: sitting chair _____, stool _____, table _____, other _____
   Behavior, if any: acute facet _____, acute disc _____, ligamentous_____, other _____

3. **HISTORY and INTERVIEW**
   Present History
   1. Where precisely did the pain start (draw it in with an "X")
   2. Where did it spread to (draw it in): _____
   3. Where is it now / currently / today: _____
   _____
   4. What makes it hurt worse: _____
   _____
   _____
   5. Does it hurt at night: yes _____, no _____,
      5b. If yes, can the pain be affected by a change in position or
         activity of any kind: yes _____, no _____
   6. What its like first thing <u>in the morning</u>: better____, stiff ____, sore ____,
   7. What its like by <u>mid-day</u>: same _____, better _____, worse _____,
   8. What its like by <u>late afternoon</u>: same ____, better _____, worse _____,
   9. What its like <u>in the evening</u>: same _____, better _____, worse _____,
   10. Pain Level 0-10: at best _____, worst _____, present _____
   11. What have you learned that makes your back better: _____
   _____

   Neurological
   12. Do you have any tingling, numbness or loss of skin sensation: no _____, yes _____, if yes, where _____
   13. Do you have any altered sensation, pain / numbness in the S4 region: no____, yes____, explain_____
   14. Do you experience any dizziness with change in neck positions? _____
   15. What treatments have you had: none_____, or_____
         Did they help: yes_____, no_____, other _____
   16. Presently, are you getting better_____, worse_____, or staying much the same_____,
   Previous History
   17. Have you had anything similar before: yes_____, no_____, if yes, describe _____
   _____
      If yes, are they increasing in **frequency**: yes_____, no_____, **severity**: yes_____, no_____,
   Miscellaneous
   18. Are you taking any medications: yes_____, no_____, if yes, describe _____
   19. When do you see your physician next: _____
   Behavioral
   20. What concerns you most: your pain_____, or restriction of activities_____, both_____, n.a._____,
   21. What are your goals in coming to me: n.a._____, (*define some goals starting with functional goals*) n.a._____,
   _____
   22. Now, is there anything else you would like to tell me before I examine your back / neck: no____
   _____

STRUCTURAL EXAMINATION n.a. _____, bed ridden _____, other _____

Patient is Typically   Comments: _____

   endomorph _____   _____

   mesomorph _____   _____

   intermediate _____   _____

   ectomorph _____   _____

Pelvis   _____

   neutral   _____   _____

   Ant. tilt   _____   _____

   Post. tilt _____   _____

   R side down _____   _____

   L side down _____

Head Position and Bearing: good _____, forward head _____, suspect S/C fault _____, _____

5. **ACTIVE MOVEMENTS**   n.a. _____, too acute _____, other

Key	Range of motion	I
	Location of block	II
	Limited by pain	X

Area _____ _____ _____

Comments: _____

6. NEUROVASCULAR ASSESSMENT unnecessary _____ , other _____

Key
0 = no contraction
1 = trace
2 = poor
3 = fair
4 = good
5 = normal

Lower Quarter

Muscle	Left	Right
L1, 2 Psoas		
L3 Quads		
L4 Tib Ant		
L5 E.H.L.		
S1 F.H.L.		
S2 Hams		

Reflexes
0 = absent
1+ = diminished
2+ = normal
3+ = increased
4+ = clonus

Reflexes	Left	Right
Knee Jerk		
S1 Ankle Jerk		
Babinski		
Clonus		

Reflexes
0=absent
1+=diminished
2+=normal
3+=increased
4+=clonus

Upper Quarter

	Left	Right
C1-2 apr chin in		
C1-2 ppr chin up		
C3 lat. nk. press		
C4 upper trapezius		
C5 biceps		
C6 wrist ext.		
C7 triceps		
C8 thumb extensors		
T1 intrinsics		

	Left	Right
C5-6 biceps		
C5-6 brachio-radialis		
C7 triceps		

Sensation   not tested _____, area tested _____, findings _____

Lumbar - additional tests performed _____,

   SLR tested _____, L_____ R_____

                cm_____ _____

   Passive Kernig: tested_____, normal____, limited____, _____

   Compression/distraction and quadrant: tested ____,normal____, positive____, _____

Cervical - additional tests performed ____,

   Compression/distraction and quadrant: tested____, normal____, positive____, _____

7. UPPER AND/OR LOWER QUARTER ASSESSMENT n.a _____,

   Upper Quarter,   performed _____, normal _____, n.a._____, _____

   Shoulder

    Left: limited____, painful____, capsular____, non-capsular____, _____

    Right: limited____, painful____, capsular____, non-capsular____, _____

   Craniomandibular

    Left: limited____, painful____, capsular____, non-capsular____, _____

    Right: limited____, painful____, capsular____, non-capsular____, _____

   Thoracic outlet findings: none____, comments, _____

Lower Quarter: performed ____, normal____, n.a. ____,

   Hip (*Faber, Thomas, Hip Joint Distraction*)

    Left: limited____, painful____, capsular____, non-capsular____, _____

    Right: limited____, painful____, capsular____, non-capsular____, _____

Sacroiliac: examined____, nothing significant____, n.a.____,

Test: ASIS compression,   positive left____, right____, comments _____

      ASIS gap,   positive left____, right____, comments_____

      Anterior torsion,   positive left____, right____, comments_____

      Post torsion   positive left____, right____, comments_____

      Post. Gap/Shear painful positive left____, right____, comments_____

      Post. Gap/Shear limited positive left____, right____, comments_____

      Faber Test,   positive left____, right____, explain:_____

      Supine to Sit Test,   positive _____, negative _____

Other sacroiliac tests/comments: _____

_____

_____

_____

_____

_____

PALPATION:

CONDITION   n.a._____,

9. POSITION   n.a._____,

10. MOBILITY   n.a._____,

Segment	FB	SBL	SBR	RL	RR	Other

Key:

X   Tender

⊗   Center Pain

⇌   Spasm

////   Guarding

↕   Reflex Contr.

Key:

0 - Ankylosed

1 - Considerable Restriction

2 - Slight Restriction

3 - Normal

4 - Slight Increase

5 - Considerable Increase

6 - Unstable

11. RADIOLOGIC AND OTHER MEDICAL DATA

Radiographs have been taken_____, reports are to hand_____,

Findings to relate _____

_____

Other medical data: _____

_____

_____

_____

PROGRESS, REASSESSMENT, AND TREATMENT NOTES:

_____

_____

_____

_____

_____

_____

_____

_____

_____

_____

_____

_____

_____

NAME: _____

Where is your pain?
Please mark on the drawings below the areas where you feel your pain.

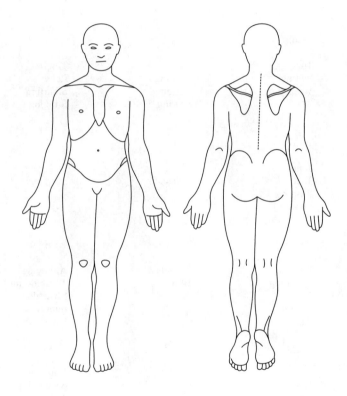

This we have already presented under Neuroanatomy, Pain, and Pain Management in the FCO seminar.

Here are many words that describe pain. Some of these are grouped below. Check (✓) any words that describe the pain you have these days.

1.	2.	3.	4.
Flickering	Jumping	Pricking	Sharp
Quivering	Flashing	Boring	Cutting
Pulsing	Shooting	Drilling	Lacerating
Throbbing		Stabbing	
Beating			
Pounding			

5.	6.	7.	8.
Pinching	Tugging	Hot	Tingling
Pressing	Pulling	Burning	Itchy
Gnawing	Wrenching	Scalding	Smarting
Cramping		Searing	Stinging
Crushing			

9.	10.	11.	12.
Dull	Tender	Tiring	Sickening
Sore	Taut	Exhausting	Suffocating
Hurting	Rasping		
Aching	Splitting		
Heavy			

13.	14.	15.	16.
Fearful	Punishing	Wretched	Annoying
Frightful	Gruelling	Blinding	Troublesome
Terrifying	Cruel		Miserable
	Vicious		Intense
	Killing		Unbearable

17.	18.	19.	20.
Spreading	Tight	Cool	Nagging
Radiating	Numb	Cold	Nauseating
Penetrating	Drawing	Freezing	Agonizing
Piercing	Squeezing		Dreadful
	Tearing		Torturing

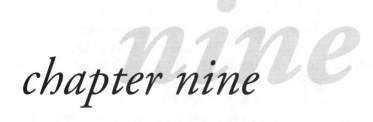

chapter nine

The Osteopathic Approach

Maria Meigel, PT, DPT, CFMT, OCS

Osteopathy is a medical practice that is based in the principles of Dr. Andrew Taylor Still. In the late 1800s, Still developed a medical model that incorporated not only pharmaceuticals and traditional medicine, but also manual techniques that drew on the body's innate ability to heal itself. The foundation of osteopathy is manipulative therapy that incorporates a number of unique techniques including muscle energy techniques, myofascial release, craniosacral therapy, strain-counterstrain, visceral manipulation, and a number of other manual approaches.

For the student interested in advanced training in these approaches we recommend looking into the continuing education courses offered through the Michigan State University College of Osteopathic Medicine http://www.com.msu.edu/cme/index.html or courses from the group Integrative Manual Therapy Solutions http://www.imtsglobal. com/index.jsp.

BACKGROUND

The osteopathic approach to treatment of lumbar spine disorders is widely accepted as a valid approach to the treatment of somatic dysfunction.[1–4] Greenman[2] defines somatic dysfunction as "impaired or altered function of related components of the body framework system; skeletal, arthrodial, and myofascial structures and related vascular lymphatic and neural elements." Not exactly synonymous with, but taken from a term coined in 1874 by Andrew Taylor Still, the father of osteopathic medicine, somatic dysfunction has recently superseded the term osteopathic lesion in accord with the World Health Organization International Classification of Diseases. Osteopathic lesion was the first term that described the possibility that dysfunction in the musculoskeletal system could occur without the presence of disease.[3,5] This idea was revolutionary and it took many years for the medical profession to accept that it is possible to have altered function in the spine or peripheral joints and that, in fact, these dysfunctions could be treated successfully with manual techniques.[2,3,5–7]

Structure Governs Function[2]

Osteopathic philosophy espouses the interrelationship between structure and function. The dictate of this philosophy is the oft-stated "structure dictates function." Andrew Taylor (A.T.) Still believed that structure governed function and function influenced structure. Integral to this thought is the use of manual therapy, an approach that addresses the structure to restore the body's maximal functional capacity to enhance the level of wellness and assist in recovery from injury and disease.

Some osteopathic schools of thought still describe structural dysfunctions by their position of fixation or the altered positional relations while others focus on the inability of a dysfunctional segment to move in certain directions.[2] A dysfunction or lesion may be classified as primary or secondary. A primary dysfunction can be due to trauma, either a single incident or a series of microtraumas that occur over time. A secondary dysfunction is a compensatory or response-driven lesion. Oftentimes there is a primary lesion at one or more sites with a palpable dysfunction elsewhere that has been dependent on the primary for its production.

Although asymmetry is the rule when dealing with the human structure,[3,8] asymmetry that is dysfunctional is significant as it is considered in the osteopathic approach to be a source of symptoms or a stressor. It is important when assessing a patient for somatic dysfunction that both position (asymmetry) and motion (range of motion/mobility) dysfunctions are addressed. Additionally, as manual therapists, it is important to discern the limiting factor (quality of motion/end-feel; what is limiting the motion) and the quantity of motion that has been lost. This is completed through the extensive clinical exam that is described following the mnemonic ART or Asymmetry, Range of motion, and Tissue tension abnormalities.

Traditional Osteopathic Examination

"A" in the mnemonic stands for the asymmetry of related parts of the musculoskeletal system, either structural or functional. This is usually discerned by observation and palpation. Grossly, a patient's posture is assessed from the front, back, and sides, evaluating alignment, weight-bearing status, and pelvis and shoulder height in relation to plumb line position. In the lumbar spine and pelvic girdle, specific bony landmarks palpated bilaterally for symmetry include the spinal transverse processes, iliac crests, posterior superior iliac spine, anterior superior iliac spine, pubic rami, ischial tuberosities, sacral bases, and inferior lateral angles (ILAs). The goal of palpation is to discern if positional dysfunction is present.

"R" in the mnemonic represents the range of motion (ROM) abnormalities indicated by alteration in range of motion of a singular joint or region of the musculoskeletal system. Restricted motion is the most common component of somatic dysfunction, but other abnormal range findings that include hypomobility, or hypermobility can also be classified as motion dysfunction. When assessing ROM abnormalities, the therapist should evaluate both anatomic and physiologic limitations and determine the quality and quantity of motion lost (or hypermobility). The therapist should ascertain if there is a major or minor motion loss. Traditionally, in the osteopathic evaluation, if greater than 50% of the motion has been lost, it is described as a major motion loss and would be seen also as a positional dysfunction (appearing in the neutral position). Likewise, if less than 50% of the motion has been lost, the motion dysfunction is considered minor. Jeffrey Ellis, PT, MTC, FFCFMT, a therapist who studied at Michigan State and taught the osteopathic approach to many physical therapists, also identified the importance of noting an end range motion loss, which is defined as loss of the last 10% of range.[9]

CONTRACTION: guarded, hypertonic, muscular
COHESION/CONGESTION: boggy, sticky, congested
CONTRACTURE: fibrotic, stiff, capsular

Once the motion dysfunction is identified, the therapist must note what the "barrier" is to this motion. These barriers (end-feels) have been described extensively in the orthopedic physical therapy literature and may include descriptions such as empty (painful), muscular, capsular, and joint (bony).[10] The relevant end-feels are outlined in the box and are important as a guide to the choice of intervention in the osteopathic approach.

"T" is the final letter of the mnemonic and it is used to prompt the therapist to examine for tissue tension abnormalities. Alteration in the characteristics of the soft tissue of the musculoskeletal system (skin, fascia, muscle, ligament, and even neural) is ascertained by observation and palpation. When evaluating the soft tissues related to somatic dysfunction, it is imperative to address tissue tone, texture, extensibility, and mobility. Mobility should include muscle play, deformation, and length. Tonal abnormalities should include decreased or increased tone, tenderness, and trigger points. The muscle should be able to move both perpendicular to the underlying tissues and parallel; lengthening and shortening efficiently as well.

Somatic dysfunction includes all the elements of the musculoskeletal system—this includes the nervous system. The therapist should not forget about the tunnels that neural tissue passes through in the pelvis and lower quadrant and syndromes that may arise. These include lumbosacral tunnel syndrome, gluteal nerve syndrome, iliacus muscle syndrome, obturator tunnel syndrome, piriformis muscle syndrome, and myralgia parasthetica. These syndromes result from tunnels where peripheral nerves could be entrapped, causing peripheral neural symptoms that may mimic radiculopathy.[11]

In the late 1980s, Ellis added three headings to the traditional osteopathic examination paradigm.[9] These criteria are, in today's physical therapy world, imperative, and will help to identify red flags where needed and guide treatment. These are "C," "H," and "S," which stand for Chief complaint, History, and Special tests. This addition creates a new examination mnemonic of "CHARTS."

The "C" for chief complaint is the first thing assessed during a patient examination. The therapist needs to assess the reason the patient is seeking treatment. After getting the patient's subjective complaint, the therapist then needs to decide if the complaint is consistent with a musculoskeletal/somatic dysfunction, or if it could be a radicular, viscerogenic, neurogenic, or psychogenic dysfunction. The therapist must also rule out an organic cause for this patient's complaint; that is, one that does not fall under the physical therapy plan of care. Additionally, the therapist needs to ascertain if the nature of the chief complaint is sharp, shooting, and electric in a distinct dermatomal pattern above the knee or into the calf, or if it is a diffuse, aching, extrasegmental pain somewhere into the buttock and posterior thigh. These qualities aid in distinguishing somatic from radicular pain (Table 9–1). A patient who is losing weight rapidly, having night sweats and unrelenting pain is relating a definite set of red flag symptoms that need to be referred out to the appropriate medical professional.[12] Likewise, a patient who is having no pain but

Table 9–1 Comparison of Somatic and Radicular Dysfunction

Somatic vs. Radicular Dysfunction	
Somatic	*Radicular*
Deep, dull aching	Sharp, shooting, radiating
Extrasegmental representation with no myotomal, dermotomal pattern	Dematomal, myotomal correlation
Reflexes intact	Diminished reflexes
Negative nerve root tension signs	Positive nerve root tension signs
Objective somatic findings	Positive radiologic findings of dysfunction

feels progressively weaker in the lower extremity is also exhibiting a red flag type condition (Exhibit 9–1). These types of complaints are all important clues to our clinical diagnosis of the patient.

The "H" for history helps to determine many aspects of the patient's dysfunction. For instance, when considering family history there are many genetic and familial dysfunctions that are common in the lumbar spine and pelvis, including rheumatologic conditions such as ankylosing spondylitis. Medical/surgical history is important as an abdominal surgery or lower

Exhibit 9–1 Red Flag Signs and Symptoms. *Source:* Greenhalgh S, Selfe J. *Red Flags: A Guide to Identifying Serious Pathology of the Spine.* Philadelphia, PA: Elsevier Churchill Livingstone, 2006.

Red flags for the lumbar spine and pelvis from the history[12]
Cancer, Tuberculosis, HIV/AIDS
Smoking
Cauda equina syndrome
Systematically unwell, trauma, bilateral pins and needles, previous failed treatment
Constant progressive abdominal pain with changed bowel
Severe night pain with disturbed sleep
Age < 10
Age > 51
Weight loss within 3–6 month period < 5%

extremity injury will disrupt the muscle and fascial balance of the kinetic chain and trunk. Pharmacologic history can confirm if the patient is taking anti-inflammatories and if so, if they are working. If not, perhaps the dysfunction is not inflammatory in nature, but is a mechanical compression that will not respond to anti-inflammatory medication. The therapist should find out if there is a history of long-term steroidal use that could weaken the connective tissue.

Finally, the addition to the mnemonic of the letter "S" is for the addition of a series of special tests (Table 9–2). These include medical testing such as lab values or radiologic examination, as well as an array of clinical tests that are typical of the osteopathic approach. In the lumbar spine and pelvis these include gait observation, forward bend test, Gillet test, seated flexion test, and sit slump. To confirm that the sacroiliac joint (SIJ) is a component of back pain, provocation tests that may be used include FABER, pelvic compression and distraction testing, the thigh thrust, Gaenslen's test, and the sacral thrust.[7,13] Recent studies indicate the importance of provocation tests in the pelvic girdle and more importantly, clustering of sacroiliac joint testing to improve the specificity and sensitivity of the clinical findings.[7,14–19]

Lumbar Spine Motion/Dysfunction Classification

Traditional osteopathy relies on an understanding of Fryette's Laws of spinal motion to define spinal dysfunction. These are a set of three laws that define how the spinal segments move. Law one states that in the neutral spine, side bending and rotation occur in opposite directions. The neutral spine is defined as the spine that is neither flexed nor extended, this would be observed by the therapist during a standing posture examination. Law two stipulates that once the facets have been engaged and are out of neutral (opened or closed/flexed or extended), then side bending and rotation occur in the same direction.

Table 9–2 Osteopathic Approach Special Tests for Lumbar Spine and Pelvic Girdle Dysfunction

Tests that Detect Movement or Position	Provocation Tests
Standing forward bend	FABER
Gillet test	Gaenslen's test
Seated flexion test	Thigh thrust
Sit slump test	Sacral thrust
Sacral spring	Compression/distraction

Lastly, law three clarifies that once motion is introduced in one plane, motion in all other planes is reduced.[3] These laws, while dictating much osteopathic manipulative effort, have been challenged by some biomechanical research. There is controversy about the true nature of the coupling patterns of motion in the spine, and this continues to be a topic of heated discussion.[9,20] Nonetheless, Fryette's Laws create a consistency in osteopathic thought in describing the ways a facet joint may become dysfunctional. For an overview of osteopathic defined facet dysfunctions based on Fryette's Laws, the reader is directed to Table 9–3. Generally, a facet joint in dysfunction will become stuck, opened (restricted closing), closed (restricted opening), or both. If the facet becomes unable to open, it is considered stuck closed or extended side bent and rotated toward that side. This, in traditional osteopathic terms, is called an ERS (extended, rotated, and side bent) dysfunction. The motion limitation is to flexion, side bending, and rotation away from the dysfunctional facet. Likewise, if the facet gets limited in its ability to close, it is unable to extend or is stuck flexed. This is sometimes called an FRS (flexed, rotated, and side bent)

Table 9–3 Vertebral Motion Dysfunction: Pelvic Girdle Motion Dysfunction Classification

Dysfunctions at a Single Vertebral Level/Single Facet (Type II)		*Physical Exam*
Extended, rotated, and side bent right (ERSR)	Unable to flex rotate and side bend to the left	Found when the patient forward bends by palpating a prominent transverse process on one side indicating dysfunction and inability to move symmetrically
Extended, rotated, and side bent left (ERSL)	Unable to flex, rotate and side bend to the right	
Flexed, rotated, and side bent right (FRSR)	Unable to extend rotate and side bend to the left	Found when the patient backward bends by palpating a prominent transverse process on one side indicating dysfunction and inability to move symmetrically
Flexed, rotated, and side bent left (FRSL)	Unable to extend, rotate and side bend to the right	

Dysfunctions of Multiple (3 or More) Vertebrae (Type I)	*Physical Exam*
Neutral, rotated right side, bent left (NRRSL)	Found during the neutral standing postural exam
Neutral, rotated left side, bent right (NRLSR)	

dysfunction and the limitation is to extension, side bending, and rotation toward the dysfunctional facet.[21,22]

The sacrum moves within the innominates at the sacroiliac joint, around three distinct axes; the transverse axis, the left oblique axis, and the right oblique axis. The motion that occurs about the transverse axis is flexion or extension, also known as nutation and counternutation. The oblique axes are named for the side of the sacral base from which they originate. Since the axis itself can't move, the base on the opposite side will rotate about the axis. Therefore the right base will rotate about the left oblique axis and the left base will rotate about the right oblique axis. The base is capable of rotating forward or backward, which may be seen as left or right rotation. The sacral motion characteristics are listed in Exhibit 9–2.[2,22]

Like all other parts of the body, sacral motion is normal motion that exists, and is driven by lumbar spine motion, breathing, and gait. If this normal motion becomes restricted, we name it by the position in which it is stuck. If the sacrum is unable to rotate right, we name it a rotated (torsioned) left sacrum. If the sacrum is unable to flex, we name it an extended sacrum. If the sacrum cannot move backward we call it a forward sacrum.

On the other side of the sacroiliac joint are the innominates, which move at the sacroiliac joint about the axis of the pubic symphysis. The innominates can rotate anterior or posterior. Additionally, the pubic symphysis moves by sheering upward and downward, mostly with weight-bearing activities.

The evaluation of the sacroiliac joint is controversial in that there is no real gold standard for dysfunction. While recent studies suggest that clustering of provocation tests improves the sensitivity and specificity of our findings considerably,[15–19] the traditional position/motion tests for the sacrum and innominate are necessary in the osteopathic approach for categorizing the patient's dysfunction and will be discussed later in the examination.

Exhibit 9–2 Sacral motion

Sacral Motion Characteristics
Nutation: Flexion about a transverse axis
Counternutation: Extension about a transverse axis
R/L backward sacral torsion: Right rotation on a left oblique axis, sacrum rotates backward
L/R backward sacral torsion: Left rotation on a right oblique axis, sacrum rotates backward
R/R forward sacral torsion: Right rotation on a right oblique axis, sacrum rotates forward
L/L Forward Sacral Torsion: Left rotation on a left oblique axis, sacrum rotates forward

---

Traditional Osteopathic Treatment Modalities

Once an accurate diagnosis of somatic dysfunction is obtained (including location of dysfunction, nature, and type), specific manual medicine therapeutic intervention is indicated. The goal of manipulation as defined by Greenman is the "use of the hands in a patient-management process using instructions and maneuvers to achieve maximal, painless movement of the musculoskeletal system in postural balance."[2] Many different manual therapy procedures are used in the osteopathic arsenal. They are, in traditional osteopathy, classified as soft tissue procedures, articular procedures, and specific joint mobilization. The specific joint mobilization category includes direct technique; exaggeration, indirect, and combined methods; and physiological response method. In addition, in conjunction with any of these procedures, activating forces can be used, including springing, thrust, gravity, respiration, and muscle energy. In more current terminology, these procedures are placed into three main groupings 1) rhythmic techniques, 2) thrust techniques, and 3) low velocity stress techniques.

It is important to note that all osteopathic techniques are typically mixed together and used according to the response from the tissues and structures being worked.[6] This approach to the use of the techniques requires a continuous cycle of palpatory examination of tissue and bony position, reevaluation, and change of treatment technique in response to the changes noted in the patient. The rhythmic techniques are used very effectively alone for treatment or as a preparatory treatment for a low velocity or thrust technique. Rhythmic techniques include kneading, stretching, articulation, effleurage, inhibition, springing, traction, and vibration. Thrust technique provides an application of force using high velocity, low amplitude movement. Low velocity stress techniques encompass techniques such as muscle energy technique, functional technique, strain-counterstrain technique, myofascial technique, harmonic technique, specific adjusting technique, gentle therapeutic manipulation, neuromuscular technique, and craniosacral technique.

APPLICATION OF THE OSTEOPATHIC APPROACH TO JOE LORES

Examination/Evaluation

The results of the additional tests and measures needed for the osteopathic approach examination are found in Table 9–4 organized according to the CHARTS mnemonic.

Table 9–4 Additional Examination Data for the Osteopathic Approach

Element from the Examination	Additional Tests/ Measures and Results	Results
Chief complaint	Is pain worse on waking in the AM?	No pain; not worse in the morning; the pain is at its lowest, rated 2 on a visual analog scale (VAS) but he feels stiff
	Does patient use shoe inserts/orthotics or any lumbar orthoses/supports? If so, please clarify if uses with work-related activities.	No
History	Results of X-ray and any other imaging	Mild degenerative changes at L5–S1; no evidence of fracture
Asymmetry and symmetry	Check alignment of the ankle/feet	Neutral subtalar joint position, feet are toed outward (4 toes visible when you look at him from behind)
	Assess for presence of leg length discrepancy	Not a true leg length difference, but an apparent Shortened left leg
	Assess for presence of side bending (scoliotic) curve in spine and compensatory curve	His "fullness" on the right is present in a neutral position, but diminishes in flexion or extension, suggesting that he does have a neutral dysfunction with a compensatory curve above
	Prone: side-to-side comparison of PSIS, sacral sulcus, infero-lateral angle (ILA)	PSIS even Right sacral sulcus is deeper Left ILA is more posterior and inferior
	Supine: side-to-side comparison of ASIS, medial malleolus, pubic tubercle	ASIS even Short left medial malleolus Pubic tubercle is even
	Tender points or trigger points bilateral Lumbosacral region and tenderness of either sacroiliac joint, piriformis muscles, gluteus medius muscles, quadratus lumborum	Sacrotuberous ligament is tender Trigger point palpation of the gluteus medius (TrP2) produced tenderness, referred pain into the right buttock with a local twitch response Trigger point palpation of the piriformis (TrP1) produced tenderness, referred pain into the right buttock with a local twitch response Trigger point palpation of the quadratus lumborum (both deep TP) produced tenderness, referred pain into the right buttock with a local twitch response

(continued)

Table 9–4 Additional Examination Data for the Osteopathic Approach (continued)

Element from the Examination	Additional Tests/ Measures and Results	Results
Range of motion	Segmental motion (PROM) of the lumbosacral spine	He is hypomobile at L4 and L5 on the R via accessory mobility testing In extension (sphinx position), L5 appears rotated right (the right transverse process is prominent); it is not apparent in the flexed position
	Pain with gross active oblique extension bilaterally?	Symptoms reproduced with active oblique extension to the right Mild discomfort on active oblique extension to the left
	PROM bilateral hips (flexion, extension, internal rotation, external rotation)	Flexion: Right = 0–130°/Left = 0–130° Extension: Right = 0–5°/Left= 0–10° IR (measured prone): Right = 0–35°/ Left = 0–40° ER(measured prone): Right = 0–50°/ Left = 0–50°
Tissue tension	Myofascial restrictions (PROM) of the lumbosacral region	Present; increased muscle tension was noted on the right, and banding was palpated from L3–S1 on the right.
Special tests	Standing flexion test	Negative
	Seated flexion test	Positive on left
	Sacral spring test	Positive
	Sphinx test	Right sulcus deepens further
	Bilateral straight leg raise (SLR)	Negative
	Pain of the inguinal regions or low back with FABER testing bilaterally	Negative
	Gaenslen's test bilaterally	Negative
	Extensibility of bilateral hip flexors and hamstrings	Thomas test: Slightly restricted on the right Hamstrings tested supine with hip flexed at 90°with passive extension of knee: Bilaterally symmetrically restricted

C: *This patient complained of pain in his low back that started 2 weeks ago. This pain was sudden in onset and is described as an aching over the right posterior lumbar spine to crest.* Because of the nature of his pain (aching), one might conclude that the problem is somatic in nature and not radicular. Radicular pain would be sharper and he would experience shooting pain, numbness, and weakness. Joe's pain is worsened with sitting, bending, getting up from sitting, and lifting. It is made better by lying down and rest. Symptoms that are worse with activities and relieved with rest oftentimes are related to mechanical dysfunction.

H: *The patient reported that 2 weeks prior to this evaluation he was lifting a heavy sink and had immediate low back pain (LBP)*. This is indicative of a mechanical dysfunction, as it was "traumatic" in nature. He does, however, report a prior history of incidental LBP, which resolved in one week. This history in conjunction with the mechanism of injury could make one suspect extreme stress on/injury to the posterior structures, namely the muscular system and disc. His past medical history of a knee surgery is most likely unremarkable to this evaluation. His systems review was also negative.

A: *Evaluation of posture revealed that his iliac crests, ASIS, and PSIS were all symmetrical, he presented with a flattened lumbar lordosis and a lumbar side bend left type I scoliosis*. These findings are noted during visual observation. On palpation he would have had asymmetry of three or more levels and subsequently this would have been confirmed with movement. The type I scoliosis, by definition, is considered a secondary or compensatory curve. When the therapist sees a type I curve, the question that should come to mind is: Why is it there? There are at least 20 reasons for a type I compensatory curve to exist (Exhibit 9–3).

Joe has a few of the dysfunctions listed in Figure 9–3, which could be causing this type I scoliosis. On further palpation, his sacral base was found to be deeper on the right and shallow on the left, and his left inferior lateral angle of the sacrum was also shallower. These findings are consistent with a sacrum that is rotated to the left. Because it is there as a positional dysfunction, it would be considered a major motion loss.[9] This is certainly something that could cause a left lumbar side bending right rotation compensation. While his innominates appear symmetrical to palpation, he does have an apparent leg length dysfunction with a shorter left leg. Because this is noted in supine by looking at the levelness of the malleoli, the leg length discrepancy could be due to innominate rotation or due to true leg length discrepancy (which was ruled out with palpation and measurement), an upslip (which is not likely due to chief complaint and history and because the symmetry of bony landmarks in standing), or a type I side bend left scoliosis in the lumbar spine.

R: *There is a limitation to flexion and extension of 50% with increase in symptoms during active movement in both directions. Side bending right is 25% limited and rotation left is 20% limited*. These findings are consistent with a side bend left type I neutral dysfunction. Side bend left and rotation

Exhibit 9–3 Twenty Reasons for a type I compensatory dysfunction

1. Idiopathic scoliosis with vertebral wedging
2. Structural leg length discrepancy
3. Functional leg length discrepancy
4. Type II lesion above
5. Type II lesion below
6. Myofascial dysfunction present in the trunk
7. Myofascial dysfunction present in the lower extremity
8. herniated nucleus pulposus (HNP)
9. Instability
10. Sacral dysfunction
11. Innominate dysfunction
12. Structural rib dysfunction
13. Atlanto-occipital dysfunction
14. Temperomandibular joint dysfunction
15. Upper quarter adverse neural tension
16. Lower quarter adverse neural tension
17. Visceral dysfunction
18. Vertigo—peripheral causes
19. Vertigo—central causes
20. Vertigo—systemic causes

right in the lumbar spine is 100% and pain free. The patient's symptoms are reproduced with active oblique extension to the right (quadrant) and there is mild discomfort on active oblique extension to the left. Right rotation is full and pain free; most likely because this patient's lumbar spine is already rotated right. *Hip passive range of motion is most notably limited in internal rotation on the right, which is 35° (left = 40°).* This can be due to a number of factors; namely a shortened or tonic piriformis, which is an external rotator, will limit hip internal rotation in prone. If the therapist finds this limited internal rotation in prone, it should be compared with internal rotation in a flexed hip position (e.g., quadruped). If it is indeed the piriformis that restricted the motion, it will not feel limited in quadruped (the piriformis changes actions to an internal rotator beyond 90° of flexion). If it continues to be tight in other positions, it is more likely a hip capsular tightness. Because this limitation due to piriformis tension is an important bit of information, it prompts the therapist to check tissue tension.

T: Because of its broad origination on the anterior sacrum, a tonic or shortened right piriformis will hold the right sacrum forward, creating left rotation. If the more inferior fibers are dysfunctional, they will hold the right inferior lateral angle forward, and in conjunction with a tonic multifidus on the left, will provide the environment for a left rotation on right oblique axis backward sacral torsion to occur. (Superior fibers could hold the right base forward into left rotation on left oblique axis forward sacral torsion FST). Figure 9–1 shows a sacrum, which could be rotated to the right via the left piriformis inferior fibers in conjunction with the right multifidus, or the left piriformis superior fibers.[9]

Likewise, if there is a mechanically induced left rotation on a right oblique axis backward sacral torsion (from flexion rotation with a load, Joe's mechanism of injury), the right piriformis will tend to become reactive. *Joe's right piriformis, gluteus medius, and quadratus lumborum produced tenderness, referred pain into the right buttock, and a twitch response. The right sacrotuberous ligament is tender.* These findings are consistent with sacroiliac joint dysfunction secondary to its origin on the sacral inferior lateral angle. Additionally, the right hip flexors are slightly limited in the Thomas test position, as are bilateral hamstrings.

S: When assessing a patient with lumbar and buttock pain, it is essential to do special tests related to the lumbar spine and pelvic girdle. As is the case with any radiating pain, it is imperative to clear the neurologic system through a screen of muscle strength by myotomes, sensation by dermatomes,

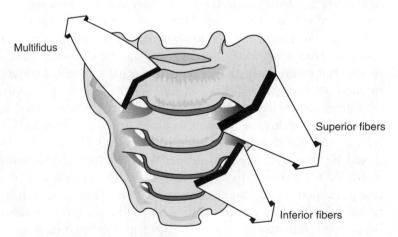

Figure 9–1 Role of piriformis and multifidus in sacral torsion dysfunction.

and reflex testing. This testing was all negative in Joe's case. In the osteopathic paradigm, the tests included standing extension/quadrant, standing forward bend, Gillet test, and leg swing. In supine, tests could include Gaenslen's as well as the innominate spring testing for end-feel and motion loss, as well as provocation, compression, and distraction. Performance of the seated flexion test is used to determine the sacral base that is dysfunctional, the sit slump test is used to assess sacral base motion in relation to lumbar flexion/extension, and sacral spring tests, once again, for motion and provocation testing. Gait is an important indicator of pelvic girdle dysfunction as well. Backward sacral torsional dysfunctions are apparent during midstance on the opposite extremity.

Additionally, X-rays, MRIs, and any other radiological testing would fall into the special tests component of the exam. In Joe's' case, his X-rays showed mild degenerative changes at L5–S1.

Diagnosis

The osteopathic clinical diagnosis for this patient would, based on the CHARTS evaluation first and most importantly, rule out a radicular dysfunction. There are clearly no dermatomal, myotomal, or DTR changes. Additionally, there are significant objective findings of somatic dysfunction. Because of this and the additional findings the patient is classified with the clinical diagnosis of spondylogenic or somatic dysfunction. The key dysfunctions include the following:

1) **Myofascial dysfunction, right gluteus medius, piriformis, and quadratus lumborum.** Although the case did not describe the iliopsoas, one would expect that the left iliopsoas complex might have excessive tone, trigger points, and/or be shortened. Based on clinical experience, the iliopsoas has been proposed to be a primary motion restrictor in extension dysfunctions (flexed segment) in the lower lumbar spine.

2) **Flexed rotated side bent right (FRSR) at L5; Limited extension side bending and rotation left at L5.** This may also be described as limited closing of the left facet. This is confirmed by sphinx position worsening the asymmetry of right side shallow, left side deep, and flexion completely correcting the asymmetry. Additionally, the mild discomfort with active oblique extension to the left, as well as the 50% limitation to passive extension would help to confirm this clinical diagnosis.

3) **Type I side bent left, rotated right in the lumbar spine; limited right side bending, left rotation**. The patient had limited active side bending right by 75% and an apparent short leg in supine at the malleoli. This is likely secondary to the type I side bending curve. Additionally, on examination he had a fullness within the right paravertebral region with marked muscle guarding on the right. Type I dysfunctions are compensatory in nature and this type I is typically driven by a type II below (L5) and/or a sacral rotational dysfunction. Joe presents with both objective findings.

4) **Sacral left rotation on a right oblique axis backward sacral torsion (L/R BST); limited right forward sacral rotation (limited forward rotation of left base)**. This diagnosis with the use of position, motion, and provocation tests; namely, palpatory asymmetries of left sacral based shallow, right inferior lateral angle deep, more asymmetrical with extension, and improved with flexion. Because this is a major (MA) motion loss, there is a resultant slightly flexed lumbar lordosis (flattened lumbar spine) as noted in the postural assessment. Additionally, because of the origin of the sacrotuberous ligament, the rotation of the sacrum would most certainly tension this ligament, which is a sacral stabilizer.

Intervention

Treatment begins with addressing the soft tissue dysfunctions.[5,9,14,21–24] In addition to preparing the environment for articular and muscle energy techniques, the tissue work will improve mobility, blood flow, length, tone, and play of the affected structures. Soft tissue involvement for sacral torsional dysfunctions, namely the left rotated sacrum that Joe presents with, must include normalization of piriformis tone and length.[14] For Joe, the therapist needs to address the right piriformis. The piriformis can be a primary motion restrictor in a sacral backward rotation. Specifically, the right piriformis would potentiate a left rotation on a right oblique axis dysfunction as previously noted. Furthermore, Joe's buttock achiness is consistent with piriformis dysfunction, either through trigger point referral or a neurovascular compression.[11] The next soft tissue to be addressed would be the left and the right psoas muscles. The psoas tension would perpetuate the limited extension of the lower lumbar spine via its origin on the anterior transverse processes, bodies, and disc of the lumbar vertebrae.[14] Specifically, the left psoas could hold the left L5 segment forward and flexed, limiting extension or closing of the facet on the left side.

Major motion loss (MA) > 50% of the motion of the segment has been lost. It can't get to neutral.

Minor motion loss (MI) 50% of the motion has been lost. The segment can get to neutral but asymmetry becomes apparent as the patient begins to move.

Finally, the left quadratus lumborum would need to be lengthened and softened, and bilateral quadratus lumborums and paraspinals treated for imbalances due to the type I neutral compensatory dysfunction. One might expect trigger points associated with stretch stress on the right and shortening/tone on the left. Techniques to address soft tissue dysfunction include myofascial release and strain-counterstrain techniques.

Joe would then be treated with a muscle energy technique for his FRSR at L5. Muscle energy techniques use principles of proprioceptive neuromuscular facilitation to accomplish the goal of gaining normal joint and segmental movement. In a muscle energy technique, the therapist positions the joint that is in dysfunction at the barrier position in three planes of movement. The patient is then instructed to voluntarily contract a specific muscle from this position against a gentle but unyielding force exerted by the therapist. This sequence is repeated 3–5 times until the barrier is cleared and motion is normalized.

For Joe, treating his L5 FRSR is achieved by placing him in right side lying (Figure 9–2), finding the extension barrier, and then rotating down to

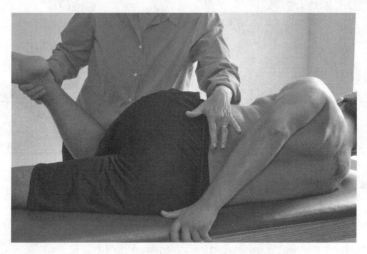

Figure 9–2 Position to treat a flexed rotated side bent lesion (FRSR).

the left rotation barrier. The muscle energy technique is performed by having the patient contract into rotation right against an unyielding counterforce. After a new rotation barrier is achieved, the side bending barrier is gained by abducting the left leg and having the patient adduct until a new side bending barrier is achieved.

Next, the L/R BST is treated by relocalizing to the sacroiliac joint barrier and having the patient perform a lower extremity abduction (Figure 9–3). These techniques are followed by neuromuscular re-education to regain motion into L5 extension side bending and rotation of the trunk to the left, sacral right rotation on a right axis forward torsion. Neuromuscular re-education would include anterior elevation patterns of the pelvic girdle and/or pelvic clock in the "6–9" range. True to the osteopathic sequence, the lumbar spine would be treated and cleared first because one would not want to treat the sacrum through a so-called "dirty lever." Finally, the patient would be reassessed in standing to see if the type I neutral dysfunction has resolved. If not, the therapist must treat this type I via muscle energy techniques including side bending to the right and rotation to the left. The patient will be sent home with a home exercise program consisting of prescriptive and corrective exercises for the specific structural dysfunctions, as well as stabilization and functional exercises for return to normal activities.

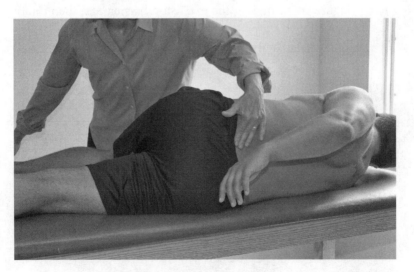

Figure 9–3 Position to treat a backward sacral torsion (L/R BST).

Prognosis

In predicting the outcome for Joe's case, one must look at the nature of his dysfunction. Because there are specific objective palpable somatic dysfunctions, these limitations and motion restrictions have a good prognosis for resolution. Additionally, the negative radiologic findings and the negative neurologic exam would contribute to a good prognosis. Joe had no complaints of radiating pain, no lower extremity weakness, and his reflexes were intact. The patient will continue to be reassessed at each visit to determine if indeed the structural findings of hypomobility are improving. In fact, because the patient is given a home exercise program consisting of prescriptive exercises for his specific somatic dysfunctions (FRS, L/R BST, type I), corrective exercise for the associated tissue and ROM limitations (piriformis, psoas, quadratus lumborum, paraspinals) and generic exercises to focus on core strength, stability, mobility, and function, the somatic dysfunction based on outcome studies should normalize in 6–8 visits. However, because of both the mild degeneration at L5–S1 in association with the length of time Joe's symptoms have been present and his active job duties, it is quite possible that the resolution of the symptoms associated with this dysfunction may take a bit longer to resolve.

Supportive Evidence

There is strong evidence favoring manipulation/mobilization with exercise in reducing pain, improvement in function, and global perceived effect for subacute and chronic spinal disorders; mobilization is a viable option for the treatment of both LBP and neck pain.[5,9,21] In fact, in a recent case series that classified patients into categories based on clinical findings, the patient in the mobilization manipulation classification had a pain reduction from 6.5/10 to .5/10 within 6 visits.[23] Additionally, Lenehan et al. studied the effect of muscle energy technique on gross trunk range of motion with the result being the attainment of improved range of motion.[25]

Huijbregts[26] editorialized on the importance placed on clinical prediction rules to identify patients with LBP most likely to benefit from manipulation. Joe does indeed meet many of the criteria necessary to be placed in a manipulation group based solely on the clinical prediction rule developed by Childs et al.[27] Huijbregts states that while he is in favor of this approach to a treatment-based classification system, one must not let go of the importance of segmental level, direction of perceived restriction, and end-feel, although there is some evidence against segmental specificity.[8] One reason for being as specific as possible (for instance treating the L5 level in Joe's case) is that the degenerative disc undergoes positive changes following joint mobilization. In fact, the stimulus provided by lumbar joint mobilization may influence the diffusion of water in degenerative intervertebral disc disease at L5–S1.[21,28] Additionally, the zygapophyseal joints are thought to be a source of LBP and these joints are mobilized during manipulative therapy of the lumbar spine. Wilde[29] identified 12 signs and symptoms that indicate the presence of zygapophyseal pain:

1 — positive response to intra-articular facet joint injection
2 — localized unilateral back pain
3 — pain relieved by fluoroscopically guided double-anesthetic blocks of the medial branch of the dorsal ramus supplying the lumbar zygapophyseal joint
4 — replication or aggravation of pain by unilateral pressure over lumbar zygapophyseal joint or transverse process
5 — lack of radicular features
6 — pain eased in flexion
7 — pain, if referred to the leg, is above the knee
8 — palpation, local unilateral passive movement shows reduced range of motion or increased stiffness on the side of lumbar zygapophyseal joint pain
9 — unilateral mm, spasm over the affected lumbar zygapophyseal joint
10 — pain in extension
11 — pain in extension, lateral flexion or rotation to the ipsilateral side
12 — radiology is unreliable and cannot dx lumbar zygapophyseal joint pain

The evidence for evaluation and treatment modalities for the sacroiliac joint remains relatively controversial, yet recent studies suggest that manual therapists can improve our reliability of implicating the sacroiliac joint as the source of dysfunction through the use of a multitest regimen.[7,13,14,16–19] In fact, a multi-test approach can reduce the need for more invasive procedures such as injection in the treatment of sacroiliac joint dysfunction.[18] In addition to sacroiliac joint provocation tests, other important tests were used to evaluate the side of dysfunction, the restriction presented, and the direction limited.[9,17,21,22] Joe's key dysfunction of a L/R BST would be treated with tissue work, muscle energy techniques, and possible manipulation to promote form closure, or stability through the improved joint congruency.

Almost as important in treatment of the pelvic girdle is the need to provide force closure, or the stabilization of the pelvic girdle through balance of the muscular system surrounding girdle.[22,30] This force closure is imperative for the patient's future ability to perform his work activities and is gained via vigorous trunk and pelvic stabilization exercises. Recent studies suggest that manual therapy in conjunction with specific adjuvant exercise is effective in treating LBP.[5]

SUMMARY

The osteopathic approach as presented here uses a format for examination summarized in the CHARTS mnemonic. All the elements of the mnemonic that drive intervention decisions, but in particular through the assessment of symmetry, range of motion, tissue tension, and special tests decisions, were rendered about the most appropriate course for Joe. The approach uses a combination of tests that provoke pain and tests that rely on therapist palpation and skill to determine the presence of dysfunction. Treatment is directed to both the spine and pelvic girdle in an attempt to normalize the structures so that function can improve. This method is fully in line with the traditional osteopathic tenet that structure governs function.

REFERENCES

1. Bronfort G, Haas M, Evans RL, Bouter LM. Efficacy of spinal manipulation and mobilization for low back pain and neck pain: a systematic review and best evidence synthesis. *Spine J.* 20044(3):335–56.
2. DeStefano L. *Greenman's Principles of Manual Medicine.* 4th ed. Philadelphia, PA: Lippincott Williams and Wilkins, 2010.
3. Fryette HH. *Principles of Osteopathic Technic.* Indianapolis, IN: American Academy of Osteopathy, 1954.
4. Nelson KE, ed, Glonek T associate ed. *Somatic Dysfunction in Osteopathic Family Medicine* Philadelphia, PA: Lippincott Williams and Wilkins, 2007.
5. Geisser ME, Wiggert EA, Haig AJ, Colwell MO. A randomized, controlled trial of manual therapy and specific adjuvant exercise for chronic low back pain. *Clin J Pain.* 2005;21(6):463–470.
6. Hartman L. *Handbook of Osteopathic Technique.* 3rd ed. Cheltenham, UK: Nelson Thomes Ltd, 2002.
7. Laslett M. Evidence-based diagnosis and treatment of the painful sacroiliac joint. *J Man Manip Ther.* 2008;16(3):142–152.
8. Fritz JM, Whitman JM, Childs JD. Lumbar spine segmental mobility assessment: an examination of validity for determining intervention strategies in patients with low back pain. *Arch Phys Med Rehabil.* 2005;86(9):1745–1752.
9. Ellis, Jeffrey, Lumbo-Pelvic Integration, course manual, 1993/2006.

10. Cyriax J. *Textbook of Orthopaedic Medicine.* 8th ed. London, England: Baillière Tindall, 1982.

11. Pécina MM, Krmpotić-Nemanić J, Markiewitz AD. *Tunnel Syndromes.* 3rd ed. Boca Raton, FL: CRC Press, 2001.

12. Greenhalgh S, Selfe J. *Red Flags: A Guide to Identifying Serious Pathology of the Spine.* Philadelphia, PA: Elsevier Churchill Livingstone, 2006.

13. Laslett M, Aprill CN, McDonald B, Young SB. Diagnosis of sacroiliac joint pain: validity of individual provocation tests and composites of tests. *Man Ther.* 2005;10(3):207–218.

14. Cibulka MT, Koldehoff R. Clinical usefulness of a cluster of sacroiliac joint tests in patients with and without low back pain. *J Orthop Sports Phys Ther.* 1999;29(2):83–89

15. Robinson HS, Brox JI, Robinson R, Bjelland E, Solem S, Telje T. The reliability of selected motion- and pain-provocation tests for the sacroiliac joint. *Man Ther.* 2007;12(1):72–79.

16. Stuber KJ. Specificity, sensitivity, and predictive values of clinical tests of the sacroiliac joint: a systematic review of the literature. *J Can Chiropr Assoc.* 2007;51(1):30–41.

17. Tong HC, Heyman OG, Lado DA, Isser MM. Interexaminer reliability of three methods of combining test results to determine side of sacral restriction, sacral base position, and innominate bone position. *J Am Osteopath Assoc.* 2006;106(8):464–468.

18. van der Wurff P, Buijs EJ, Groen GJ. A multitest regimen of pain provocation tests as an aid to reduce unnecessary minimally invasive sacroiliac joint procedures. *Arch Phys Med Rehabil.* 2006;87(1):10–14.

19. Vincent-Smith B, Gibbons P. Inter-examiner and intra-examiner reliability of the standing flexion test. *Man Ther.* 1999;4(2):87–93.

20. Barnes D, Stemper BD, Yogananan N, Baisden JL, Pintar FA. Normal coupling behavior between axial rotation and lateral bending in the lumbar spine–biomed 2009. *Biomed Sci Instrum.* 2009;45:131–136.

21. Beattie PF, Donley JW, Arnot CF, Miller R. The change in the diffusion of water in normal and degenerative lumbar intervertebral discs following joint mobilization compared to prone lying. *J Orthop Sports Phys Ther.* 2009;39(1):4–11.

22. Lee DG. *The Pelvic Girdle: An Integration of Clinical Expertise and Research.* 4th ed. Edinburgh: Churchill Livingstone, 2010.

23. Pinto D, Cleland J, Palmer J, Eberhart SL. Management of low back pain: a case series illustrating the pragmatic combination of treatment- and mechanism-based classification systems. *J Man Manip Ther.* 2007;15(2):111–122.

24. Mitchell FL, Moran PS, Pruzzo NA. *An Evaluation and Treatment Manual of Ostopathic Muscle Energy Procedures I.* Valley Park, MO: Mitchell, Moran and Pruzzo Assoc., 1979.

25. Lenehan KL, Fryer NDG, McLaughlin P. The effect of muscle energy technique on gross trunk range of motion. *Journal of Osteopathic Medicine.* 2003;6(1):13–18.

26. Huijbregts P. Clinical prediction rules: time to sacrifice the holy cow of specificity? *J Man Manip Ther.* 2007;15(1):5–8.

27. Childs JD, Fritz JM, Flynn TW, Irrgang JJ, Johnson KK, Majkowski GR, Delitto A. A clinical prediction rule to identify patients with low back pain most likely to benefit from spinal manipulation: a validation study. *Ann Intern Med.* 2004;141(12):920–928.

28. Beattie PF. Current understanding of lumbar intervertebral disc degeneration: a review with emphasis upon etiology, pathophysiology, and lumbar magnetic resonance imaging findings. *J Orthop Sports Phys Ther.* 2008;38(6):329–340.

29. Wilde VE, Ford JJ, McMeeken JM. Indicators of lumbar zygapophyseal joint pain: survey of an expert panel with the Delphi technique. *Phys Ther.* 2007;87(10):1348–1361.

30. van Wingerden JP, Vleeming A, Buyruk HM, Raissadat K. Stabilization of the sacroiliac joint in vivo: verification of muscular contribution to force closure of the pelvis. *Eur Spine J.* 2004;13(3):199–205.

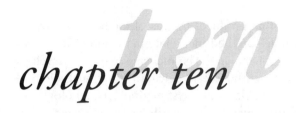

chapter ten

Movement System Impairment Syndromes Approach

Shirley Sahrmann, PT, PhD, FAPTA

The Movement System Impairment Syndromes approach was conceptualized by Dr. Shirley Sahrmann with additional development and refinement in collaboration with her associates at Washington University School of Medicine. Dr. Sahrmann was an early advocate for the development of classification systems that would direct physical therapy treatment and the first to categorize pain disorders into movement impairment syndromes. The underlying tenet of the Movement System Impairment Syndromes approach lies in the identification and correction of faulty alignment and movement patterns in order to treat and prevent musculoskeletal pain. Dr. Sahrmann's first book entitled Diagnosis and Treatment of Movement Impairment Syndromes *was published in 2002 and was followed by* Movement System Impairment Syndromes of the Extremities, Cervical and Thoracic Spines, *published in 2010. Dr. Sahrmann is currently professor of Physical Therapy, Neurology, Cell Biology, and Physiology at Washington University School of Medicine in St. Louis, Missouri. For more information on this approach and opportunities for continuing education please visit http://physical therapy.wustl.edu.*

BACKGROUND

Movement System Syndromes

An important physiological system of the body is the human movement system (MS). Unfortunately this system has not gained the amount of recognition that is consistent with its role in human functioning. The movement system is defined as the system that produces motion of the body as a whole or of its component parts. It relies on the functional interaction of the structures that contribute to the act of moving. The movement system develops dysfunctions that are induced by pathokinesiological or kinesiopathological problems.[1] Pathokinesiological problems are dysfunctions or pathologies of body systems such as the neurological or the cardiovascular systems that induce impairments in movement. A pathology of the nervous system such as Parkinson's disease or multiple sclerosis causes impairments in movement. A cardiovascular event such as a cerebral embolism or aneurysm can affect the central nervous system or the cardiac system itself. The resulting pathologies also cause alterations in movement. A kinesiopathological problem is one in which movement induces a pathology in a tissue or the function of another physiological system. For example, repeated or sustained wrist flexion can cause carpal tunnel syndrome. Another example is repeated lumbar extension that causes spondylolisthesis. Physical therapists are the health professionals who should be responsible for developing programs for optimal development of the tissues and other systems that are affected by movement and exercise. Those tissues include bone, muscle, blood vessels, etc., and systems such as the nervous, cardiovascular, pulmonary, and metabolic. In addition to guiding the optimal development of all the components of the MS, the PT is also responsible for monitoring the maintenance, diagnosing dysfunctions, and developing appropriate and effective treatment programs. Movement system syndromes describe the dysfunctions of the system. An important concept is that there are signs of movement impairments before the onset of symptoms and addressing the signs can be a means of prevention. Just as the signs of hypertension, high cholesterol and high glucose levels can be addressed to prevent the onset of stroke, myocardial infarction or diabetes.

Implicit in this concept is that because the movement system has components from other anatomical systems (e.g., muscular, skeletal, and nervous) the dysfunctions arise from alterations in the interactions of these other systems. When a dysfunction occurs as indicated by pain and difficulty with mobility, a factor believed to be a *cause* is altered precision of joint movement. Therefore all of the components contributing to the altered movement need to be assessed. The focus is not on the painful tissue, the *source* of the pain, but on the multiple factors that *caused* the tissues to become painful and/or continue to irritate tissues. The underlying cause is believed to be accessory motion hypermobility, which is usually loss of precise motion. In simplistic terms, the alteration in movement, subtle as that alteration may be, is the cause of the pain because of the associated tissue microtrauma that eventually becomes macrotrauma. As is well known from kinesiology, any type of activity involves movement of multiple segments of the body whether for actual participation in the chain of movement or for stabilization of various segments upon which the movement of a limb is to take place. We propose that the repeated movements and prolonged postures of daily activities establish a pattern of muscular or joint participation such that a joint gradually begins to move more readily and easily in one direction.[1] Because the human body follows the rules of physics and takes the path of least resistance for movement, a pattern is established that eventually results in a vicious cycle. The more frequently the joint moves, the more readily and easily the associated tissue changes contribute to the movement occurring at the affected joint rather than at other joints along the kinesiological chain. For example, during forward bending, movement occurs in the thoracic and lumbar spines as well as in the hip joint. A multiplicity of factors contributes to the joint where the movement will occur the most readily. Men have a higher center of gravity than women, so to keep the line of gravity in the base of support, men tend to flex their lumbar spine more than women. If the man also has a tall pelvis, which is associated with low back pain (LBP),[2] where the height of the pelvis is a greater percentage of the overall trunk height than in other men, the degree of lumbar flexion is even greater than in other men. These men usually have a flat spine with the iliac crests being located at L3 or higher and not L4. During forward bending these men tend to use their hamstrings to control their upper body as they bend forward. The prolonged activity of the hamstring muscles further contributes to excessive lumbar flexion and reduces the amount of hip flexion during the forward bend. Repeated motion of this joint, which is evident in increased frequency as well as altered motion, causes microtrauma and eventually macrotrauma. This trauma can not only induce tissue damage but can be combined with the degenerative process that occurs in all or most tissues. The challenge of any form of motion or exercise is to find the balance of activity that enhances the health of the tissues versus activity that can cause tissue injury. As with all mechanical systems, the more precise the motion the longer the system will function, without injury of the components, and the greater the efficiency. That is why there is the science of tribology, which is designed to understand and optimize the maintenance of precise motion in mechanical systems. Because of this appreciation of kinesiology, our examination focuses on whether spinal alignment is appropriate for a given patient, the quality of spinal movement, and the behavior of symptoms during movement. In addition, the patient is instructed in how to correct the altered movement and the effect on symptoms is reassessed. Because of the interactions of the entire body, movements of the limbs are also assessed for an effect on both associated movement of the spine and the effect on symptoms. If movement of the spine is detected, then the spine is stabilized, either passively or actively, while the limb movement is repeated and the effect on symptoms reassessed. Observations based on the results of these tests result in the identification of a movement direction or directions that most consistently cause pain and that when corrected reduce or alleviate the symptoms. This is the direction of movement in which the spine moves the most readily during activity. The diagnosis is the syndrome described for the offending movement direction. In addition to the specific exam of spine and limb movements, functional activities such as rolling, supine to sitting, sitting to standing, walking, sitting, and standing alignment are assessed. Work and fitness activities are also reviewed as are any other specific activities that cause pain such as getting in and out of the car or walking stairs. As with other components of the exam, the movement pattern and the affect on symptoms are also assessed and corrected.

The examination is designed not only to arrive at a diagnosis but also to identify the contributing factors. In a general manner, contributing factors can fall into two major categories, motor pattern coordination deficit and/or force production deficit. Patients with a motor pattern coordination problem have adequate muscle strength but the pattern of muscle participation is the primary factor contributing to the movement imprecision and the pain problem. The patients with force production deficit have a primary problem of muscle weakness usually in the trunk or proximal girdle muscles that is contributing to the imprecise movement. As might be expected the problems identified in most patients are somewhere in between these two categories of motor pattern coordination deficit and force production deficit. What the practitioner should keep in mind is that identifying a muscle deficiency should be viewed as an indicator of the movement deficit, not the cause. In other words, strengthening the muscle will not correct the problem because *the muscle deficiency is caused by the movement pattern* instead of being the reason for the movement pattern. Obviously, the strength deficit of the muscle just further contributes to the development of a vicious cycle. An example is the patient with a swayback posture causing the line of gravity to be markedly posterior to the hip joint. These individuals usually have poor development of their gluteal muscles because the external moment is keeping the hip extended and minimizing the use of the hip extensor muscles. When these patients do bend forward and return to standing they use the ankle (hip) strategy minimizing the activation of the gluteal hip extensor muscles. Strengthening the gluteal muscles will not change the patient's alignment or muscle use pattern, but changing the patient's alignment will change the muscle use pattern.

The description of syndromes serves as a basis of pattern recognition upon which diagnosis is based. The physical examination is used to make a diagnosis and to identify the contributing factors, which need to be addressed in the treatment program. Importantly the contributing factors for a specific diagnosis can vary. The contributing factors are the multiple impairments that contribute to the alteration in precise joint motion.

In summary, the basic premise is that the cause of a condition is a subtle alteration in the precision of joint motion that is causing microtrauma that leads to macrotrauma and eventually pain. The subtle alteration is believed to be hypermobility evident in both quality and frequency of arthrokinematic (accessory) joint motion. This hypermobility is the cause versus the source of the pain problem. The source is the pathoanatomical structure that is painful. Stopping the movement also stops the pain because the movement irritating the tissue is ceased.

The underlying factor in the development and maintenance of the hypermobility is that the body takes the path of least resistance. The site of the path of least resistance is a function of the relative flexibility/stiffness of the soft, contractile, and supporting tissues about a joint. Musculoskeletal pain is a part of the progressive degeneration of the human body that is affected by lifestyle. Thus alleviation of the pain is not correction of the problem. Slowing of the progression of the problem, the tissue microtrauma, and the degeneration is achieved by stopping the hypermobility of the accessory motion, which is accomplished by identifying the direction of pain inducing motion and the contributing factors. Based on the premise that there is a relatively consistent kinesiological relationship to the pain, patients are classified into groups. The classification is designed to provide direction for treatment and for understanding the kinesiopathology. The classifications or syndromes are extension-rotation, extension, rotation, flexion-rotation, and flexion. The syndrome is named for the movement direction that most consistently causes symptoms, that most often is associated with a movement impairment, and that when the movement impairment is corrected, the symptoms are decreased or eliminated. A specific physical exam is used to identify the syndrome that consists of movements of the spine and of the extremities with the focus on how the movements affect the spine and the symptoms.

Based on research and clinical experience, the lumbar flexion (LF) and flexion-rotation (LF-R) syndromes are more common in younger and taller subjects often with an initial acute onset of pain than in older and shorter individuals. The flexion syndrome is present in the younger patient because of greater tissue flexibility and a minimum of degenerative changes. These are patients that are susceptible to the development of herniated discs. Contributing factors are greater stiffness of the hip extensor muscles than the lumbar extensor muscles. These patients can also have well developed abdominal muscles that not only contribute to the lumbar flexion but also to the lumbar compression from the passive stiffness of the abdominal muscles. These patients usually have increased lumbar flexion range of motion and sit in lumbar flexion.

Patients with lumbar extension (LE) and extension-rotation (LE-R) syndromes are older, shorter in stature, and have chronic pain. This condition is usually associated with degenerative changes such as changes in disc height and alignment as found in spondylolisthesis or spinal stenosis. Contributing factors in these syndromes are usually the opposite of the flexion syndrome but not always. The typical patient with an extension-rotation syndrome has poor abdominal musculature, hypertrophied back extensors, and short or stiff hip flexor muscles. Another variant is a patient with a marked thoracic kyphosis but who is swayed back such that the lumbar spine is extended or, at a minimum, the alignment of the thorax increasing the posterior loading of the lumbar spine. In the swayed back posture the abdominal muscles can become the antigravity muscle group in the standing position that then decreases their length and increases their stiffness. These patients also demonstrate an asymmetry in the size of the paraspinal area and in the characteristics of trunk rotation and side bending. The lumbar rotation (LR) syndrome is also usually present in patients with chronic back pain and the characteristics are similar to the extension-rotation syndrome but are usually more symmetric in rotation and have pain with both flexion and extension motions.

Evidence for the Model

The evidence for this model has come from the clinical and laboratory studies of Linda Van Dillen, PT, PhD.[23–25] Dr. Van Dillen, her graduate students, and fellow investigators have demonstrated the reliability of the test items of the examination[6,25] and the validity of the examination in defining specific classifications.[20] Evidence has been obtained for the extension, extension-rotation, and rotation syndromes. [17,20,23] Because the majority of patients in

Dr. Van Dillen's studies have had chronic pain, she has not had adequate subjects to support the flexion or flexion-rotation classifications except for a case report.[19] Clinical studies have also demonstrated that two therapists performing the examination on individuals with LBP make the same diagnosis 73% of the time.[25] Laboratory studies have demonstrated that both hip rotation and knee flexion in prone cause lumbopelvic rotation earlier and to a greater degree in patients with LBP than in control subjects.[9] Hip lateral rotation in prone also caused pain more often in men with LBP than in women with LBP.[11,18] The majority of the lumbopelvic motion in men with LBP occurred during the first 60% of their hip lateral rotation range of motion.[18] Laboratory studies also indicated that patients who were diagnosed with the extension-rotation syndrome had asymmetrical lumbopelvic motion during hip lateral rotation and side bending while patients with the rotation syndrome had symmetrical motion with these tests.[10,12,14,15] Clinical studies also demonstrated that LBP that was associated with limb movements can be eliminated or reduced by preventing the lumbar motion.[13,21] Currently a randomized control trial of generic treatment versus classification-based treatment is in the final stages thus additional information will be available in the not too distant future.

Overview of the Examination

As stated, the underlying premise is that movement of the spine in a specific direction is the cause of the pain and that movement occurs directly during motions of the trunk and indirectly during motions of the limbs. In addition to the offending motion direction of the spine, the tissue and motor control impairments that are considered contributing factors are also identified. The tests also provide the basis for the corrective exercise program and the modification of functional activities. Basically, when the patient fails a test, correction of that test motion becomes the exercise. It is important that the patient is instructed in what is believed to be the pain causing movement direction and how to modify the movement and thus control the symptoms. The same strategy is applied to functional activities.

The systematic examination consists of tests of trunk motion and limb motions performed in the standing, supine, side lying, prone, quadruped, and sitting positions. In addition to the tests assessing the precision of motion; the effect on symptoms; and the muscle performance, length, and stiffness; functional activities are also assessed. Again, clinical experience and research support the belief that the most important aspect of the treatment program is correcting the way the patient performs daily activities and the alignments that are maintained during the course of the day.

The examination consists of primary tests in which the patient moves in the self-selected preferred pattern while the symptoms and the quality or pattern of motion are assessed. The secondary test is correction of the movement pattern and reassessment of symptoms. The examination format consists of:

Standing

Symptoms, alignment, forward bending, return from forward bending, rotation to each side, side bending, single leg standing, back to wall with back relaxed, back to wall with shoulder flexion.

Supine

Hip flexor length test, supine position, passive and active hip/knee flexion, passive and active hip abduction/lateral rotation from hip flexion, passive straight-leg raise, active bilateral shoulder flexion; Note: the performance of the abdominal muscles is inferred by the behavior of the lumbopelvic area during the tests and, if necessary, specific abdominal muscle testing is performed.

Side lying

Symptoms during the change in position and the pattern used to change position, symptoms in the position, passive and active hip lateral rotation/abduction from hip flexion, passive and active hip abduction/adduction. Manual muscle testing of the hip abductor muscles.

Prone

Symptoms in the position, passive and active knee flexion, passive and active hip rotation with the knee flexed. If the patient has a working diagnosis of flexion syndrome, then passive and active hip extension with the knee flexed and/or extended are tested.

Quadruped

Symptoms and alignment, rocking backward, shoulder flexion.

Sitting

> Symptoms and alignment, knee extension, unloading the spine by pushing into the seat of the chair with hands.

Gait

> Symptoms, lumbopelvic pattern of motion.

APPLICATION OF MOVEMENT SYSTEM IMPAIRMENT SYNDROMES MODEL FOR JOE LORES

Patient Examination/Evaluation

History

> The patient is a 39-year-old male who works as a plumber. He had arthroscopic knee surgery in 1986 and his knees are painful and swollen. He had a previous incident of LBP that resolved with rest. He is receiving medication for high blood pressure but is otherwise in good health. His physician's exam did not identify any systemic conditions and his screening form was also negative for red flag conditions. His current problem of LBP developed 2 weeks ago when he was installing a sink. He has pain with most activities associated with his job as well as with his activities of daily living (ADLs). He complains of pain in both sitting and standing with the greatest relief when recumbent. His symptoms have improved since the onset of the problem. He rates his pain level as ranging from 3–6/10. His weight is 195 lbs. and his height is 5′ 9″ giving him a BMI of 29, which places him in the overweight range. He has pain with bending, twisting, flexion, extension, and going from sit to stand.
>
> Based on this information, his movement system working diagnosis is rotation, with lumbar flexion being a major contributing factor. The diagnosis of rotation is indicated by the presence of symptoms with both flexion and extension as well as by side bending. In addition, Hispanics are generally very flexible and his job requires a great deal of bending and working in awkward positions. His height and flexibility suggest that he will be flexing primarily in his lumbar spine rather than in his hips. The knee pain most likely further contributes to excessive motion of his lumbar spine in order to avoid knee flexion and kneeling. The pain with lumbar extension is consistent with a slight rotational problem in which the structures of the spine

aren't perfectly aligned and thus are subjected to stress when a motion that requires appropriate approximation of the posterior structures is required. He does not have any radiating symptoms, so nerve entrapment does not seem to be the issue, rather mechanical soft tissue irritation seems most likely. Correcting the flexion and enabling the facet joints to appropriately align and maintain their positions would seem to be a feasible rationale for correcting this problem. The reduction of symptoms when recumbent and minimal spinal compression is consistent with this proposed mechanical aspect of his problem.

Tests and measures

Alignment

The patient has a tall pelvis, thus his iliac crests are at least 1 inch higher than his belt line. This is consistent with his relatively flat lumbar spine. He has a slight thoracic kyphosis with a prominent abdomen. The poor definition of his gluteal muscles is consistent with the swayback posture in which the weight line is posterior to the hip joint. With this type of posture during forward bending the motion is to sway posterior from the ankles and the return to standing also with hip sway rather than hip extension. He has well developed back extensor muscles. The right side of his lumbar area is bigger than the left, which could be from lumbar rotation. These characteristics predispose him to lumbar flexion and rotation (LF-R) except for well developed back extensor muscles. The tendency for Hispanics to be flexible and the tall pelvis also contribute to lumbar flexion during bending and sitting. During forward bending, because of his flat back, to avoid lumbar flexion his hips must flex almost immediately. Usually the tall pelvis is associated with a long trunk in proportion to the lower extremities. To keep his center of gravity in his base of support he has to flex his trunk rather than his hips unless he bends his knees. As noted previously he may be avoiding knee flexion because of the knee pain and swelling.

Forward bending

He has increased symptoms and his lumbar spine flexes faster than his hips and he has excessive lumbar flexion with failure to achieve 80° of hip flexion. The asymmetry of his lumbar spine is still evident in the prominence of the right side when he is in the flexed position. Correction of his forward bending by having him support his upper body with his hands on a high plinth while he flexes his hips eliminates his symptoms during forward bending. These findings are consistent with lumbar flexion syndrome. He was instructed in returning from forward bending by using hip extension rather than lumbar extension. He did not have any symptoms when performing the motion in this manner.

Side bending

The patient has pain with side bending to the right and his movement is at the iliac crest level as indicated by this being the point of the axis of rotation. The rest of the spine does not change its orientation, suggesting a lack of shared movement in other vertebral segments during the motion. Manual support of his spine at the level of the iliac crest eliminates his symptoms, supporting the belief that lumbar rotation in this region is contributing to his pain problem. Side bending to the left did not cause symptoms and the lumbar spine had a curve when moving in this direction. The lack of a curve bending to the right and a normal curve going to the left is consistent with his spine being slightly rotated to the right (LR).

Rotation

The patient has a greater range of rotation to the right than to the left, which is further support for rotation being a factor in his condition. He also rotates off of axis by having his trunk shift to the right when rotating to the left. This is another sign of rotational dysfunction (LR).

Single-leg standing

He has lumbopelvic rotation during single-leg standing on the right, another indication of a lumbar rotation problem (LR).

Trunk unloading

Because his symptoms decrease with unloading his thorax by lifting his trunk with the therapist's hands in his axilla, compression appears as a factor contributing to his symptoms. This partial unloading of his trunk did not totally eliminate his symptoms

Standing with back to wall:

The lack of change in symptoms does not support a lumbar extension (LE) condition. Similarly, contraction of his abdominal muscles does not notably affect his symptoms, also failing to support an extension problem (no LE).

Supine tests

Hip flexor length test:

He has pelvic anterior tilt during the leg lowering indicating that he has a relative flexibility problem with his back too flexible into extension relative to his hip flexors. The improvement in range and reduction in anterior tilt when the test is performed with his hip is abducted indicates that his tensor fascia lata iliotibial band (TFL-ITB) is the stiff and/or short muscle. His right TFL-ITB is short because when his pelvis is manually stabilized, his hip will not extend unless his hip is abducted. The shortness of the TFL-ITB combined with his lumbar spine flexibility could contribute to lumbopelvic rotation during walking. Instead of hip extension and lateral rotation at the end of stance phase, he would have lumbopelvic rotation as a compensation (LR).

Supine position:

The patient's symptoms increase in this position when his hips and knees are extended and are reduced with a pillow under his head and shoulders to accommodate to his thoracic kyphosis and a pillow under his knees that would alleviate the stretch on the hip flexors. Though both of these changes can be consistent with a lumbar extension problem they can also indicate a lumbar rotation problem particularly when there is asymmetry in the stiffness and shortness of the hip flexor muscles. (LR)

Passive hip/knee flexion:

The weight of the patient's lower extremity is consistent with an individual with a job that requires physical activity but he does not have any notable stiffness, or passive resistance, to hip/knee flexion but at the end of the hip flexion range of motion his lumbar spine flexes (LF).

Active hip/knee flexion:

He does not have any symptoms with active motion of either the right or left lower extremity, but he does have more than 0.5 inch of movement of his anterior superior iliac spine during lumbopelvic rotation with right lower extremity motion but not left. The motion occurs early in the range of motion (LR).

Hip abduction/lateral rotation from flexion:

He has lumbopelvic rotation during the first 50% of the motion and increase in symptoms with right lower extremity motion but not with the left. If his pelvis is stabilized, either passively or actively his symptoms are slightly reduced (LR).

Bilateral shoulder flexion:

Does not affect his symptoms but he has an increase in his lumbar curve. This is indicative of lumbar spine that is flexible into extension and a latissimus dorsi muscle that is stiffer than his abdominals and that may be short (no LE).

Rolling:

He has symptoms when rolling to his side but performs the motion by moving his lower extremities first, causing lumbopelvic rotation. When instructed and given adequate verbal and tactile cues to roll from hooklying by leading with his arm and rolling "like a log," he does not have any symptoms. The most important modification besides rolling with all segments moving at the same time is being sure the patient only minimally contracts his hip flexors and does not try to lift his lower extremities. This basic movement pattern and the associated symptoms are consistent with a rotation problem (LR).

Side lying:

He has symptoms when in this position on both the left and right sides. A folded towel just above the iliac crest eliminates his symptoms. A pillow between his knees slightly reduces his symptoms. The positive effect of the support at the level above the iliac crest is another indication of a rotation problem. In side lying, his spine is going into a slight side bend and the support prevents this change in position of his spine (LR).

Hip abduction/lateral rotation from flexion in side lying:

The patient has lumbopelvic rotation during the early phase of hip motion another indication that his lumbar spine is more flexible than his hip joint. He needs both verbal and tactile cues to correct the motion so that the motion is confined to the hip joint. His range of hip joint motion is also reduced when he performs the motion correctly (LR).

Hip abductor manual muscle test:

The patient did not have any difficulty being positioned in the correct test alignment nor did he have pain during the performance of the test. He did have some slight weakness of his right hip abductors (4+/5), but not left hip abductor muscles (5/5). Because he was not able to maintain the hip at the end range of hip abduction but was able to hold well after the hip adducted a few degrees, his hip abductor muscles were judged as long rather than weak from atrophy. He did not have any lateral pelvic tilt during performance of hip abduction and adduction.

Active hip abduction/adduction:

Palpation of the lateral abdominals when the patient performs this motion indicated that he was not recruiting these muscles to stabilize the pelvis during the active hip motion. This means he is using his contralateral hip abductors and pushing into the plinth to stabilize his pelvis. He is instructed to "stop" pushing down with the opposite hip and to try to contract his lateral abdominals.

Prone:

In this position the patient has symptoms and is more comfortable with a pillow under his abdomen. This is consistent with lumbar extension problems but also the presence of the asymmetry in his lumbar spine can be another reason he has symptoms when his spine is somewhat extended and more comfortable when his spine is flat.

Passive knee flexion:

There is notable resistance to passive knee flexion and associated anterior pelvic tilt. That is consistent with stiffness of his quadriceps and TFL-ITB. Because his lumbar spine is flexible into rotation, the stretch of the quadriceps and TFL-ITB is causing anterior pelvic tilt and lumbopelvic rotation that was greater on the right than on the left. The lumbar motion is associated with increased symptoms. Manual stabilization of the pelvis decreases the symptoms. These findings are consistent with LR-E.

Hip rotation:

Hip lateral rotation with his knee flexed caused early lumbopelvic rotation on the right but not on the left. There was no change in the symptoms. There was no lumbopelvic rotation during hip medial rotation and no change in symptoms. Hip lateral rotation range of motion was 50° on both the right and the left. The medial rotation was 35° on the right and 40° on the left. These findings of good or normal range of motion indicate that the lumbopelvic motion is not because of restriction of motion at the hip joint but because of the relative flexibility of the lumbar spine.

Quadruped:

Alignment: slight lumbar flexion with the right paraspinal area more prominent than the left. His hips are flexed to about 75°. If he allows his lumbar spine to move toward neutral and out of flexion, his symptoms improve (LF-R). The patient was able to tolerate this position with pads under his knees. The excursion of rocking backward was limited to avoid pain in his knees.

Rocking backward:

When he rocks backward his hips flex and the flexion of his lumbar spine increases. His symptoms increase slightly during this motion. The right side of his back also becomes more prominent than the left, which is consistent with rotation to the right. He was instructed to relax his back and hips so that they do not flex and to come backward by pushing with his hands. When the movement was performed by pushing with his hands rather than using his hip flexors to move back toward his heels, he does not have the lumbar flexion and he no longer has symptoms. This finding is consistent with the iliopsoas contributing to the lumbar flexion and to the symptoms. With approximately 10 repetitions of the rocking while preventing the lumbar flexion, the patient was able to perform the motion easily and without any symptoms. The rapid change in his condition supports the belief that he will be able to change the relative flexibility of his hips versus his spine and alleviate the symptoms (LF-R).

The relaxation of the spine and the cessation of hip flexor muscle activity during the rocking backward allows the lumbar spine to develop a slight inward curve. As the lumbar spine alignment becomes more extended, the facet joints overlap more than when the lumbar spine is flexed. The overlapping of the facet joints helps to reduce the rotation of the lumbar vertebrae and thus correct one of the major contributing factors to the patient's back pain (LR).

Shoulder flexion:

In the quadruped position, when the patient flexed his right shoulder the lumbar spine maintained a constant position but during left shoulder flexion his lumbar spine rotated clockwise or to the right. This is another contributing factor to the rotation problem. He was then asked to perform isometric shoulder extension with the right upper extremity as he flexed his left shoulder. The strategy is to use the right latissimus dorsi muscle to prevent the clockwise rotation (LR).

Sitting:

Unsupported sitting on the edge of the plinth with his feet unsupported. The patient has symptoms in this position. He is sitting in lumbar flexion. Factors contributing to his symptoms are the compression on his spine and the pull on his spine from his feet being unsupported.

Knee extension:

During right knee extension, his pelvis tilts posterior, the lumbar spine flexes and rotates clockwise, and symptoms increase slightly. Right knee extension is −45° of full excursion and the left is −35°. During left knee extension there is pelvic posterior tilt and lumbar rotation but not an increase in symptoms. When the motion of the lumbar spine is prevented by manual stabilization, the symptoms do not increase but he does report pulling in the posterior thigh, consistent with stretch of the hamstring muscles.

Manual muscle testing of the iliopsoas muscle:

Because his symptoms were not severe, the effect of iliopsoas muscle contraction and the performance of the muscle was assessed bilaterally. He did not have any increase in symptoms during the testing but the muscle groups tested 4/5 bilaterally.

Sitting in a chair with a back rest and arm supports with his hips and knees at the same level and his feet on the floor:

If he supports his body with his arms and relaxes his trunk muscles, his symptoms decrease. When he pushes his extended arms into the seat of the chair to unload his trunk his symptoms are slightly alleviated. These findings suggest that loading or compression of his spine contributes to his problem.

Sit to stand:

When the patient came to standing by sliding to the front of the chair and pushes up from the arm rests avoiding any lumbar flexion, his symptoms did not change.

Gait:

During gait he was observed to have lumbopelvic rotation at the end of terminal stance on the right but no other gait faults were observed.

Squatting:

When asked to squat at approximately 60–70° of hip flexion there was posterior tilt of his pelvis and associated lumbar flexion.

When asked to perform 1 leg kneeling (the hip extended and knee flexed on limb that is going down, while the other hip and knee are both flexed and are forward of the other leg) going to a 6-inch high step, he had increased left side bending when he goes down on the right knee. He had difficulty performing this motion but there was not an increase in his symptoms.

Diagnosis

The diagnosis for this patient is lumbar rotation-flexion. As stated previously, when the patient has symptoms with both flexion and extension, rotation is believed to be the cause of the problem. The patient had a prevalence of both symptoms and signs with flexion and rotation. An additional contributing factor is compression.

The test results supporting the diagnosis are:

Table 10–1 Test Results

Test	Flexion	Extension	Rotation
Alignment: flat back Right side > left	sign		sign
Forward bend	sign – symptom		
Side bending			sign – symptom
Rotation			sign
Single-leg standing			sign
Supine: Hip flex length			sign
Position			symptoms
Passive hip flexion	sign		
Active hip flexion			sign
Hip abd/lat rot			sign – symptom
Rolling			sign – symptom
Side lying: position			sign – symptom
Hip lat rot/abd			sign
Prone: position		symptom	symptom
Knee flexion			sign – symptom
Hip rotation			sign
Quadruped	sign – symptom		sign – symptom
Rocking backward	sign – symptom		sign – symptom
Sitting: position	sign – symptom		
Knee extension	sign – symptom		sign – symptom
Gait			sign

Lumbar compression is considered an additional factor. The patient's symptoms were decreased in the recumbent position, the therapist manually unloading his trunk, and the patient unloading his trunk by pushing into the seat of the chair when sitting. Clearly those tasks required by his job contribute to his lumbar problems such as the way he forward bends, side bends, rotates, and the limitations imposed by his knee joint problems.

Intervention

Initial treatment

The examination provides the information necessary to develop both the corrective exercise program and the appropriate modification of functional activities. The contributing factors are not specific muscle weakness as much as movement pattern coordination problems. Thus he has to learn how to move at specific joints in an optimal way as well as perform functional motions in an optimal manner. Typically when the patient has a positive test result, that same motion is used as the therapeutic exercise. Thus the patient is instructed in the correct performance of the exercises used during the examination, which means that there are no symptoms when performing the exercise. This also enables the patient to be "in charge" of his symptoms by understanding what motions cause or increase the symptoms and how to modify the motion to reduce or eliminate the symptoms. The emphasis is not on repetitions but on precise performance. Most often the patient is to perform between 6–10 repetitions of each exercise. The program is designed not to take more than 20 minutes. Usually as the patient learns how to perform the exercises correctly, he can do them more rapidly and add repetitions without adding to the time required to complete the program. The exercises are considered helpful in optimizing control of segments but are not expected to correct the performance of daily and functional activities. Considering the patient's occupation, he is instructed in forward bending at the hips and allowing his knees to flex as he bends forward. He will also practice the return from forward bending. He is instructed to side bend by tilting his shoulders rather than moving in his lumbar spine. Similarly he is encouraged to rotate his whole body by pivoting on the supporting surface or to move in his thoracic spine and not in his lumbar spine. The patient is to practice one leg kneeling to be used in his work. A 6-inch-high pad that he can use to kneel on is recommended. He is also told to wear loose pants in order to enable him to flex more easily in the hips rather than in the lumbar spine and to be able to flex his knee more easily than if the pants are tight and restrictive. The patient practices rolling without pain and walking with his hands on his hips to stop the lumbopelvic rotation. When he gets his symptoms, he is to get on his hands and knees and let his lumbar spine relax toward extension and then rock backward by pushing with his hands. He has to be sure the motion is hip flexion and not lumbar flexion. The patient is also instructed in correct sitting with a support behind his back and his hips back in the chair. The purpose is to avoid lumbar flexion rather than to increase lumbar extension. He should have supports under his arms and he should stand up every 30 minutes to change the loading on his spine. He is also encouraged to walk in the corrected manner for 15–20 minutes several times a day. When sleeping he is to use a folded towel at his waist and a pillow between his knees in side lying. He is also told that if any of the exercises cause pain he is to stop the exercise. The patient is told that he is to try to decrease or eliminate his symptoms as soon as they become exaggerated and not wait for them to increase in intensity until he has to cease his activity. The rationale is that if he keeps his symptoms to a minimum, the tissue irritability is minimized and healing is expedited. He is also correcting the cause of the tissue irritation.

Treatment progression

The patient will return in one week. His status will be assessed by asking about his symptoms and having him demonstrate his exercises. If his symptoms are decreased in intensity and frequency as is expected, he would start practicing movements involved in his occupation. He will be asked to describe the most common positions he uses when working so that any appropriate modifications can be made. The manner in which the patient picks up and carries his tools will be assessed. The weight of his tools will be incorporated into his practice motions. He will also be observed getting in and out of his car to be sure he is not rotating or flexing his back either when entering or leaving his car and that his car seat is keeping him out of lumbar flexion. The patient will be encouraged to lose weight because of the positive value for his lumbar spine problem but also for his knee pain.

Because of the requirement for him to work in a variety of positions, assessment of movement at his knees is also indicated. The shortness of his iliotibial band could be contributing to tibiofemoral rotation and he may be rotating in the knee joint while going up and down stairs as well as during sit to stand.

The patient will return again in a week at which time his exercise program will be reviewed and he will demonstrate his functional and work activities. If he continues to improve, he will return in 2 week intervals for 2 more visits and then in 1 month.

Prognosis

The patient is expected to do well because his symptoms are relatively low level and do not radiate into his lower extremities. His symptoms can be modified by correcting his movement impairments. His symptoms and signs fit a pattern.

His total number of visits is expected to be about 6, extending over about a 3 month period.

SUMMARY

LBP can be considered part of a progressive condition that is associated with tissue changes arising from mechanical stress and the tissue degeneration that occurs with aging. Mechanical stress on the lumbar spine can be the result of the pattern of movement of the spine as well as from demands imposed on the spine by the motion of the extremities. A variety of external and internal factors affect the rate and extent of the degenerative process that is associated with mechanical stress in addition to aging. This understanding of LBP means that the physical therapist's knowledge of kinesiology, anatomy, and motor control provides the basis to identify the tissue and movement impairments causing the LBP. As an expert in the movement system, the Movement System Impairment Syndromes approach dictates that the physical therapist perform an exam that identifies the movement direction that most consistently causes pain, the associated movement impairments, and the contributing factors (tissue adaptations). Support of the diagnosis is derived by correcting the impaired movement pattern and noting the affect on the symptoms. A systematic exam involving movement of the spine itself and importantly the extremities is used to make the diagnosis and to guide the treatment program.

REFERENCES

1. Sahrmann S. *Diagnosis and Treatment of Movement Impairment Syndromes.* St. Louis, MO:Mosby; 2002.
2. Merriam WF, Burwell RG, Mulholland RC, Pearson JC, Webb JK. A study revealing a tall pelvis in subjects with low back pain. *J Bone Joint Surg Br.* 1983:65(2):153–156
3. Hoffman SL, Harris-Hayes M, Van Dillen LR. Differences in activity limitation between 2 low back pain subgroups based on the movement system impairment model. *PM R.* 2010;2(12):1113–1118.
4. Scholtes SA, Norton BJ, Lang CE, Van Dillen LR. The effect of within-session instruction on lumbopelvic motion during a lower limb movement in people with and people without low back pain. *Man Ther.* 2010;15(5):496–501.
5. Harris-Hayes M, Holtzman GW, Earley JA, Van Dillen LR. Development and preliminary reliability testing of an assessment of patient independence in performing a treatment program: standardized scenarios. *J Rehabil Med.* 2010;42(3):221–227.

6. Harris-Hayes M, Van Dillen LR. The inter-tester reliability of physical therapists classifying low back pain problems based on the movement system impairment classification system. *PM R*. 2009;1(2):117–126.

7. Harris-Hayes M, Sahrmann SA, Van Dillen LR. Relationship between the hip and low back pain in athletes who participate in rotation-related sports. *J Sport Rehabil*. 2009;18(1):60–75.

8. Van Dillen LR, Bloom NJ, Gombatto SP, Susco TM. Hip rotation range of motion in people with and without low back pain who participate in rotation-related sports. *Phys Ther Sport*. 2008;9(2):72–81.

9. Scholtes SA, Gombatto SP, Van Dillen LR. Differences in lumbopelvic motion between people with and people without low back pain during two lower limb movement tests. *Clin Biomech* (Bristol, Avon). 2009;24(1):7–12.

10. Gombatto SP, Norton BJ, Scholtes SA, Van Dillen LR. Differences in symmetry of lumbar region passive tissue characteristics between people with and people without low back pain. *Clin Biomech* (Bristol, Avon). 2008;23(8):986–995.

11. Scholtes SA, Van Dillen LR. Gender-related differences in prevalence of lumbopelvic region movement impairments in people with low back pain. *J Orthop Sports Phys Ther*. 2007;37(12):744–753.

12. Gombatto SP, Klaesner JW, Norton BJ, Minor SD, Van Dillen LR. Validity and reliability of a system to measure passive tissue characteristics of the lumbar region during trunk lateral bending in people with and people without low back pain. *J Rehabil Res Dev*. 2008;45(9):1415–1429.

13. Van Dillen LR, Maluf KS, Sahrmann SA. Further examination of modifying patient-preferred movement and alignment strategies in patients with low back pain during symptomatic tests. *Man Ther*. 2009;14(1):52–60.

14. Gombatto SP, Collins DR, Sahrmann SA, Engsberg JR, Van Dillen LR. Patterns of lumbar region movement during trunk lateral bending in 2 subgroups of people with low back pain. *Phys Ther*. 2007;87(4):441–454.

15. Van Dillen LR, Gombatto SP, Collins DR, Engsberg JR, Sahrmann SA. Symmetry of timing of hip and lumbopelvic rotation motion in 2 different subgroups of people with low back pain. *Arch Phys Med Rehabil*. 2007;88(3):351–360.

16. Van Dillen LR, Sahrmann SA, Caldwell CA, McDonnell MK, Bloom N, Norton BJ. Trunk rotation-related impairments in people with low back pain who participated in 2 different types of leisure activities: a secondary analysis. *J Orthop Sports Phys Ther*. 2006;36(2):58–71.

17. Harris-Hayes M, Van Dillen LR, Sahrmann SA. Classification, treatment and outcomes of a patient with lumbar extension syndrome. *Physiother Theory Pract*. 2005;21(3):181–196.

18. Gombatto SP, Collins DR, Sahrmann SA, Engsberg JR, Van Dillen LR. Gender differences in pattern of hip and lumbopelvic rotation in people with low back pain. *Clin Biomech* (Bristol, Avon). 2006 Mar;21(3):263–271.

19. Van Dillen LR, Sahrmann SA, Wagner JM. Classification, intervention, and outcomes for a person with lumbar rotation with flexion syndrome. *Phys Ther*. 2005;85(4):336–351.

20. Van Dillen LR, Sahrmann SA, Norton BJ, Caldwell CA, McDonnell MK, Bloom NJ. Movement system impairment-based categories for low back pain: stage 1 validation. *J Orthop Sports Phys Ther*. 2003;33(3):126–142.

21. Van Dillen LR, Sahrmann SA, Norton BJ, Caldwell CA, McDonnell MK, Bloom N. The effect of modifying patient-preferred spinal movement and alignment during symptom testing in patients with low back pain: a preliminary report. *Arch Phys Med Rehabil*. 2003;84(3):313–322.

22. Van Dillen LR, Sahrmann SA, Norton BJ, Caldwell CA, Fleming D, McDonnell MK, Bloom NJ. Effect of active limb movements on symptoms in patients with low back pain. *J Orthop Sports Phys Ther*. 2001;31(8):402–413.

23. Maluf KS, Sahrmann SA, Van Dillen LR. Use of a classification system to guide nonsurgical management of a patient with chronic low back pain. *Phys Ther.* 2000;80(11):1097–1111.

24. Van Dillen LR, McDonnell MK, Fleming DA, Sahrmann SA. Effect of knee and hip position on hip extension range of motion in individuals with and without low back pain. *J Orthop Sports Phys Ther.* 2000;30(6):307–316.

25. Van Dillen LR, Sahrmann SA, Norton BJ, Caldwell CA, Fleming DA, McDonnell MK, Woolsey NB. Reliability of physical examination items used for classification of patients with low back pain. *Phys Ther.* 1998;78(9):979–988.

appendix one

Lower Quarter Examination

(*key test for low back diagnosis)

    A. STANDING
1. Appearance (size, structural proportions)
2. Alignment
3. Forward bending: corrected forward bending*
4. Return from forward bending: corrected return from forward bending*
5. Side bending; corrected side bending*
6. Rotation*
7. Back bending*
8. Single leg stance
9. Hip and knee flexion (partial squat) (LE)

    B. SITTING
1. Alignment (corrected vs. flexed or extended)*
2. Knee extension with dorsiflexion
3. Hip flexion (iliopsoas) muscle performance (LE)
4. Hip rotation (muscle performance and ROM) (LE)

    C. SUPINE
1. Bilateral hip and knee flexion (passive)*
2. Hip flexor length test
3. Position of hips and knees extended vs. hips and knees flexed*
4. Unilateral hip and knee flexion (passive and active)
5. Hip abduction/lateral rotation from flexion*
6. Lower abdominal muscle performance

Source: Shirley Sahrmann.

    7. Upper abdominal muscle performance (optional)

    8. SLR (passive and active)

    9. Iliopsoas muscle performance (LE)

  10. TFL-ITB muscle performance (LE)

D. SIDE LYING

    1. Position

    2. Hip lateral rotation/abduction

    3. Hip abduction

    4. Hip adduction (top LE and bottom LE)

    5. Modified Ober (LE)

    6. Hip abd/LR/ext (post. gluteus med.) muscle performance

E. PRONE

    1. Position (pillow vs. no pillow)*

    2. Knee flexion*

    3. Hip rotation*

    4. Hip extension with knee extended*

    5. Hip extension with the knee flexed (gluteus maximus) muscle performance

F. QUADRUPED

    1. Alignment (preferred vs. corrected)

    2. Rocking backward*

    3. Rocking forward*

    4. Shoulder flexion*

G. STANDING WITH BACK TO WALL

    1. Flatten back*

    2. Shoulder flexion

H. BASIC MOBILITY

    1. Rolling

    2. Supine to sit

    3. Sit to stand

    4. Gait

    5. Stairs

    6. Positions or movements specific to job or sport

LE: test item for hip, knee or foot syndrome

appendix two

Movement System Lower Quarter Examination

Source: Shirley Sahrmann.

Patient: _____ DOB: _____ Date: _____

PT with a diagnosis of _____

Referred by Dr. _____ on _____ for physical therapy.
Pt scheduled at his/her earliest convenience.

S: Pt is a _____ y/o M F with complaints of _____ that began _____.

Precipitating event _____ Previous episodes _____

Occupation _____ Fitness activity _____

Pain: Most common location: _____ Severity ___/10 Numbness/tingling Y N location _____
Rate: (0–10) Night _____   Supine _____   Prone _____   Sidelying _____
Rolling _____   Sitting _____   Standing _____   Walking _____
Upon arising _____   Morning _____   Afternoon _____   Evening _____

O: Past Medical History:
Surgeries: Accidents/injuries:

Medications: Precautions:

Body Type: Height: _____ Weight: _____ Build: _____

Posture: Thoracic: Normal _____ Kyphosis _____ Flat _____ Scoliosis _____ Asymmetry _____
Lumbar: Normal _____ Lordosis _____ Flat _____ Scoliosis _____ Asymmetry_____
Iliac crest level: Y N Higher: R L Symmetrical: Y N Describe: _____
Pelvic tilt: Y N Anterior _____ Posterior _____ Lateral Pelvic rotation: Y N Toward: R L
Genu varus: Y N Genu valgus: Y N

Standing Tests:
Forward bending: Pain: Y N lumbar flexion > < hip flexion
Hip flexion only: Pain: decreased - increased - same
Return from forward bending: Pain: Y N lumbar extension > < hip extension hip sway: Y N
Hip extension only: Pain: decreased - increased - same
Side bending: L- Pain: Y   N Asymmetry: Y N L > R Corrected: decreased - increased – same
R- Pain: Y   N Asymmetry: Y N R > L Corrected: decreased - increased – same
Rotation: L- Pain: Y N Asymmetry : Y N L > R Off axis: Y N
R- Pain: Y N Asymmetry: Y N   R > L Off axis: Y N
Stand on one leg: L- Trunk lateral bend: Y N Pelvic rotation: Y N Hip drop: Y N Med rot: Y N
R- Trunk lateral bend: Y N Pelvic rotation: Y N Hip drop: Y N Med rot: Y N

Supine Tests:
Hip flexor length: L-TFL ____ RF____IP____ R-TFL ____ RF____ IP____ Normal (n) Short (sh) Stiff (st)
Direction of susceptibility to movement: L-extension: Y N rotation: Y N
R-extension: Y N rotation: Y N
Hips and knees extended: Pain: Y N   L ____ R ____ Both ____
knee/lumbar support: decreased - increased – same
Hip extensor length: L - (n) (sh) (st) angle ____ Pain: Y N Groin pain: Y N Axis of rot faulty: Y N
R - (n) (sh) (st) angle ____ Pain: Y N Groin pain: Y N Axis of rot faulty: Y N
Active hip and knee flexion; L- Pain: Y N comp rotation: Y N Corrected: decreased - increased – same
R- Pain: Y N comp rotation: Y N Corrected: decreased - increased – same

Lower abs ____ / 5   Upper abs ____ / 5

Hip abd/lat rot from flexion: L- Pain: Y N Limited hip mvmt: Y N Compensatory rot.: Y N Groin pain: Y N

                        R- Pain: Y N Limited hip mvmt: Y N Compensatory rot.: Y N Groin pain: Y N

SLR: L ____ Neural Tension: Pain Y N active hold: Pain Y N axis of rotation faulty : Y N

       R ____ Neural Tension: Pain Y N active hold: Pain Y N axis of rotation faulty : Y N

Rolling: Pain: Y N Corrected: decreased - increased – same

Supine to sit: Pain: Y N Corrected: decreased - increased – same

Side Lying Tests:

Position: Pain: Y   N   Corrected: decreased - increased - same

Hip Lat.Rot./bent knee: L - Pain Y N Compensatory pelvic rot: Y N Corrected: decreased - increased - same

                        R - Pain Y N Compensatory pelvic rot: Y N Corrected: decreased - increased - same

Hip Abduction: L - Strength: ____/5 Pain: Y N Lateral pelvic tilt: Y N

              R - Strength:____/5 Pain: Y N Lateral pelvic tilt: Y N

Prone Tests:

Position: Pain: Y N corrected with pillow(s): decreased – increased - same How many? ____

Knee flexion: L - Pain: Y N ant. tilt: Y N pelvic rot.: Y N femoral rot: Y N Correct: decreased-increased-same

             R - Pain: Y N ant. tilt: Y N pelvic rot: Y N femoral rot: Y N Correct: decreased –increased-same

Hip rot: L- Pain: Y N Range: mr ____ lr____Wide arc: Y N comp.rotation: Y N

      Corrected: decreased-increased-same

      R- Pain: Y N Range: mr ____ lr____Wide arc: Y N comp.rotation: Y N

      Corrected: decreased-increased-same

Hip extension- knee extended: L- Pain: Y N lumbar ext.: Y N comp.rotation: Y N

                    Corrected: decreased- increased-same

                   R- Pain: Y N Lumbar ext: Y N comp.rotation: Y N

                    Corrected: decreased- increased-same

Hip extension- knee flexed: L- Pain: Y N lumbar ext: Y N Glut max strength: L ____/5

                  Hamstring dominance: Y N

                 R- Pain: Y N lumbar ext: Y N Glut max strength: R ____/5

                  Hamstring dominance: Y N

Hands-Knees:

Preferred Alignment : lumbar flex: Y N Lumbar rot: L R thoracic flex: Y N Thoracic rot: L R

In preferred position: Pain: Y N Corrected: decreased- increased-same

Rocking backward: Pain: Y N lumbar flex: Y N Lumbar rot: Y N Corrected: decreased- increased-same

Arm lifts: L- Pain: Y N lumbar rot: Y N thoracic rot: Y N Corrected: decreased- increased-same

         R-Pain: Y N lumbar rot: Y N thoracic rot: Y N Corrected: decreased- increased-same

Sitting:

Lumbar spine: flat   flexed extended Pain: Y N Corrected: decreased- increased-same

Knee extension: L-: Pain: Y N Hamstring Length: ____ Calf muscle length: ____ medial rot: Y N

          compensatory lumbar flexion: Y N lumbar rotation: Y N

          Corrected: decreased - increased - same

          R-: Pain: Y N Hamstring Length:____ Calf muscle length: _____ medial rot: Y N

          compensatory lumbar flexion: Y N lumbar rotation: Y N

          Corrected: decreased - increased - same

Iliopsoas strength: L- ____/5 hip rotation range: mr ____ lr ____ strength: mr ____/5 lr ____/5

             R- ____/5 hip rotation range: mr ____ lr ____ strength: mr ____/5 lr____/5

Sit to stand: Pain: Y N corrected: decreased - increased - same

Standing:

      Back to wall: Pain: Y N preferred position of lumbar spine: flat flexed extended fatten back: decreased-increased-same

               shoulder flexion: Pain: Y N compensatory lumbar ext.: Y N Corrected: decreased- increased-same

               chest expansion: at least 2 inches: Y N decreased with shoulder flex.: Y N

    Stairs: Pain: Y N Location:_____ Corrected: decreased- increased-same

    Compression symptoms: Y N Relief with decompression: Y N

Walking:

      Primary faults: _____ Corrected: decreased- increased-same

Other Observations: _____

A: Patient's signs, symptoms, test results consistent with a diagnosis for physical therapy of:

Lumbar: Extension   Rotation   Flexion   Rotation-Extension Rotation-Flexion Movement System

Impairment resulting in _____ with without radiating symptoms _____.

Femoral: anterior glide superior glide medial rotation lateral rotation accessory hypermobility adduction

Movement System Impairment resulting in _____ with muscle strain of _____ and/or weakness of _____.

Contributing Factors: _____.

Rehab Prognosis: poor fair good   excellent depending upon patient compliance.

Problem #1) Decreased function due to _____.

P: Pt to be seen ___ x/week/month for ___ weeks/ months: D/C: F/U: undetermined

        STG: 1.) Pt will be independent in HEP ×1 in 1 week

              2.) Pt will report ____% decrease in pain during _____ in _____ weeks.

        LTG: 1) Upon discharge pt will report min pain during _____ in _____ months.

Treatment Plan: HEP (see attached sheet) and education regarding correct movement patterns.

Patient participated in establishment of the above plan.   Treatment time: _____

Addendum: Treatment initiated. Problem #1 addressed with exercise and education.   Eval time: _____

                                                              Total time: _____

appendix three

Movement System Syndromes of the Low Back

Source: Shirley Sahrmann.

---

*No permission needed to duplicate

Name _____ M F   Hgt _____ Weight _____ Age _____ Date _____

Occupation _____   Fitness Activity _____

Structural Characteristics _____

Pain Location: _____

Position	Test	Segment	Impairment	Ext	Rot	Flex
Standing		spine	Pain			
	Alignment	Thoracic	Kyphosis	E		
			Flat			F
			Swayback	E		
			Asymmetry R L		R	
		Lumbar	Lordosis	E		
			Flat/flex			F
			Asymmetry R L		R	
		Pelvis	Anterior tilt	E		
			Posterior tilt			F
			Lateral tilt		R	
	Forward bend (Fb)	Spine	Pain			F
	Corrected F b		Pain Y N <			F
	Return F b		Pain	E		
			Lumbar ext	E		
	Corrected return		Pain Y N <	< E		
	Side bending		Pain		R	
			Asymmetry		R	
	Rotation		Pain		R	
			Asymmetry		R	
	Single-leg Stand		Spine rotation		X	
			Hip drop		X	
Total						

Comments:

_____
*No permission needed to duplicate

Position	Test	Segment	Impairment	Ext	Rot	Flex
Supine	Hip flexor lgth compensation	Lumbopelvic	Anterior tilt	E		
			TFL short/stiff		R	
			Flex short/stiff	E		
			R L asymmetrical		R	
	Position	LE extended	Pain < = >	> E		<**F**
		LE flexed	Pain < = >	< E		>**F**
		Support L spine	Pain < = >	>E		<**F**
	Hip-knee flexion	Lumbopelvic	pain	E	R	
			Pelvic rotation		R	
	Hip abd/lateral rot	Lumbopelvic	Pain		R	
			Pelvic rotation		R	
	Abdominal muscles	Pelvis	< 2/5	E		
			> 2/5			
Sidelying	Position	L spine	Pain		R	
	Support at waist	L spine	Pain < = >		R	
	Hip lateral rotation	Lumbopelvic	Pain		R	
			Pelvic rotation		R	
	Hip abductor MMT	lumbopelvic	Pain		R	
			Weak/long			
	Hip abd/add active	lumbopelvic	Lateral pelvic tilt		R	
Total						

Comments:

---

*No permission needed to duplicate

Position	Test	Segment	Impairment	Ext	Rot	Flex
Prone	Position	Lumbopelvic	pain	E		
	Support under abdomen		Pain < = >	<E		>F
	Knee flexion	Lumbopelvic	Pain	E		
	Hip lateral rotation	Lumbopelvic	Pain		R	
			Pelvic rotation		R	
	Hip medial rotation	Lumbopelvic	Pain		R	
			Pelvic rotation		R	
Quadruped	Position	Lumbopelvic	Pain			
		Alignment	Lumbar flexion			F
			Lumbar rotation		R	
			Thoracic flexion	E		
			Thoracic rotation		R	
	Rocking backward	Lumbar	Pain			F
			Flexion			F
			Rotation		R	
			Extension	E		
	Shoulder flexion	Lumbar	Pain		R	
			Rotation		R	
Sitting	Flexed	Lumbar	Pain			F
	Flat		Pain			F
	Extended		Pain	E		
	Knee extension	Lumbopelvic	Pain			F
			Flexion-rotation		R	F
Standing	Resting L-spine on wall	Lumbopelvic	Pain < = >	<E		>F
	Shoulder flexion		Pain < = >	>E		
Gait	gait	Lumbopelvic	Pain		R	
			Pelvic rotation		R	
			Hip drop		R	
			L-spine extension	E		
Total						

Comments:

---

*No permission needed to duplicate

Diagnosis for Physical Therapy: flexion; extension; rotation; rotation-extension; rotation-flexion

Contributing factors:

Functional activities needing modification

Walking

Standing

Sitting

Recumbent
Position

Rolling

Work arrangement

Recreational/fitness activities

Symptom modification activities

Contract abdominals

Back against wall

Sitting

Quadruped

Recumbent: supine   prone

Key exercises

---

*No permission needed to duplicate

chapter eleven

A Treatment-Based Classification Approach

Paul E. Mintken, PT, DPT, OCS, FAAOMPT
Mark D. Bishop, PT, PhD

The treatment-based classification approach is an evidence-based approach that was originally conceived and described by Anthony Delitto, Rick Bowling, and Dick Erhard in 1995. These researchers and clinicians developed a scheme for management of low back pain through a systematic examination and subsequent classification of patients. Since it was first proposed, the approach has been the basis of a substantial body of research and has been applied across a number of clinical settings.

Students interested in learning more about this approach are encouraged to explore the continuing education offerings of a group called Evidence in Motion at www.evidenceinmotion.com.

BACKGROUND

The Treatment Based Classification (TBC)[1] and staging system incorporates differential diagnosis, identification of red and yellow flags that may require referral, and aims to identify specific subgroups of patients that respond to specific physical therapy interventions. The beauty of this system is that it is fluid, patients can move between classifications as their presentation changes, and the approach is constantly evolving as new evidence emerges. This approach evolved as a result of the limitations of the pathoanatomical model's inability to determine a definitive diagnosis in patients with low back pain (LBP). The medical model has failed miserably when it comes to LBP, as identifying relevant pathology is only possible 10–15% of the time.[2,3] LBP is a heterogeneous condition. If research has taught us anything, it is that it is not reasonable to expect any one intervention to be useful for all patients with LBP.

The classification system proposed by Delitto et al.[1] was developed for "stage I" patients with moderate to high levels of disability, including acute LBP. It is not intended for patients with chronic LBP, although it can still be a useful model for guiding initial interventions. If the patient does not have a moderate level of pain and disability, they are put into "stage II" or "stage III" and the therapist focuses on treating identified impairments and functional limitations. See Table 11–1 for a brief description of the staging criteria for the TBC. The patient is initially screened for red flags (potential medical or systemic issues that may require referral) and yellow flags (potential medical or psychosocial issues that may require referral) (See Figure 11–1).

It is beyond the scope of this chapter to review potential red flags that would contraindicate treatment, but a brief review of the biopsychosocial model of LBP and yellow flags are important, as many of these variables have direct impact on the classification and treatment of patients with LBP.

Biopsychosocial Model of Low Back Pain

Waddell[4] proposed a biopsychosocial model for the management of LBP. This model took into account the influence of physical, psychological, and social factors in patients with LBP and recognized that LBP is more like an illness than a pathoanatomic diagnosis (Figure 11–2). The identification of a "pain generator" is an exercise in futility as many asymptomatic people have pathoanatomy on imaging.[5–9] Successfully treating patients with LBP requires that the clinician take into account both physical and psychosocial factors.

Table 11–1 Staging of Patients Based on the Treatment-Based Classification

Stage I	Stage II	Stage III
Oswestry > 30%	Oswestry 15–30%	Oswestry < 15%
Unable to sit > 30 minutes	Able to sit, stand, walk	Able to perform complex tasks
Unable to stand > 15 minutes	Unable to perform complex tasks	Unable to perform demanding tasks
Unable to walk > 0.25 mile	No stage I findings	

Source: Adapted from Delitto A, Erhard RE, Bowling RW. A treatment-based classification approach to low back syndrome: identifying and staging patients for conservative treatment. *Phys Ther.* 1995;75(6):470-485; discussion 485-479.

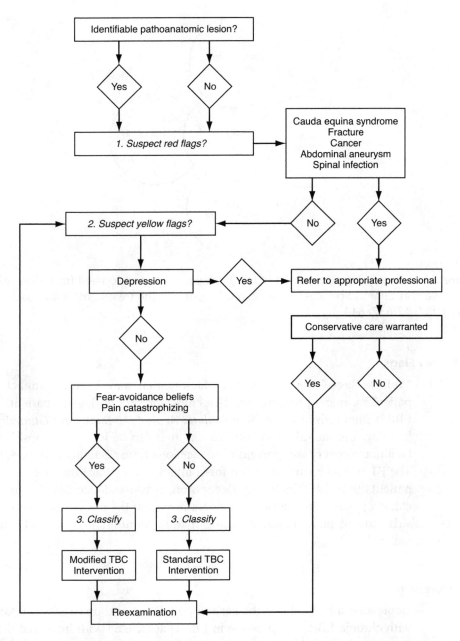

Figure 11–1 Overview of differential diagnosis and classification process for low back pain. *Source:* Modified with permission from Magee, D., Zachazewski, J., and Quillen, W., *Pathology and Intervention in Musculoskeletal Rehabilitation,* 1st Edition. Saunders Book Company, 2008.

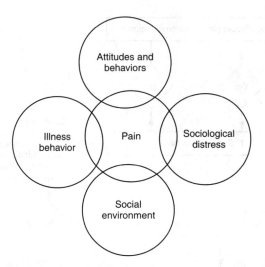

Figure 11–2 Biopsychosocial model of low back pain. *Source:* Modified from Waddell G. Volvo Award in Clinical Sciences: A new clinical model for the treatment of low-back pain, *Spine,* 1987; 12:632–644.

Yellow Flags

"Yellow flags," are psychosocial factors that may have an impact on a patient's clinical presentation. Screening for yellow flags in patients with LBP is summarized in the *New Zealand Acute Low Back Pain Guide:*[10] Yellow flags are identified to "find factors that can be influenced positively to facilitate recovery and prevent or reduce long-term disability and work loss." The PT should routinely screen for common yellow flags that are present in patients with LBP, including depression, fear-avoidance beliefs, and pain catastrophizing. In addition, consideration about the presence of central sensitization of pain should be made if the symptoms are more chronic in nature.[11,12]

Depression

Depression affects 6% of the general population and up to 20% of patients with chronic LBP.[13] Depression in LBP is associated with increased disability, pain, medication use, and unemployment.[14] Effective screening for depression involves more than clinical intuition, as research has shown this approach is not sensitive enough to identify depression in patients with

LBP.[15] Two specific questions from the Primary Care Evaluation of Mental Disorders Patient Questionnaire are extremely sensitive for screening patients for depression.[15] The questions are (1) "During the past month, have you often been bothered by feeling down, depressed, or hopeless?" and (2) "During the past month, have you often been bothered by little interest or pleasure in doing things?" Arroll et al.,[16] reporting on the use of the 2 question screen in patients seeing a primary care provider, found that the 2 screening questions had a sensitivity of 97%, a specificity of 67%, a likelihood ratio for a positive test was 2.9, and the likelihood ratio for a negative test was 0.05. An answer of yes to either question should raise the suspicion of depression while answering no to both questions lowers the probability of depression.

Fear-avoidance beliefs

Fear-avoidance beliefs relate to a patient's fear related to the LBP condition and how work and physical activity affects the condition, and how the patient feels the condition should be managed.[17–20] Patients with elevated fear-avoidance beliefs tend to take a conservative approach to managing back pain, and avoid any activities that they think will make the pain worse. This leads to the development of an exaggerated perception of pain and chronic disability.[17] Waddell[20] stated that the "fear of pain and what we do about it may be more disabling than pain itself." Fear-avoidance beliefs can be predictive of the development of chronic LBP.[21–24] The Fear-Avoidance Beliefs Questionnaire (FABQ) is the current gold standard for assessing fear-avoidance beliefs.[20] Multiple studies have shown that the FABQ is a reliable, valid, and responsive measure in clinical settings.[25–32] The FABQ has 16 items, which are scored on a scale from 0 (strongly disagree) to 6 (strongly agree). Five of these items are designed as distracters in the questionnaire and are not included in the scoring. The FABQ has two subscales: a seven-item (items 6, 7, 9–12, and 15) work subscale (FABQ-W; score range, 0–42) for fear-avoidance beliefs about work, and a four-item (items 2–5) physical activity subscale (FABQ-PA; score range, 0–24) for fear-avoidance beliefs about physical activity. Higher scores represent higher levels of fear-avoidance beliefs.

Fritz et al.[21] reported that the work subscale of the FABQ is an effective screen for return to work in patients with work-related LBP. Patients who scored higher than 34 on the FABQ-W were less likely to return to work by 4 weeks (positive likelihood ratio 3.3) while patients who scored lower than

29 on the FABQ-W were more likely to return to work (negative likelihood ration 0.08). Crombez et al.[33] suggest that a FABQ-PA of greater than 15 should be considered an elevated score, but this requires further validation. George et al.[24] reported that general orthopedic patients with elevated an FABQ-W score greater than 29 reported higher self-reported disability at 6-months scores, and were more likely to have reported no improvement in disability. If a patient presents with elevated fear-avoidance beliefs, treatment should shift from a traditional management model to one of teaching the patient to confront their fears using a cognitive behavioral approach with graded exercise and graded exposure.[34–45]

Pain catastrophizing

Pain catastrophizing in LBP is a belief that doing activities that cause pain will lead to the worst possible outcome.[46] Sullivan et al.[46] defined catastrophizing as an "exaggerated negative 'mental set' brought to bear during painful experiences." Catastrophizing leads to increased emotional distress and a more intense pain experience. Pain catastrophizing during acute LBP predicted self-reported disability at 6 months and 1 year.[47,48] Pain catastrophizing is commonly measured using a reliable and valid scale, the 13-item Pain Catastrophizing Scale (PCS).[49,50] The scale includes questions such as "I worry all the time about whether the pain will end," and the scale ranges from 1 (not at all) to 4 (always) with scores ranging from 0–52. Since no cutoffs have been defined for the PCS, we use a score of greater than 31 as a cutoff, as this has been reported to exceed the 75th percentile and suggests that a patient may be at risk for having chronic disability from musculoskeletal pain (http://pdp-pgap.com/en//index.html).

Central sensitization

Chronic pain and psychosocial distress can lead to a condition known as a central sensitized pain state.[12,51–53] "Central sensitization" is defined as a condition in which peripheral noxious inputs into the central nervous system lead to an increased excitability where the response to normal inputs is greatly enhanced.[51] The central nervous system becomes "hyperexcitable" due to a combination of increased responsiveness and decreased inhibition.[54] This is analogous to the volume being turned up on the system such that normally innocuous stimuli generate painful sensations and noxious stimuli cause an exaggerated pain response.

Central sensitization has been described as a change in both the software and the hardware of the central nervous system[54] such that the cellular depolarization threshold is reduced.[55] Cellular activity continues after peripheral nociception stops and this cellular activity spreads to other neighboring cells.[56] In a person with central sensitization of pain, nociceptive cells may begin to depolarize with input from primary afferent mechanoreceptors, which are normally low threshold.[57] In other words, pain is perceived in the presence of input that is normally not perceived as noxious. In the "centrally sensitized" patient with chronic LBP this may lead to the perception of LBP, even in the presence of normal stimuli such as movement or pressure.

PTs can have an impact on pain sensitivity through ion channels. Although the complexity of ion channel regulation is not completely understood, and most of the research has been conducted on animal models, clinicians are using the information known about ion channels to improve care for patients with chronic pain.[58,59] Ion channels are basically proteins lumped together with a gate to allow ions to flow in/out of a membrane.[60,61] Ion channels do not have a uniform distribution along the axolemma, as certain areas have higher concentrations, including the DRG, nodes of Ranvier, axon hillocks, and regions of the axon that have lost myelin.[60–64] There are countless types of ion channels; some are sensitive to movement, temperature, pressure, blood flow, etc. From a survival perspective, this is an effective means for the nervous system to become "sensitive" to various stimuli. The type and amount of ion channels found in the axolemma is in a constant state of change.[60,61,63] The half-life of some ion channels may be as short as 2 days,[59] and ion channels that disappear are not always replaced by the same type. In fact, ion channel synthesis is directly impacted by the environment,[59] such that lowering the temperature around an animal with experimentally removed myelin produces higher concentrations of "cold-sensing" channels in that area; while animals in stressful environments produce higher concentrations of adrenosensitive channels, and animals that have joints with restricted movement cause upregulation of movement sensitive ion channels.[60,61,63,64] Higher concentrations of similar ion channels in an area increases the likelihood that a nerve will depolarize and create an action potential, and these areas become abnormal impulse generators.[61,65–68] The nervous system then becomes sensitized to all types of stimuli (movement, pressure, temperature, anxiety, stress) and these normally nonpainful stimuli now evoke a pain experience.[58,64] Suggestions for clinically identifying central sensitization in patients with persistent pain have been developed.[69]

Central sensitization commonly manifests clinically as widespread hypersensitivity to touch, temperature, sound, light, smell, and mechanical loading of tissues. Clinical tests to assess for this hypersensitivity include assessment of pressure pain thresholds, manual palpation, neurodynamic tests, temperature, accessory motions, and vibration at sites remote from the symptomatic site.[69] The key point for clinicians to keep in mind is that ion channels can turn over every few days. If we can get the patient with chronic pain moving in a nonpainful and nonthreatening way, we may be able to change the amount and type of ion channels and hence have an impact on activities that may evoke a pain response. For further information, the reader is directed to the work of David Butler.[58,70,71]

Identification of Subgroups

Identifying the yellow flags will allow the clinician to identify patients that may be appropriate for referral because of depression, elevated fear, or those who have an increased risk of experiencing chronic disability. Missing these signs may lead the patient down the road to a chronic pain state. If the patient is a candidate for PT, the therapist completes an examination that includes the history and tests and measures, and based on key signs and symptoms, places the patient into one of four classification categories: specific exercise, manipulation, stabilization, or traction. The specific criteria for placing a patient into one of these classifications has evolved over the years with the emergence of newer evidence. The current criteria along with proposed interventions are outlined in Table 11–2.[72] The current algorithm for examination and classification is outlined in Figure 11–3.[72]

Several LBP classifications have been described in the literature, for a detailed review the reader is directed to an article by Riddle[73] in which he compares the Quebec Task Force on Spinal Disorder (QTFSD) system, the Bernard and Kirkaldy-Willis classification, the McKenzie approach, and the TBC.

The interrater reliability of the TBC has been reported to be low ($\kappa = 0.14–0.45$)[74] to moderate ($\kappa = 0.56$).[75] The predictive, prescriptive and discriminant validity of the TBC has also been investigated.[75–79] Several randomized controlled trials have also reported prescriptive validity for the TBC in that classification based treatment resulted in better short term outcome compared to generic exercise prescription[76,80] or guideline-based treatment.[77]

Table 11-2 Proposed Classification Criteria and Interventions for the Treatment-Based Classification

Classification	Current Classification Criteria	Proposed Intervention Procedures
Manipulation	• No symptoms distal to the knee • Recent onset of symptoms (< 16 days) • Low FABQ-W score (< 19) • Hypomobility of the lumbar spine • Hip internal rotation ROM (35° for at least 1 hip)	• Manipulation of the lumbopelvic region • Active ROM exercises
Stabilization	• Younger age (< 40 y) • Greater general flexibility (postpartum, average SLR ROM 0.91°) • "Instability catch" or aberrant movements during lumbar flexion/extension ROM • Positive findings for the prone instability test • For patients who are postpartum: • Positive posterior pelvic pain provocation (P4), and ASLR and modified Trendelenburg tests • Pain provocation with palpation of the long dorsal sacroiliac ligament or pubic symphysis	• Promoting isolated contraction and cocontraction of the deep stabilizing muscles (multifidus, transversus abdominus) • Strengthening of large spinal stabilizing muscles (erector spinae, oblique abdominals)
Specific Exercise Extension	• Symptoms distal to the buttock • Symptoms centralize with lumbar extension • Symptoms peripheralize with lumbar flexion • Directional preference for extension	• End-range extension exercises • Mobilization to promote extension • Avoidance of flexion activities

(continued)

Table 11–2 Proposed Classification Criteria and Interventions for the Treatment-Based Classification (continued)

Classification	Current Classification Criteria	Proposed Intervention Procedures
Flexion	• Older age (> 50 y) • Symptoms centralize with lumbar flexion • Directional preference for flexion • Imaging evidence of lumbar spinal stenosis	• Mobilization or manipulation of the spine and/or lower extremities • Exercise to address impairments of strength or flexibility • Body weight-supported treadmill ambulation
Lateral shift	• Visible frontal plane deviation of the shoulders relative to the pelvis • Directional preference for lateral translation movements of the pelvis	• Exercises to correct lateral shift • Mechanical traction
Traction	• Presence of sciatica • Signs of nerve root compression • Positive crossed straight leg raise test • Failure to demonstrate centralization on clinical examination (especially peripheralization with extension)	• Mechanical traction • Progress to exercises favoring directional preference when symptoms stabilize

Source: Modified with permission from Fritz JM, Cleland JA, Childs JD. Subgrouping patients with low back pain: evolution of a classification approach to physical therapy. *J Orthop Sports Phys Ther.* 2007;37(6):290–302.

Classification of Specific Low Back Pain Subgroups

Manipulation classification

Manipulation has been used to treat back pain for thousands of years.[81] Several randomized controlled trials have reported that manipulation is an effective treatment for back pain,[80,82–87] while others have found that manipulation is not more effective than other treatments.[88–91] Systematic reviews and meta-analyses are also mixed on the effectiveness of manipulation for LBP.[92–100] The inconsistency of the research evidence suggests that manipulation may be most effective for a subgroup of patients.[93] The TBC approach attempts to identify the patients who may benefit from manipulation. Prior to recent evidence, determining if a patient was a candidate for manipulation relied on expert opinion and the identification of structural asymmetries.[101–104] Unfortunately, many of the theories and clinical tests

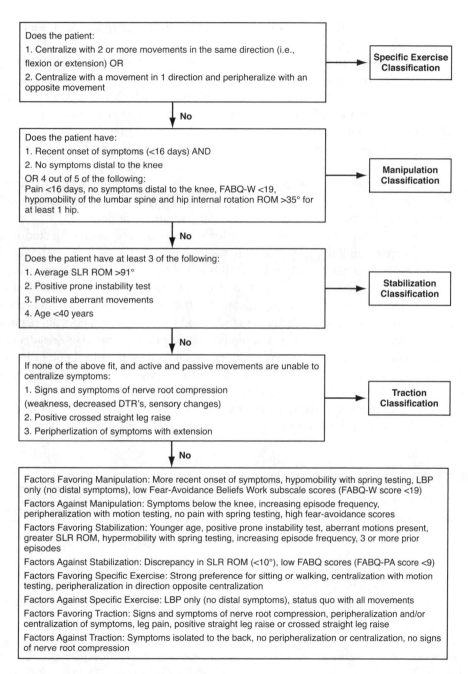

Figure 11–3 Algorithm for determining subgroup.

used to identify patients that may benefit from manipulation are either not valid or are unreliable.[84,105–113] Flynn et al.[84] developed a clinical prediction rule (CPR) purported to accurately identify a subgroup of patients likely to benefit from manipulation using an extensive history and physical examination. Five variables were reliable predictors of which patients would experience at least a 50% improvement in their scores on the Oswestry Disability Index. A patient with at least four out of five of these variables has over a 95% chance of success. The five variables included a duration of symptoms < 16 days, no symptoms distal to the knee, a Fear-Avoidance Beliefs Questionnaire Work (FABQ-W) subscale score of less than 19, at least one hip with > 35° internal rotation, and hypomobility in the lumbar spine assessed via central posterior-anterior vertebral pressures (Table 11–3).[84]

CPRs are not recommended for widespread use until subjected to prospective validation.[114] This CPR was subsequently tested and validated in a randomized controlled trial.[83] Childs et al.[83] reported that patients with LBP who were positive on the CPR and were treated with the manipulation combined with exercise had significantly better outcomes than patients receiving exercise alone, while the patients who had two or fewer factors almost always failed to respond to the manipulation intervention. To put these results in perspective, if a patient presents with at least 4 factors, the likelihood of improvement increases to above 92%, while patients with 2 or less of the identified variables would only respond dramatically to manipulation 9% of the time.

Clinical implementation of the five item CPR may be limited, as it requires the use of the FABQ as well as an inclinometer. Fritz et al.[115] subsequently

Table 11–3 Validated clinical prediction rule for manipulation classification

Examination Finding	Positive Definition
Duration of current low back pain episode	Less than 16 days
Presence of leg pain	Symptoms proximal to knee
Fear-avoidance beliefs questionnaire (work scale)	Less than 19/42
Lumbar spine mobility testing (prone)	One or more hypomobile segments
Hip internal rotation	At least one hip with internal rotation greater than 35°

*At least 4/5 positive examination findings constitute a positive clinical prediction rule (+likelihood ratio = 13.2) and fewer than 3/5 positive examination findings constitute a negative clinical prediction rule (−likelihood ratio = 0.10).

Source: Flynn T, Fritz J, Whitman J, et al. A clinical prediction rule for classifying patients with low back pain who demonstrate short-term improvement with spinal manipulation. Spine. 2002;27(24):2835-2843.

developed a "pragmatic" two factor rule. The 2 factors included a symptom duration of less than 16 days and no symptoms distal to the knee (patients must also not have signs of nerve root compression). In this retrospective review, 29% of 141 subjects who received manipulation presented with these 2 criteria, and 85.4% of those had greater than a 50% reduction in their ODI at 1 week. The high specificity of 0.92 and positive likelihood ratio of 7.2 suggest that patients with these 2 criteria and no contraindications to lumbopelvic manipulation should have this intervention. The presence of these two factors accurately predicts status on the five criteria rule.[116]

Fritz et al.[117] went on to further strengthen the validity of the rule by reporting that patients who had less than three out of five predictors were much less likely to experience a successful outcome. Cleland et al.[86] supported the generalizability of the CPR by comparing the outcomes of patients who were randomly assigned to receive one of three manual therapy techniques for two consecutive treatment sessions followed by a strengthening program for an additional three sessions. Pair-wise comparisons revealed no differences between the Flynn et al.[84] supine manipulation and a side-lying rotational manipulation[118] at any follow-up period. Significant differences existed in the ODI and NPRS at every follow-up between the thrust manipulation groups and an oscillatory mobilization group at 1 week and 4 weeks. A significant difference was also noted in ODI scores at 6 months in favor of the manipulation groups. The results of this study support the generalizability of the CPR to different patients and settings from which it was derived and validated. This supports the previous findings of a case series by Cleland et al.[118] in which 11 of the 12 patients (92%) who satisfied the CPR and were treated with a side-lying rotational manipulation had a 50% reduction in ODI scores in 2 visits. Based on these studies, patients with LBP who satisfy the CPR may be expected to have a significant reduction in disability with either manipulation technique, and it may be a neurophysiological mechanism that results in these changes.[119–123]

Traditionally, determining which patients needed manipulation has relied heavily on biomechanical theory, mobility assessments, and detailed treatment paradigms. When Flynn et al.[84] set out to develop the CPR, they hypothesized special tests based on the osteopathic model would be important classification criteria. This did not turn out to be the case, and many of these special tests lack reliability and validity. One of the strongest predictors for the CPR was duration of symptoms and absence of leg pain,[84,124] and this correlates well with research from chiropractic studies.[125,126] Biomechanical theories have also traditionally supported the use of specific techniques for specific regions or dysfunctions.[101,127] The notion that a specific technique is required for a specific dysfunction has recently been challenged.[86,128–130] Practitioners, may try to target interventions to specific areas, but evidence shows that this is not as accurate as is popularly believed.[131,132,133]

Stabilization classification

Spinal instability was originally described as a condition in which adjacent vertebra move excessively, and the proposed treatment was surgery or immobilization.[134–136] Lumbar instability is purported to be determined by measuring excessive amounts of motion, such as > 4.5 mm sagittal plane translation or $> 15\%$ translation of the vertebral body width in the sagittal plane during flexion/extension X-ray films.[134,135,137] The validity of the radiographic classification of instability is questionable, as there is significant variation in spinal motion in asymptomatic individuals.[138,139] The original TBC proposed in 1995[1] included a classification labeled "immobilization," embracing the definition of excessive vertebral movement. As "instability" is an elusive and hard to define term, research is moving away from the concept of instability and moving towards the concept of spinal stabilization. Panjabi[140] originally described three subsystems responsible for stability of the spine. The bones, discs, and ligaments comprise the passive subsystem, while the muscles and tendons comprise the active subsystem. The central and peripheral nervous system comprises the neural subsystem, which is purported to direct the active subsystem to provide the needed stability. Physical therapists have been guilty of labeling patients as "unstable," when, in fact, it may simply be that the neural subsystem is not doing its job of telling the active subsystem how and when to turn on.[141] Hodges et al.[141] reported that early activation of transversus abdominis (TrA) and obliquus internus abdominis (OI) occurred prior to activation of the deltoid during rapid arm movement in patients without LBP, while subjects with LBP failed to recruit TrA or OI. This would suggest that patients with LBP have an altered neural subsystem and may benefit from stabilization exercises. Unfortunately, numerous randomized controlled trials report conflicting results.[142–146] As with manipulation, there may be a subgroup of patients that may benefit from stabilization exercises.

The initial TBC of Delitto et al.[1] proposed that the history of patients in the stabilization subgroup would include items such as trauma, pregnancy, frequent episodes of LBP, and short-term success with manipulation or immobilization of the spine with belts or corsets. Expert opinion at that time recommended avoiding end-range positions of the spine and bracing for more severe cases, along with spinal muscle stabilization exercises.

Controversy exists as to what constitutes a "state-of-the-art" lumbar stabilization program. It is clear that this classification has evolved from avoiding motion (immobilization) to controlling motion (stabilization). A significant body of work has arisen out of Australia focusing on the importance of the local lumbar stabilizers such as the transversus abdominus and the lumbar multifidus.[141,147–155] These authors have reported that impaired firing of these muscles is almost universal in patients with LBP, and the ability of these muscles to fire normally does not spontaneously recover.[141,145,147,150,153] This line of thinking has support from randomized clinical trials that have demonstrated that this exercise approach leads to better outcomes.[143,152,156–158]

This approach is in contrast to the theories of Stuart McGill and others[142,145,159–163] who believe that exercises focused on improving the strength and endurance of larger spinal muscles is more functional and optimizes outcomes. Koumantakis et al.[142] reported on 67 subjects with LBP who were randomized to either a specific retraining group or a general strengthening group. Superior outcomes were reported for the general strengthening group at 8 weeks, with no between-group differences at 5 months. Cairns et al.[145] reported on 97 subjects with LBP who were randomized to receive specific muscle retraining or conventional physical therapy. The specific muscle retraining group also received instruction in firing the transversus abdominus and multifidus combined with real-time ultrasound feedback. There were no significant differences between groups at 3 and 12 month follow ups. The proponents of the specific retraining approach would counter with an article by Hides et al.[152] in which 39 subjects were randomized to either a control group or a specific retraining program targeting the transversus abdominus and multifidus. Two to 3 years after treatment, the subjects in the specific exercise group had a recurrence rate of 35% while the control group had a recurrence rate of 75%. It is unknown whether the general strengthening program would result in the same decrease in recurrence rates. At this time, it is unclear which stabilization approach, specific versus general, is best for patients with LBP.

A CPR has been derived in an initial attempt to identify stabilization classification patients who may benefit from a stabilization program.[160] The rule is composed of variables that predicted a 50% improvement in disability from LBP. Four examination findings were identified (Table 11–4): aberrant movements during sagittal plane lumbar ROM; age < 40 years; average straight-leg raise (SLR) range of motion (ROM) greater than 91° and a positive prone instability test (PIT). Patients were considered positive on the rule if they had 3 of the 4 variables (+LR, 4; 95% CI, 1.6–10). The presence of 3 variables shifted the post-test probability of success to 80%

Table 11–4 Preliminary Clinical Prediction Rule for Stabilization Classification*

Examination Finding	Positive Definition
Age	Less than 40 years old
Lumbar flexion observation (standing)	Aberrant movement pattern noted
Straight leg raise range of motion (supine)	Average (R + L)/2 is greater than 91°
Prone instability test	Decrease in pain when posteroanterior pressure is applied during muscle contraction

*At least 3/4 positive examination findings constitute a positive clinical prediction rule (+likelihood ratio = 4.0).

(assuming a pretest probability of 50%). The predictive ability of this CPR is not as strong as the manipulation CPR, and it has not yet been validated. A negative CPR was also derived that identified which patients would not achieve the minimal clinically important difference on the ODI following a stabilization intervention. Twenty five percent of the subjects in this trial failed to meet the minimal clinically important difference. The negative CPR is defined as the presence of 3 of the following findings: 1) absence of aberrant movements, 2) a negative prone instability test, absence of lumbar hypermobility, and 3) a score of less than 9 on the FABQ physical activity subscale. If the patient has 3 of the 4 variables in the negative CPR, this shifts the pretest probability of failure from 25% to a post-test probability of failure of 86%. Thus these patients may not be good candidates from the lumbar stabilization intervention described by Hicks et al.[160]

Further work has been done that identifies women who are postpartum and experiencing posterior pelvic girdle pain who are likely to benefit from lumbopelvic stabilization interventions.[164–166] A composite of tests has been proposed, including the active SLR,[166] a positive posterior pelvic pain provocation test,[165,166] pain in the symphysis pubis with palpation,[165] pain to palpation in the long dorsal sacroiliac ligament,[166] and a positive modified Trendelenburg test[165] (Table 11–5).[72]

The findings of the mentioned studies make sense from a "stabilization" standpoint. Patients who need spinal stabilization exercises tend to be more flexible with increased intervertebral active and passive motions with compromised dynamic stabilization. While these findings are encouraging and can help clinicians postulate who might need this intervention, this classification requires further research and refinement.

Table 11–5 Additional Examination Items Proposed to Identify Postpartum Women with Posterior Pelvic Girdle Pain Who May Benefit from Stabilization Interventions

Examination	Description of the Test
Posterior pelvic pain provocation (P4) test[165,166]	The patient is supine. The therapist passively flexes the patient's hip to 90° and applies a posteriorly directed force through the longitudinal axis of the femur. The test is positive if the patient reports a deep pain in the gluteal area during the test.
Active straight-leg raise test[166]	The patient is supine with straight legs and feet 20cm apart. The patient is instructed to lift the legs one after the other approximately 20 cm above the table without bending the knee. The patient is asked to score the difficulty of the task on a 6-point scale (0, no difficulty at all; 1, minimally difficult; 2, somewhat difficult; 3, fairly difficult; 4, very difficult; 5, unable to do). Any score greater than 0 is a positive test.
Provocation of the long dorsal sacroiliac ligament[166]	The patient is supine. The therapist palpates the long dorsal sacroiliac ligament bilaterally. A positive test occurs if at least 1 side is painful, and the pain persists at least 5 seconds after the removal of the therapist's hand.
Provocation of the pubic symphysis with palpation[165]	With the patient in supine the entire front side of the pubic symphysis is palpated gently. If the palpation causes pain that persists more than 5 seconds after the removal of the therapist's hand, it is recorded as positive.
Modified Trendelenburg test[165]	The therapist is behind the standing patient. The patient is asked to stand on one foot while flexing the opposite knee and hip to 90°. The test is positive if the hip descends on the flexed side.

Source: Modified with permission from Fritz JM, Cleland JA, Childs JD. Subgrouping patients with low back pain: evolution of a classification approach to physical therapy. *J Orthop Sports Phys Ther.* 2007;37(6):290–302.

Specific-exercise classification

The specific exercise classification is an evidence-based synthesis of the pioneering work of McKenzie.[167,168] Delitto et al.[1] used the Mckenzie principles to develop a classification that identified those patients that responded well to repeated exercises to relieve their symptoms. In the initial TBC, the presence of centralization with repeated movements was the primary criteria for inclusion into the specific exercise classification. Centralization is a concept with numerous operational definitions.[23,169–179] In the TBC approach, centralization occurs "when a movement or position results in abolishment of pain or paresthesia, or causes migration of symptoms from an area more distal or lateral in the buttocks and/or lower extremity to a location more proximal or closer to the midline of the lumbar spine."[72] The movement that centralized symptoms became the primary mode of treatment for the patient in the specific exercise classification. This approach was later refined to include the concept of "directional preference"[180,181] (DP), which is defined as "an immediate, lasting improvement in pain from performing either repeated lumbar flexion, extension, or sideglide/rotation tests."[181] As was the case with manipulation, specific exercises given to heterogeneous groups of patients with LBP do not result in clinically meaningful benefit.[182–187] Once attempts were made to examine these interventions in homogenous patient populations (subgroups), evidence started to emerge supporting the use of specific exercise interventions.[169,171,172,175,178,180,181,188–190]

In the current TBC, the key factor for identifying patients that fit the specific exercise classification is still centralization. It has been shown that patients who exhibit centralization early in the course of treatment have a better prognosis.[23,169,171–179,188,189,191] Centralization is a valid and reliable examination finding, and there is substantial evidence to support the use of centralization to classify or subgroup patients with LBP.[170,180,189,192,193] Patients who experience centralization early in the course of treatment have greater reductions in pain and disability, return to work sooner and more often, experience lower levels of pain and disability at 12 months, and are less likely to experience chronic pain than patients whose symptoms do not centralize.[23,169,171–173,175,176,188,194,195] The DP may also be useful in placing a patient in the specific exercise classification.[180,181] The concept of centralization is often confused with DP, as a patient who centralizes with one movement can be said to exhibit a DP. DP, however, does not require that centralization be present. It just implies that one movement feels better than another, which would include a larger subset of patients with LBP. The tests used to determine the DP of the lumbar spine are repeatable.[170,196] Additional research is needed to examine the usefulness of centralization versus DP for identifying patients likely to respond to specific-exercise interventions.

Long et al.[181] reported on 230 patients who exhibited a DP and were randomized to receive a specific-exercise intervention that matched their DP, a specific-exercise intervention that was opposite to their DP, or a control group that received a nondirectional exercise. For 83% of the patients extension was the direction of preference. They reported significantly greater reductions in every outcome measure when the exercise matched the patient's DP compared to the unmatched group. Additionally, one-third of both the opposite DP and nondirectionally treated subjects withdrew within 2 weeks because of no improvement or a worsening of symptoms.[181]

Browder et al.[197] compared the effects an extension-oriented treatment approach (EOTA) to a lumbar spine stabilization program in a sample of patients with LBP and symptoms distal to the buttocks that centralized with extension. The EOTA included extension exercises and mobilizations to promote extension. Subjects in the EOTA group demonstrated significantly greater improvements in disability than the group that received trunk strengthening exercises at 1 week, 4 weeks, and 6 months. Based on the studies cited, the optimal intervention strategy for patients in the extension specific-exercise classification may be a combination of exercise and mobilization to promote end-range extension.[72] Petersen et al.[198,199] studied 260 patients with chronic LBP with or without sciatica, comparing an extension-oriented protocol with a general-strengthening program. In the initial study, although the sample was heterogeneous, short-term results favored the extension protocol group, but the effect size was small.[198] In the follow-up study, no differences in outcomes were found between the treatment groups at 14 months.[199]

Patients who fit the flexion-specific exercise classification tend to be older, and the most common pathoanatomic diagnosis in this group is spinal stenosis.[200,201] The exercises that were originally recommended for this subgroup included end-range flexion exercises, traction, and avoidance of extension activities.[1] Most of the research focus for this classification has been on patients with spinal stenosis, and recommended interventions include flexion based exercises, lumbar stabilization, manual therapy to the lower quarter, neurodynamic interventions and treadmill walking (with or without body weight supported).[200–206] Whitman et al.[201] conducted a randomized trial in 58 patients diagnosed with lumbar spinal stenosis who had a directional preference for flexion. Patients were randomized to one of two 6-week physical therapy programs: a manual physical therapy, exercise, and progressive body-weight supported treadmill walking group or a flexion exercise and walking group (without body weight supported). While both groups improved, more of the patients in the manual physical therapy, exercise, and walking group reported recovery at 6 weeks. At 1 year, 62% of the manual therapy, exercise, and walking group and 42% of the flexion exercise and walking group still reported improvement. It appears that both approaches improve pain and function, and additional gains may be realized with the inclusion of manual physical therapy interventions, exercise, and a progressive body-weight supported treadmill walking program. Thus patients who present with a directional preference for flexion may benefit from a multimodal intervention package.

In the original TBC, a third specific-exercise classification was included.[1] This subgroup presented with a lateral shift, and recommended interventions that included end range lateral shift movements and traction. As this subgroup is relatively rare, it is not commonly considered in most current TBC research.[72,74,75,77,78,192,193,207] Gillan et al.[208] randomized 40 patients with a "trunk list" to receive either repeated end-range lateral-shift exercises or advice and massage. The group receiving the lateral-shift exercises had greater resolution of the lateral shift, but there were no differences in disability at 3 months. Harrison et al.[209] published a nonrandomized clinical trial of 63 consecutive retrospective subjects with a lateral shift and chronic LBP and 23 volunteer control subjects. Treatment included lateral shift correction exercises and traction. The 63 subjects reported greater pain reductions and improvements in the trunk list compared to the subjects who received no treatment. Further research is needed to identify the most effective interventions for this subgroup.

Traction classification

In the original TBC, Delitto et al.[1] postulated that a subgroup of patients exists who would benefit from traction. At that time, there was no evidence to support the notion that lumbar traction was a useful intervention when applied to a heterogeneous group of patients with LBP. The authors felt that the subgroup of patients in this classification would present with signs and symptoms of nerve root compression that did not centralize with active movements. The evidence is clear that traction applied to all patients with LBP is not an effective intervention for decreasing pain and disability.[210–215] Again, it is possible that a subgroup may exist that would benefit from traction. Clinicians cite signs and symptoms of nerve root compression as the main criterion for the use of traction.[213] Buerskens et al.[211] compared 12 sessions of sham traction to 12 sessions of mechanical lumbar traction in patients with nonspecific LBP; no difference was found between groups. An attempt was made to analyze subgroups of patients who responded favorably via a secondary analysis, but none of the analyzed variables predicted success. The examination criteria proposed in the original TBC were not investigated.

Fritz et al.[216] set out to determine if a subgroup of patients with LBP exists who is likely to benefit from mechanical traction. Sixty-four subjects with LBP, signs and symptoms of nerve root compression and/or numbness extending distal to the buttock, and an ODI score $\geq$ 30% were randomized into one of two treatment groups; an extension-oriented treatment approach group (EOTA) and a traction plus EOTA group (TRACT). The TRACT group had significantly greater reductions in disability and fear-avoidance at 2 weeks, but there were no between-group differences at 6 weeks. Traction was only used for the first 2 weeks. At 6 weeks, 82.6% of the TRACT group vs. 73.1% in the EOTA group reported improvement. Success was determined as a 50% improvement in the ODI at 6 weeks, and 60.9% of the TRACT group and 61.5% of the EOTA group met the criteria for success. Two baseline examination variables were associated with short term success with traction: peripheralization with extension, and a positive crossed SLR test. Based on their results, criteria for membership in the traction classification would include the presence of sciatica, signs of nerve root compression, and either peripheralization with extension movements or a positive crossed SLR test.[216]

Cai et al.[217] studied subjects with a diagnosis related to the lumbosacral spine with a chief complaint of pain and/or numbness in the lumbar spine, buttock, and/or lower extremity. Their primary aim was to develop a CPR to determine which patients would benefit from traction. They identified 4 predictors for short-term benefit from traction: 1) FABQ-W score less than 21, absence of neurological deficit, age above 30, and non involvement in manual work. The pretest probability of short-term success with traction was 19.4%. If subjects exhibited 3 or more of the variables in the CPR, the posttest probability of success increased to 42.2%. Limitations of this study include studying a heterogeneous group of patients, an uneven distribution of male and female subjects, and a mix of acute and chronic patients. The traction was only applied for three sessions, and the force applied was below what is normally recommended.[218] Finally, the CPR only accounted for 37.2% of the variance in the study, suggesting some important predictors may have been missed.

It appears that traction is most likely to help patients with leg pain, signs and symptoms of nerve root compression, inability to centralize symptoms with active movement testing, a positive crossed straight leg raise with symptoms for less than 6 weeks.

Reliability and Validity of the TBC

The reliability of the classification system has been examined in several studies. Interrater reliability of the individual factors identified for the manipulation,[84] stabilization,[160,219] and specific-exercise[170] subgroups has been published. Heiss et al.[74] used 4 PTs unfamiliar with the TBC to classify 45 patients with acute LBP. Three out of 4 rater pairs achieved a kappa value of 0.45 (55% agreement). The fourth rater pair had a low kappa (0.15). Fritz and George[75] examined the reliability of the TBC in 120 consecutive patients with acute LBP examined by 7 PTs experienced in the TBC. They reported a kappa value of 0.56 (65% agreement) between examiners. Kiesel et al.[220] reported a higher kappa value (0.65) examining 30 patients with LBP using 8 PTs familiar with the TBC. Finally, Fritz et al.[193] examined the reliability of the TBC algorithm (Figure 11–3) with the traction classification removed and using 30 PTs with varying levels of experience with the TBC. The overall agreement between therapists was 76%, with a kappa value of 0.60 (95% CI: 0.56, 0.64). No differences in agreement existed based on experience. It has also been shown that the intervention strategies utilized in the TBC can be effectively carried out by PTs, regardless of clinical experience.[221]

Several studies have investigated the validity of the TBC. George and Delitto[78] investigated the discriminant validity of the TBC. They reported that present pain intensity, duration of LBP, total lumbar flexion, presence of leg pain, and history of LBP were useful in predicting TBC group membership. These variables correctly classified 65% for specific exercise, 45% for manipulation, and 32% for stabilization. This study provided evidence supporting the discriminant validity of TBC.

Fritz et al.[77] investigated the effectiveness of the TBC approach versus treatment according to clinical practice guidelines in patients with acute, work-related LBP. They reported statistically significant differences in outcomes (disability and return to work) at 4 weeks that favored the TBC approach. There were no significant differences at 1 year.

Brennan et al.[79] investigated the effectiveness of decision-making within the TBC approach. The authors classified 123 subjects with LBP according to the TBC. All subjects were randomized to receive direction-specific exercises, manipulation or stabilization, regardless of their classification. Outcomes were then compared between patients who had received "matched treatment" by classification and "unmatched" treatment. The authors found a statistically significant reduction in disability, favoring the matched treatment group after 4 and 52 weeks.

APPLICATION OF THE TBC APPROACH TO JOE LORES

Examination

Figure 11–4 provides the reader with a TBC-based examination of Joe while Appendix 11–1 has an abbreviated version of the TBC examination form. The TBC-based physical exam components are operationalized and described as follows by the position the patient is in for each test or measure.

Name: Joseph Lores		**Age:** 40	**Date:** ___/___/___

Diagnosis: LBP **Referred by:** _____ **Initial Numerical Pain Score:** 2–6

FDAQ Score: 14 **Initial Oswestry Disability Index:** 42% **Initial FABQW/PA** Score: 16/18

Medical History: ☒ Reviewed on Intake Form Comments: High blood pressure, clavicle fracture, knee arthroscopy

Current History: ☐ Gradual ☒ Sudden ☐ Traumatic: Back pain started when he was installing a sink; felt pain immediately. For the first week he was getting better but now in the second week he is neither improving nor getting worse. This was a work injury, but he is self-employed as a plumber. No work = no pay.

Symptom Distribution:	Symptoms	Location	Nature
Lumbar	1	3	1
Buttock	1	3	1
Thigh	0	0	0
Lower Leg/Foot	0	0	0
	0 = None 1 = Pain 2 = Stiffness 3 = Parasthesia	1 = Central 2 = Bilateral 3 = Right 4 = Left	1 = Constant 2 = Intermittent 3 = Variable

Ordering of Symptoms:

Worst __2__ 1 = Standing 2 = Sitting

Best __3__ 3 = Walking 4 = Indeterminate

Temporal Order of Symptoms:

Worst __3__ 1 = Morning 2 = Midday

Best __4__ 3 = Evening 4 = Indeterminate

Patient's Goals for This Episode (*List*):

1. work without pain

_____

_____

Prior History of Lower Back Pain:

First Episode: 2002 Number of Episodes: 2

Previous Care—Effective: Rest/Tylenol, resolved in a week

Previous Care—Not Effective _____

Standing Examination

Baseline Symptoms: 2/10 up to 6/10

**Reports directional preference for extension

Legend:

— = End of range

☐ = Pulling sensation or stretching – not painful

\> = Pain felt lateral to spine (right)

< = Pain felt lateral to spine (left)

= Symptoms felt in lower extremity

O = Reduction or ablation of symptoms on movement

'' = Symptoms in opposite extremity (right)

! = Symptoms in opposite extremity (left)

Lateral shift: yes or no

Pelvic Landmarks:

Iliac Crests:

Front: ☒ Level ☐ High Left ____° ☐ High Right ____°

Back: ☒ Level ☐ High Left ____° ☐ High Right ____°

PSIS: ☒ Level ☐ High Left ☐ High Right

ASIS: ☒ Level ☐ High Left ☐ High Right

Standing Flexion Test:

☐ Negative ☐ Positive Left ☐ Positive Right

Response to Movement:	Worsened	Improved	Status Quo
Flexion	☒	☐	☐
Extension	☒	☐	☐
Right Side-Bend	☒	☐	☐
Left Side-Bend	☐	☐	☒
Ext in Right Pelvic Transloc	☐	☐	☒
Ext in Left Pelvic Transloc	☐	☐	☒
Repeated Flex in Standing	☒	☐	☐
Repeated Ext in Standing	☐	☒	☐

Painful Arc: ☐ Yes ☒ No Catching: ☐ Yes ☒ No

Reverse Rhythm: ☐ Yes ☒ No

Notes:

Pain with flexion, extension and right side bend. Directional preference for extension.

Figure 11–4 Joe Lores TBC Examination.

Name: Joseph Lores   **Patient ID#:** _____

Seated Examination

Pelvic Landmarks:

Iliac Crests: ☒ Level   ☐ High Left   ☐ High Right

PSIS: ☒   ☐ High Left   ☐ High Right

Seated Flexion Test: ☐ Negative   ☒ Positive   ☐ Positive Right

Repeated Flexion: ☐ Status Quo   ☐ Worsens   ☐ Improves

Motor Examination:	Left	Right
Hip Flexion (L2-L3)	5/5	5/5
Knee Ext (L3-L4)	5/5	5/5
Ant. Tibialis (L4)	5/5	5/5
EHL (L5)	5/5	5/5
Peroneals (L5-S1)	5/5	5/5
Gastroc/Soleus (S1-S2)	10 rep	10 rep

(0-10 Heel Raises)

Deep Tendon Reflexes: Left   Right

Knee Jerk   2   2

Ankle Jerk   2   2

0 = Absent
1 = Diminished
2 = Normal
3 = Hyper Reflexive

Sensation: ☒ Intact

☐ Diminished: _____

☐ Absent: _____

Thoracic Spine Movement:

☒ WNL

☐ Limited: _____

Notes:

Supine Examination

Straight Leg Raise: Left   Right

Range of Motion   70°   70°

Sciatica   ☒ Neg ☒ Neg   ☐ Pos ☐ Pos

Distracted SLR   ☒ Neg ☒ Neg   ☐ Pos ☐ Pos
(Waddell)

Long Sit Test:

☒ Negative

☐ (+) Left Lengthens

☐ (+) Right Lengthens

Faber Test: Left: ☒ Negative   ☐ Pain ☐ Groin ☐ Buttock

Right: ☒ Negative   ☐ Pain ☐ Groin ☐ Buttock

Hip ROM: Left   Right

Flexion   ☒ WNL ☐ Limited   ☒ WNL ☐ Limited

Int Rot (90°)   ☒ WNL ☐ Limited   ☒ WNL ☐ Limited

Ext Rot (90°)   ☒ WNL ☐ Limited   ☒ WNL ☐ Limited

Notes:

Prone Examination

Level	WNL	Hypomobile	Hypermobile	None	Local	Distant
L1	☒	☐	☐	☒	☐	☐
L2	☒	☐	☐	☒	☐	☐
L3	☒	☐	☐	☒	☐	☐
L4	☐	☒	☐	☐	☒	☐
L5	☐	☒	☐	☐	☒	☐
Sacrum				☒	☐	☐

(Mobility columns: WNL, Hypomobile, Hypermobile; Pain columns: None, Local, Distant)

Prone Instability Test: ☒ Negative   ☐ Positive

Hip Internal Rotation ROM (0°):

Left   40°   Right   35°

Prone on Elbows:

☐ Status Quo ☐ Worsens   ☒ Improves

Femoral Nerve Stretch:

☒ Negative   ☐ Positive

Regional Disturbance (Waddell):

☒ Negative   ☐ Positive

Overreaction (Waddell)   :

☒ Negative   ☐ Positive

Notes:
• Central P-A pressures produce pain at the L4 and L5 levels
• Unilateral pressures produce pain on the right at L4 and L5 levels
• Hypomobility noted centrally at both L4 and L5
• Hypomobility noted unilaterally at L4 and L5 on the right
•

Clinical Evaluation Summary: Patient fits the *Manipulation classification* of the TBC as he has all 5 positive factors: 1. Recent onset (< 16 days), 2. o symptoms distal to the knee, 3. Hypomobility with spring testing, 4.FABQ (work scale) score < 19, and 5. Hip IR at least 35 degrees on one side. Based on this, the patient has a 92% or greater chance of having a 50% reduction in disability on the Oswestry in 7 days or less if treated with high velocity thrust manipulation and exercise.

Figure 11–4 Joe Lores TBC Examination (continued).

Standing

- Lateral shift (trunk list):[222] Visible asymmetrical alignment of the spine with the shoulders lateral to the hips in the frontal plane to the right or left.
- Active range of motion (AROM) of the lumbar spine (Figure 11–5):[223,224] Lumbar range of otion is measured with a fluid-filled inclinometer. The patient stands erect. The inclinometer is held at T_{12}-L_1 and the patient is asked to flex, extend and sidebend as far as possible. Measurements are taken with a single inclinometer, and the effect on the patient's symptoms is noted.
- Directional preference:[180,181,190] This term focuses on selecting a particular direction of exercise that exhibits a centralization of symptoms with lumbar movement testing during the initial examination. The therapist notes if patient's symptoms centralize with extension, flexion or if the patient has no directional preference.

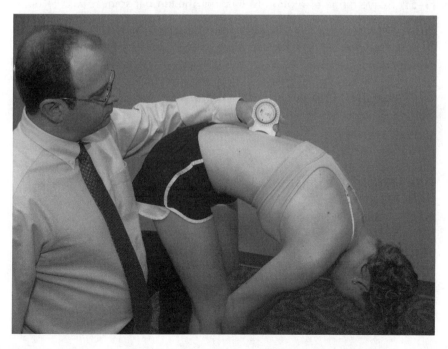

Figure 11–5A Active range of motion (AROM) of the lumbar spine. *Source:* Courtesy of David M. Weil.

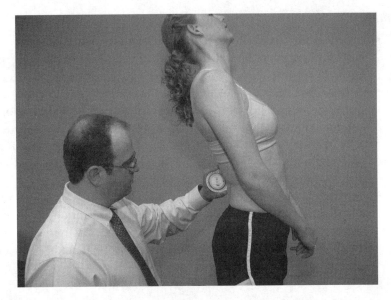

Figure 11–5B Active range of motion (AROM) of the lumbar spine. *Source:* Courtesy of David M. Weil.

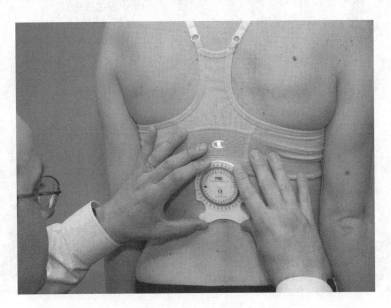

Figure 11–5C Active range of motion (AROM) of the lumbar spine. *Source:* Courtesy of David M. Weil.

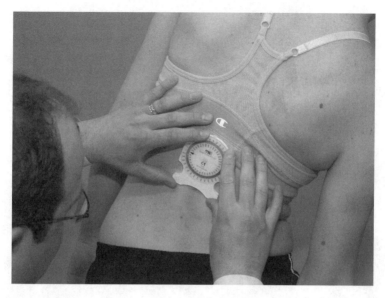

Figure 11–5D Active range of motion (AROM) of the lumbar spine. *Source:* Courtesy of David M. Weil.

- Aberrant movements (Figure 11–6):[160,207,225] The patient is asked to flex the trunk forward as far as possible and return to the starting position. The presence of any of the movement abnormalities is noted. The patient is considered to have aberrant movements if any of the following 5 findings are present.[207]
  - Instability catch: An instability catch is defined as any trunk movement outside of the plane of specified motion during that particular motion.
  - Painful arc (on descent or return): Symptoms felt during the movement at a particular point in the motion that are not present before or after this point.
  - Thigh climbing: Using the hands on thighs or some other external support to push up on when returning from flexion to the upright position.
  - Reversal of lumbopelvic rhythm: The trunk being extended first, followed by extension of the hips and pelvis to bring the body back to upright position.
- Modified Trendelenburg test:[165] The patient is instructed to raise one leg to 90° hip flexion. The test is positive if the pelvis is descending on the flexed side.

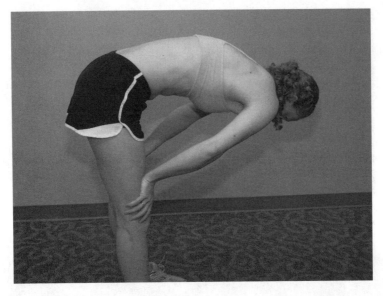

Figure 11–6 Aberrant movement of thigh climbing on return from flexion. Other aberrant motions with AROM would include an instability catch, a painful arc, or a reversal of lumbopelvic rhythm. *Source:* Courtesy of David M. Weil.

- General ligamentous mobility on the Beighton Ligamentous Laxity Scale (BLLS):[225] This scale consists of 4 bilateral tests of the extremities and one forward bending test. A point is given for each test the subject can perform. The scores range from 0 to 9. With a test result of ≥ 4, hypermobility is generally considered to be present.
  - Passive hyperextension of the knees greater than 10°
  - Passive hyperextension of the elbow greater than 10°
  - Passive hyperextension of the fifth finger greater than 90°
  - Passive abduction of the thumb to contact the forearm
  - Placing both hands flat on the floor while bending forward without flexing the knees.

Supine

- Average straight leg raise (SLR) range of motion (Figure 11–7):[224] The patient is supine with the head relaxed. The examiner holds the

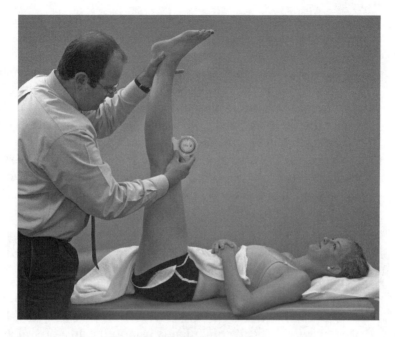

Figure 11–7. Average straight leg raise (SLR) range of motion. *Source:* Courtesy of David M. Weil.

foot with one hand to maintain the hip in neutral rotation. An inclinometer is positioned on the tibial crest just below the tibial tubercle. The leg is raised passively by the examiner, whose other hand maintains the knee in extension. The leg is raised slowly to the maximum tolerated straight leg raise and this is recorded in degrees. The opposite leg is then tested in the same manner. Average straight leg raise is computed by adding the maximum straight leg raise of the left and right legs and dividing by two.

- Pain provocation test of the pubis symphysis:[165,207] The examiner gently palpates the anterior portion of the pubic symphysis. The test is positive if the pain persists for at least 5 seconds after the examiner's hand is removed.
- Pelvic torsion or Gaenslen's test:[165,207] One leg is bent in full hip and knee flexion and the other extended with the leg over the edge of the table. The examiner simultaneously applies overpressure to the flexed hip

and a downward force on the extended leg. The test is positive if the patient experiences familiar pain in the sacroiliac region. The test is performed on both sides.

- Thigh thrust or posterior shear test (POSH):[165,207] The examiner flexes the patient's hip on the painful side to 90°. The examiner places one hand under the sacrum and applies a downward force through the line of the femur with the other hand. The test is positive if the patient experiences their familiar pain in the sacroiliac region.

- Active straight leg raise test:[165, 207] The patient lies with legs straight and feet 20cm apart, and is instructed to raise one leg 5cm above the couch without bending the knee. The test is positive if the patient notices heaviness in one or both legs.

Prone

- Spring testing with postero-anterior intervertebral pressures (PAIVMs) to the lumbar spine for mobility and pain provocation (Figure 11–8):[84,124,160,219,225–227] PAIVM testing is used to identify involved lumbar segments. Particular attention is paid to the area of symptoms, especially if a hyper or hypomobility is suspected. The central and unilateral posterior-anterior accessory motions of each segment are examined through their available range using the Australian oscillation grades of I–IV (provided that the patient can tolerate all grades of motion). Fritz et al.[219,227] have found that if mobility is decreased, the patient may be a good candidate for mobilization/manipulation, whereas if the mobility is increased, the patient may benefit from stabilization. Reliability results for interexaminer assessment of PAIVM testing are mixed.[219,225,226,228–230] Assessment of pain provocation usually results in higher reliability.[225] Among motion studies, regional range of motion was more reliable than segmental range of motion.[230]

- PAIVMs are performed by placing the hypothenar eminence of the hand over the spinous process of the segment to be tested. With the elbow and wrist extended, the examiner applies a gentle but firm, anteriorly-directed pressure on the spinous process. Interpretation of whether a segment is hypomobile, normal, or hypermobile should be based on the examiner's anticipation of what normal mobility should feel like at that spinal level and compared to the mobility detected in the spinal segments above and below the segmental level of interest.

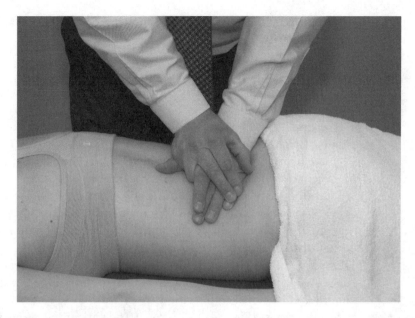

Figure 11–8 Spring testing with postero-anterior intervertebral pressures (PAIVMs) to the lumbar spine for mobility and pain provocation are performed by placing the hypothenar eminence (just distal to the pisiform) of the hand over the spinous process of the segment to be tested. With the elbow and wrist extended, the examiner applies a gentle but firm, anteriorly-directed pressure on the spinous process. Examiner identifies pain provocation and mobility at each lumbar segment. *Source:* Courtesy of David M. Weil.

The goals of performing PAIVMs are to:

1. *Identify* the spinal segment or segments involved.
2. Determine if the motion is normal, hyper or hypomobile (may help to classify the patient in the TBC).
3. Determine the *sequence of pain to resistance*; i.e., the pain occurs before resistance as evidenced by patient report or spasm, pain is identified with resistance, pain occurs after the therapist meets resistance, no pain occurs anywhere in the range.
4. Determine whether the impairment in a particular segment is primarily one of *pain or of stiffness*. If it is primarily pain, and increased motion is present, consider stabilization exercises. If stiffness is present, consider mobilization or manipulation interventions.

- ○ For the purposes of the TBC, the following options are available for each level tested:
  - ▪ Hypomobility—Passive mobility is judged to be hypomobile at ≥ 1 lumbar spine segmental level
  - ▪ Normal—Passive mobility is judged to be normal throughout the lumbar spine (L1–L5)
  - ▪ Hypermobility—Passive mobility is judged to be hypermobile at ≥ 1 lumbar spine segmental level
    - ▫ Note that some patients may have a hypomobile segment suggesting manipulation and a hypermobile segment suggesting stabilization. Research would suggest that in these patients, barring any contraindications to manipulation, that the clinician should manipulate the patient followed by lumbar stabilization exercises.[231,232]
  - ▪ If the patient has pain with PAIVMs at any level, the clinician should also perform the prone instability test to determine if symptoms improve with global stabilization.[160, 225]
- • Prone instability test (Figure 11–9):[160,225] The patient lies prone with the body on the examining table and legs over the edge and feet resting on the floor. While the patient rests in this position, the examiner applies posterior to anterior pressure (PA) to the lumbar spine. Any provocation of pain is noted. Then the patient lifts the legs off the floor (the patient may hold table to maintain position) and PA pressure is applied to the same level of the lumbar spine.
  - ○ Positive test—If pain is present in the resting position, but subsides substantially (either reduces in severity/intensity or resolves) in the second position, the test is positive. Mild improvement in symptoms does not constitute a positive test.
  - ○ Negative test—If pain is present in the resting position, but does not subside substantially in the second position, the test is negative. Further, if the patient did not have any pain provocation with P-As, then the test is negative.
- • Hip internal rotation range of motion (Figure 11–10):[84,124] The patient lies prone. The examiner places the leg opposite the leg to be measured in 30° of hip abduction to enable the tested hip to be freely moved into external rotation. The lower extremity of the side to be tested is kept in line with the body (i.e., neutral abduction/adduction), and the knee on that side is flexed to 90° with the ankle in the neutral position, and the leg in the vertical position. The inclinometer is placed on the distal aspect of the

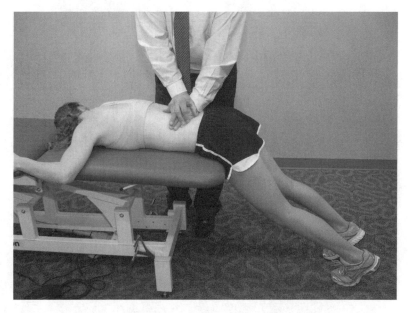

Figure 11–9A Prone instability test (PIT). *Source:* Courtesy of David M. Weil.

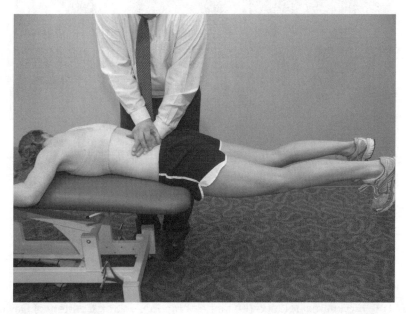

Figure 11–9B. Prone instability test (PIT). *Source:* Courtesy of David M. Weil.

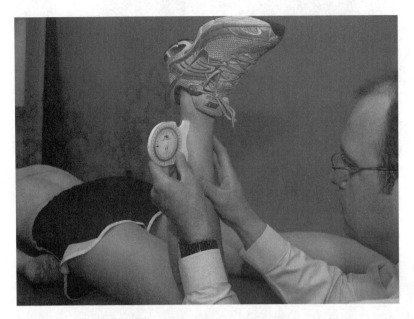

Figure 11–10A Hip internal rotation (IR) range of motion. *Source:* Courtesy of David M. Weil.

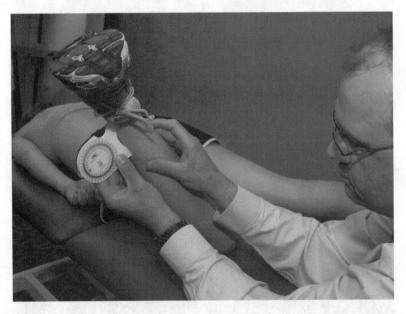

Figure 11–10B Hip internal rotation (IR) range of motion. *Source:* Courtesy of David M. Weil.

fibula in line with the bone and zeroed. Measurement of hip IR (hip rotated in a lateral direction, leg moved toward the edge of the plinth) is recorded at the point in which the pelvis first begins to move. The measurement should be recorded bilaterally. When measuring hip rotation, be sure that the knee remains in the same place.

- Test of the long dorsal sacroiliac ligament:[165] The examiner palpates the areas above both of the patient's sacroiliac joints. The test is positive if at least on one side the pain persists for a minimum of 5 seconds after the examiner's hand is removed.

Examination Findings for Joe Lores

Joe Lores is a 39-year-old male referred to physical therapy with right-sided low back and buttock pain that started suddenly about 2 weeks ago while he was installing a sink.

A systems review was performed, and it was determine that the musculoskeletal system would require further examination.[233] All other systems were within normal limits with the exception of mildly elevated blood pressure. His initial score on the modified Oswestry Disability Index was 42%, representing moderate disability.[234] See the completed TBC examination form for more details.

Evaluation and Diagnosis

There is strong evidence that this patient is appropriate for the manipulation classification of the TBC and is likely to have a favorable prognosis when managed using an intervention that includes a high velocity low amplitude (HVLA) thrust manipulation directed toward the lumbar spine and range of motion (ROM) exercises for the lumbar spine.[84,86,115,124] Patient characteristics that suggest a favorable prognosis when treated with HVLA interventions were originally identified by Flynn et al.[84] and subsequently validated by Childs et al.[124] Combined, the results indicate that patients who have at least four of the five characteristics and receive HVLA and a ROM exercise have a greater than 92% likelihood of having a 50% reduction in perceived disability in two to four days after the intervention is performed.[124] These factors are summarized in Table 11–3 and Joe exhibits five out of five of these prognostic characteristics supporting the choice of the manipulation classification.

Intervention

In the derivation and validation of the CPR, the side to be manipulated was the more symptomatic side based on the patient's self-report.[84,124] If the patient could not identify a more symptomatic side, the therapist selected a side for manipulation. After the manipulation was performed, the therapist noted whether or not a cavitation (i.e., a "pop") was either heard or felt by the therapist or patient. If a pop was experienced, the procedure was complete for that session. If no cavitation was produced, the patient was repositioned and the manipulation was attempted again. If no cavitation was experienced, the therapist attempted to manipulate the opposite side. A maximum of two attempts per side was permitted.[86]

In this case, we must be specific that the intervention technique should not be just any manual therapy intervention. It must be HVLA manipulation. Both the derivation and validation studies used the same HVLA manipulation as the primary intervention. Subsequent work to the validation of the patient characteristics has confirmed that the intervention must be HVLA manipulation to maximize outcomes. As noted earlier in this chapter, Cleland et al.[86] specifically compared the effects of three different manual therapy interventions on the pain and disability reports of patients with back pain who met the criteria for membership in the manipulation classification of the TBC. Two of those interventions were HVLA manipulations and the third was an oscillatory nonthrust mobilization technique. These authors reported that there were no differences in pain or disability outcomes between groups of patients receiving the different types of thrust intervention. However, significant differences in outcome existed between the thrust and nonthrust groups suggesting generalizability of the CPR to other thrust techniques but not to the oscillatory technique studied.[86]

Further, Hancock et al.[90,91] performed an analysis of data from an RCT of interventions for acute LBP to determine if the CPR would generalize to a variety of manual interventions including interventions directed toward the lumbar or thoracic spine, sacroiliac joint, pelvis or hip. Ninety-seven percent of the interventions were nonthrust low velocity mobilization techniques. These authors found that patients who were positive on the rule, and received some form of general manual therapy to the lower quadrant did not recover faster than patients who were positive on the rule and did not receive interventions. While not providing direct support for our choice of HVLA manipulation for the current patient case, the work by Hancock et al.[90, 91] does indicate that the intervention should not be low velocity mobilization.

Examples of the HVLA interventions used are shown in Figures 11–11 and 11–12. The two HVLA techniques that have support for their use include a supine thrust manipulation and a sidelying thrust manipulation.

We will use the terminology recommended by Mintken et al.[235,236] for describing the recommended manipulative interventions, which includes:

1. Rate of force application: Describe the rate at which the force was applied.
2. Location in range of available movement: Describe whether motion was intended to occur only at the beginning of the available range of movement, towards the middle of the available range of movement, or at the end point of the available range of movement.
3. Direction of force: Describe the direction in which the therapist imparts the force.
4. Target of force: Describe the location to which the clinician intended to apply the force.

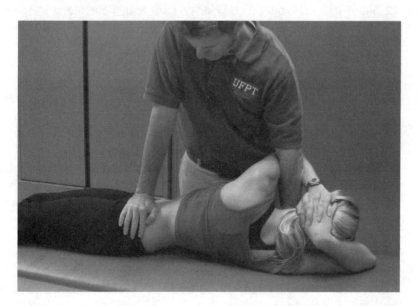

Figure 11–11 Supine technique: high-velocity, end-range, posterior-inferior force to the right innominate on the lower lumbar spine in supine, with lumbar left side-bending and right rotation. *Source:* Courtesy of Joel E. Bialosky.

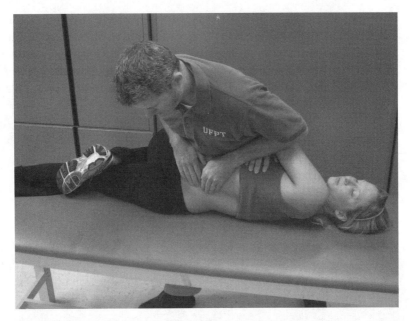

Figure 11–12 Side-lying technique: high-velocity, end-range, left-rotational force to the lower lumbar spine on the mid lumbar spine in a left side-lying, right lumbar side-bent position. *Source:* Courtesy of Joel E. Bialosky.

5. Relative structural movement: Describe which structure or region was intended to remain stable and which structure or region was intended to move, with the moving structure or region being named first and the stable segment named second, separated by the word "on."
6. Patient position: Describe the position of the patient, for example, supine, prone, recumbent. This would include any premanipulative positioning of a region of the body, such as being positioned in rotation or side bending.

Using the previous model the supine technique for the right side (Figure 11–11) would be described as a high-velocity, end-range, posterior-inferior force to the right innominate on the lower lumbar spine in supine, with lumbar right side-bending and left rotation.[235,236] This manipulation is the technique that was used in the development and validation of the CPR.[84,124] The technique is performed with the patient supine. The therapist stands on the side opposite of that to be manipulated. The patient is passively moved into side-bending towards the side to be manipulated. The patient interlocks the fingers behind his or her head. The therapist passively rotates the patient, then delivers a high-velocity, low amplitude thrust to the anterior superior iliac spine in a posterior and inferior direction (Figure 11–11).[86]

The side lying technique for the right side (Figure 11–12) would be described as a high-velocity, end-range, right-rotational force to the lower lumbar spine on the mid lumbar spine in a right side-lying, left lumbar side-bent position.[235,236] This alternate technique has been shown to produce similar outcomes in patients who are positive on the CPR.[86,118] The patient is positioned side lying with the more painful side up. The therapist flexes the top leg until movement is palpated at the selected vertebral level. The therapist then grasps the patient's bottom shoulder and arm and introduces sidebending and rotation until motion was felt at the selected level. The patient is then log rolled towards the therapist, who then applies a high-velocity, low amplitude thrust of the pelvis in an anterior direction (Figure 11–12). Similar decision-making to the supine technique is used to guide the therapist. The more painful side is identified by the patient, if there is not a side that is clearly more painful, the therapist chooses the side. While the production of a cavitation was used in the studies to determine when the procedure was completed during a session (up to 2 attempts allowed per side), it is clear from subsequent studies and data analysis that there is no relationship between an audible pop and improvements in disability, pain or ROM in individuals with LBP or neck pain.[237–240]

Currently, the dosage of this intervention that is most effective is not clear. However, as stated, the studies supporting the effectiveness of HVLA manipulation have all used a maximum of two applications to both sides.[84,124] Specifically, the decision algorithm has been to manipulate the more symptomatic side based on the patient's self-report. If the patient is unable to identify a more symptomatic side, the therapist selects a side for manipulation. In the prior studies using this intervention, if there was no cavitation (the "pop" often associated with HVLA interventions) during the first application, the intervention was repeated on the same side.[84,124] If, again, there was no cavitation, the therapist attempted to thrust the opposite side with a maximum of two attempts per side. However, recent work has suggested that the occurrence of cavitation is not associated with better pain and disability related outcomes[238–240] or with immediate neurophysiological changes in pain sensitivity.[237] Consequently, basing dosage decisions on the immediate cavitation may not be necessary. Our patient has indicated that the symptoms are predominantly on the right, therefore the suggested technique would be targeted to the right side.

In addition to the HVLA manipulation used, other concurrent interventions on the first day should include simple ROM exercises (supine pelvic tilt range of motion exercises, Figure 11–13 A and B) and instructions on the performance of these simple exercises outside of contact with the physical therapist.[84,124] In the validation study, patients were instructed to perform a set of 10 repetitions in the clinic and 10 repetitions of the exercise 3–4 times daily at home on the days in which the patient did not attend therapy.

Finally, this patient should receive an educational intervention at the first visit. Patient education should include the anatomy of the lumbar spine, biomechanical counseling and reassurance that recovery expectations are good and that a gradual return to normal activities is more effective than bed rest for treating acute low back problems.[241–243] Activity recommendations should consider the patient's age and general health (hypertension, in this case), and the physical demands of his job tasks. Additionally, he should be given advice to maintain usual activity within the limits of pain, as continuing ordinary activities within the limits permitted by the pain leads to more rapid recovery than either bed rest or back-mobilizing exercises.[187] That said, patients with an acute episode of LBP may be more comfortable if they

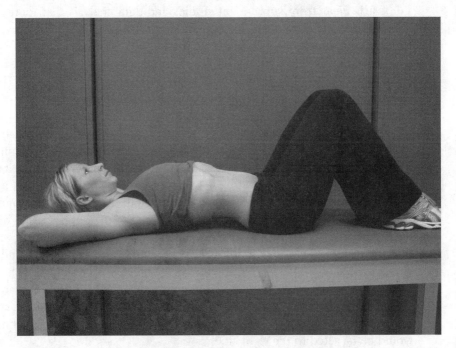

Figure 11–13A. Anterior pelvic tilt. *Source:* Courtesy of Joel E. Bialosky.

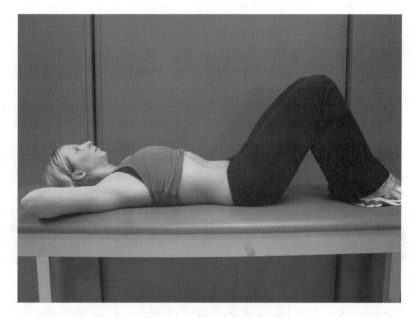

Figure 11–13B Posterior pelvic tilt. *Source:* Courtesy of Joel E. Bialosky.

temporarily limit or avoid specific activities known to increase mechanical stress on the spine, especially prolonged unsupported sitting, heavy lifting, and bending or twisting the back while lifting.[244]

Also, the need for special tests should be addressed if relevant to this patient. Specifically, some patients feel that they have been done a disservice if there has not been imaging performed.[245] Joe has had an X-ray in the past 12 months but he should be reassured that there is low need for additional imaging unless red flags (serious pathology or worsening neurological signs) are present.[3]

Prognosis and progression of intervention

At the commencement of each session, the physical therapist should review patient status to determine the best intervention for the current session. In the case of our current patient, this would consist initially of reviewing self-reports of disability and pain. There were no yellow flags to consider; therefore the progression of the intervention is not dependent on graded exposure methods.

Given this patient's presentation one would assume a very favorable prognosis and expect a 50% reduction in disability within 7 days with HVLA manipulation to the lumbar spine, advice to stay active, and simple pelvic tilt exercises (the treatment delivered in the studies investigating the CPR).[84,115,124] Once the reduction in disability is achieved, the patient should be progressed to a comprehensive exercise program to address any movement impairments and improve motor control of the deep musculature providing stability to the lumbopelvic spine. Based on the results of the studies by Long et al.,[181,190] we would also include extension exercises, as the patient reported a directional preference for extension. In a follow up case series, Long et al.[190] reported that poor outcomes from nonspecific/unmatched exercise protocols appeared to reverse when patients with directional preference were given subgroup-matched, direction-specific exercises. According to the original Long et al.[181] RCT, they recommended having the patients exercise every two waking hours, 5 to 10 minutes per session using exercises that matched the patient's directional preference. In this case, it could include extension in lying (prone press-ups, Figure 11–14) or extension in standing. We realize this is moving into interventions that are usually thought of as treatment for the specific exercise classification, but the beauty of the TBC is that it is a fluid classification, and patients may move between classifications during an episode of care.

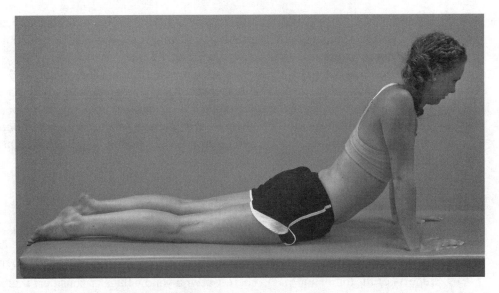

Figure 11–14 Prone press-up. *Source:* Courtesy of David M. Weil.

The evidence for treating Joe strongly suggests starting with manipulation, but we would then include other interventions for which evidence exists, including direction specific exercises and lower quarter strengthening, including motor control exercises. The efficacy of motor control exercises for the treatment of LBP is controversial. Supporters of this approach emphasize attaining independent contractions of the deep trunk muscles (transversus abdominus and lumbar multifidi) prior to performing more dynamic, functional tasks.[141,150–153,246–250] Other authors have disputed the need for such a specific focus on retraining the deep trunk muscles.[142,162,251–253]

Inhibition of the deep multifidii muscles is evident after an episode of acute LBP and a loss of motor control persists after the pain has abated.[152–154,254,255] Our current patient here shows evidence of this impact on multifidii and transverse abdominus based on the results of the clinical exam. There appears to be good evidence supporting the long-term benefits of activating these deep stabilizing muscles.[152,157] For example, a study of patients under the age of 45 who were experiencing unilateral LBP compared specific activation of multifidus and the transverse abdominus to medical management.[152] The results indicated few short-term differences between groups in recurrence of LBP but significant differences in recurrence at 2 and 3 year follow-up.

We would recommend that by the third visit, the patient should be progressed to a strengthening program for the muscles around the lumbar spine. As stated, the exact exercise prescription and dosage remains unclear. Therefore we will propose what we use clinically for patients with a similar presentation. For the transversus abdominus, abdominal bracing is used. Methods of teaching activation of the transverse abdominis are described in detail by Richardson et al.[151] An isometric co-contraction can be achieved when a patient gently draws in the lower abdomen without letting motion occur in the lumbar spine. Suggested cues include instructions like "draw your lower abdomen up and in" or "pull your navel up towards your spine."[151] Additional feedback can be provided using manual facilitation by the therapy, use of pressure biofeedback or rehabilitation ultrasound.[220,254,256–258] Four-point kneeling is suggested as the easiest position in which to experience activation of the transverse abdominis and Richardson et al.[151] advocate that a patient start in this position (Figure 11–15 A–B). These authors also indicate that the supine and prone positions be used to evaluate the activation of these muscles.

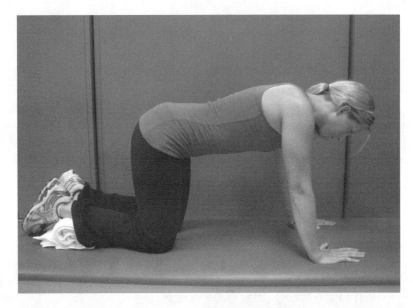

Figure 11–15A Abdominal drawing in maneuver in quadruped—starting position. *Source:* Courtesy of Joel E. Bialosky.

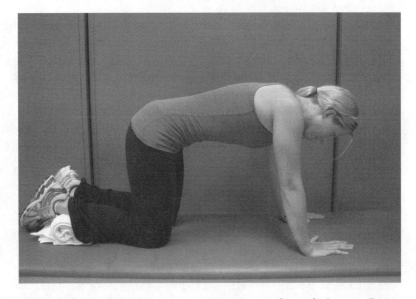

Figure 11–15B Abdominal drawing in maneuver in quadruped. *Source:* Courtesy of Joel E. Bialosky.

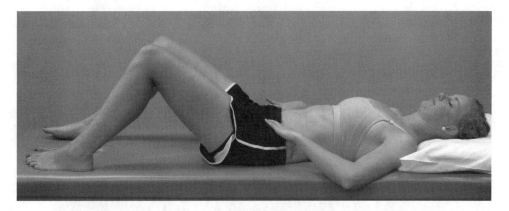

Figure 11–16 Supine position for the abdominal bracing. *Source:* Courtesy of David M. Weil.

The exercises that were used in the validation of the CPR and the subsequent trial comparing the 2 HVLA techniques to the low velocity mobilization used the supine position for the abdominal bracing (Figure 11–16).[86,124] See Table 11–6 for the exercise program utilized in the validation study for the manipulation CPR.[259] The patient is in supine with hips and knees flexed, and is instructed to draw in the abdominal wall without holding their breath (Figure 11–16). A suggested exercise goal is 10 contractions for 20 seconds. Once the patient achieves this goal, abdominal bracing in standing is added (Figure 11–17). For this exercise, the patient is standing with the lumbar spine against the wall. Abdominal bracing is performed as described and the patient is instructed to flex the hip and knees approximately 45° while maintaining the bracing. A suggested goal for this is 20 wall slides. When the patient achieves this goal, abdominal bracing during a bridge maneuver is added, without extending the lumbar spine (Figure 11–18). A suggested goal for this exercise is to hold the position for 10 second and perform 10 repetitions.

For the erector spinae and the multifidus, we would begin with quadruped single leg lifts where the patient performs the abdominal bracing maneuver (Figure 11–19). Particular attention is paid to local firing of the lumbar multifidus at the painful level. Cues are given for the patient to fire these muscles while performing the abdominal bracing (to achieve co-activation of the transversus and multifidus). Once good co-activation is achieved, the patient is then instructed to extend one hip without extend-

Table 11–6 Exercise Program Used in Childs et al. validation study[259]

Muscle Group	Exercise	Performance	Exercise Progression
Transversus abdominus	Abdominal bracing	Patient is in supine with hips and knees flexed. Patient is instructed to draw in the lateral abdominal wall without holding the breath.	Goal—10 contractions for 20 seconds each—then add bracing in standing and with bridging.
	Abdominal bracing in standing	Patient is standing with lumbar spine against a wall. Bracing performed as above, patient is instructed to flex the hip and knees approximately 45° while maintaining bracing.	Goal—20 wall slides.
	Abdominal bracing with bridging	Bracing performed as above, patient instructed to lift the hips without extending the lumbar spine.	Goal—able to hold position for 10 seconds – begin with 10 repetitions.
Erector spinae/ Multifidus	Quadruped single leg lifts	Patient is in quadruped, abdominal bracing is performed as above. The patient is instructed to ex- tend one hip	Goal—20 lifts with each hip without pain – then add. opposite arm and leg lifts
	Quadruped opposite arm and leg lifts	Exercise performed as above, except the opposite shoulder is flexed simultaneous with hip extension.	Goal—20 lifts on each side without pain.
Oblique Abdominals	Horizontal side support	Patient is side-lying with hips extended and knee flexed 900, propping on the elbow to create lumbar side-bending. Patient is instructed to lift the pelvis until the lumbar side-bending is eliminated.	Goal—10 lifts on each side, with a hold time of 10 seconds, without pain—then progress to advanced side support exercise.
	Advanced horizontal side support	Exercise is performed as above except the knees are extended	Goal—10 lifts on each side, with a hold time of 10 seconds, without pain.

Source: Courtesy of John Childs.

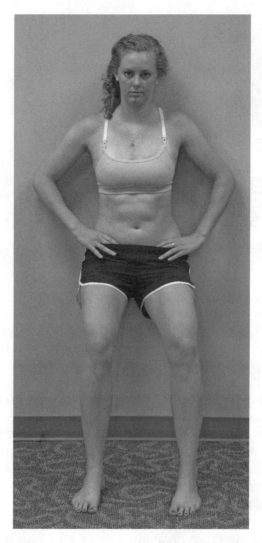

Figure 11–17 Abdominal bracing in standing. *Source:* Courtesy of David M. Weil.

ing the spine. A suggested goal for this exercise is 20 lifts with each hip without pain. Once this goal is achieved, the patient is progressed to alternate arm and leg lifts. The exercise is performed as described, except the opposite shoulder is flexed while simultaneously extending the contralateral hip (right arm, left leg and vice versa). A suggested goal for this exercise is 20 lifts on each side without pain.

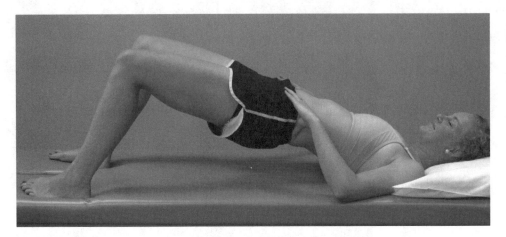

Figure 11–18 Abdominal bracing with bridging. *Source:* Courtesy of David M. Weil.

For the abdominal obliques, a horizontal side support exercise is utilized (Figure 11–20). The patient is side-lying with the hips extended and the knees flexed to 90° while propping on the elbow to create lumbar side-bending. The patient is then instructed to lift the pelvis until the lumbar side-bending is eliminated. A suggested goal for this exercise is to hold it for 10 seconds, performing 10 lifts on each side, without pain. Once this goal is achieved, the exercise is progressed to an advanced side support, where the exercise is the same as described, except that the patient's knees are extended. A suggested goal for this exercise is to hold it for 10 seconds, performing 10 lifts on each side, without pain.

In addition to emphasis on the deep stabilizing muscles, general exercise of the trunk muscles could provide long-term benefits to our patient. There are a variety of programs suggested to improve spinal stabilization. The majority of the support is generally for active strengthening exercise programs as no clear differences have been identified among the different stabilization strengthening programs studied.[142,160,162,163,260] For example, Koumantakis et al. performed a randomized controlled trial to examine the usefulness of the addition of specific stabilization exercises (transversus and multifidus) to a general strengthening approach for patients with recurrent nonspecific LBP. Fifty-five patients were randomized to a stabilization-

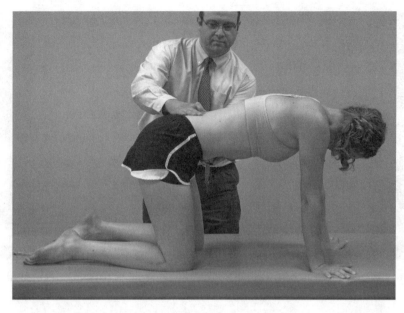

Figure 11–19A Abdominal bracing in quadruped. *Source:* Courtesy of David M. Weil.

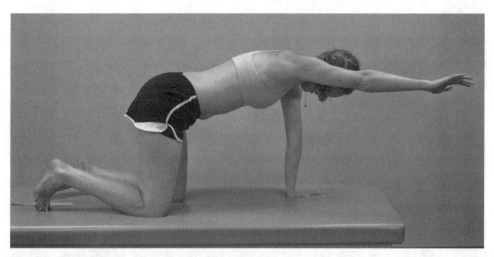

Figure 11–19B Abdominal bracing with quadruped arm lift. *Source:* Courtesy of David M. Weil.

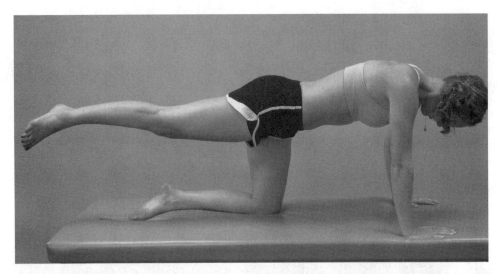

Figure 11–19C Abdominal bracing with quadruped leg lift. *Source:* Courtesy of David M. Weil.

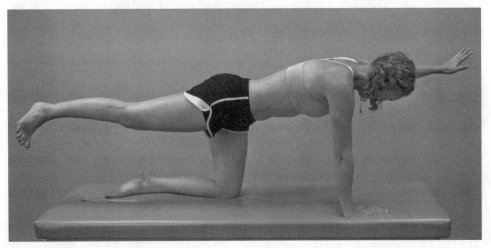

Figure 11–19D Abdominal bracing with quadruped arm and leg lift. *Source:* Courtesy of David M. Weil.

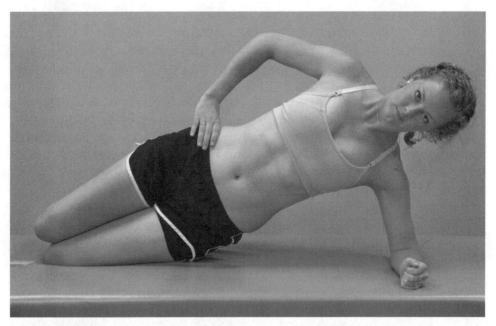

Figure 11–20A Horizontal side support exercise starting with the knees bent and progressing to knees extended. *Source:* Courtesy of David M. Weil.

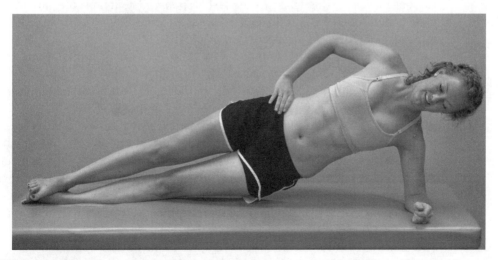

Figure 11–20B Horizontal side support exercise starting with the knees bent and progressing to knees extended. *Source:* Courtesy of David M. Weil.

enhanced exercise group (n = 29) or a general exercise-only group (n = 26). Both groups received 8 weeks of treatment along with *The Back Book*. Pain and disability improved in both groups. There were no significant differences in outcomes between groups except for decreased disability in the general exercise-only group that was present immediately after the intervention but not at a 3-month follow-up, suggesting that a stabilization-enhanced exercise approach does not appear to provide additional benefit to patients with subacute or chronic LBP.[142] Readers are encouraged to review the Koumantakis et al.[142] manuscript, as it has very detailed descriptions and figures of all the exercises interventions that were prescribed for both groups.

Measuring patient progress

We would measure progress on this individual primarily using the modified ODI, the NPRS, and the global rating of change.

We think that the modified ODI is the best outcome measure to use with Joe. The modified ODI is a 10-item questionnaire addressing different aspects of daily function that might be affected by LBP.[234,261,262] It was first published in 1980 by Fairbanks et al.[261] Patients are encouraged to respond to the items based on how they are feeling at the time of the questionnaire administration. Each item has a total of six possible responses. Each response is assigned a numeric value from 0–5 with a "0" being assigned to the first response and a "5" assigned to the last response. The item scores are summated, multiplied by 2 and reported as a percentage.[234,261] Higher scores indicate higher levels of self-reported disability.

Fritz and Irrgang[262] compared a modified version of the ODI and the Quebec Back Pain Disability Scale (QUE). In their study, they replaced the sex life item with a section regarding employment and home-making, and reported that the modified ODI was responsive and reliable.

The minimal clinically important difference (MCID) has been reported for the ODI in different populations of individuals with LBP. For individuals with LBP less than 3 weeks, the MCID for the modified ODI has been reported at 6 points. This is similar to the work by Beurkens et al.,[263] that found cut-off values of 4–6 points for the original ODI as presented by Fairbanks et al.[261] The intraclass correlation coefficient (ICC) for the modified ODI in the Fritz and Irrgang study was 0.90.[262] Kopec et al.[264] reported an ICC value of 0.91 for the modified ODI given 1 to 14 days apart.

Clinically we like to use an 11-point NPRS to measure pain intensity. The scale is anchored on the left with the phrase "No Pain" and on the right with the phrase "Worst Imaginable Pain." Numeric pain scales have been shown to be reliable and valid.[265-270] Patients rate their current level of pain and their worst and least amount of pain in the last 24 hours. The average of the three ratings or any single rating may be used to represent the patient's level of pain. We also like to utilize a pain diagram to record the location and nature of a patient's symptoms by drawing it on a human figure.[271-274] Pain diagrams have been shown to be a reliable tool to localize patient's symptoms.[275]

The 15-point global rating of change (GROC) scale described by Jaeschke et al.[276] is a useful tool to assess patient perceived changes in status. This form takes less than a minute to complete, and gives valid and reliable information on patient status. The scale ranges from -7 (a very great deal worse) to 0 (about the same) to $+7$ (a very great deal better). Intermittent descriptors of worsening or improving are assigned values from -1 to -6 and $+1$ to $+6$ respectively. We generally administer the GROC at follow-up examinations as a quick method of determining changes in patient status. It has been reported that changes of -3 to -1 or $+1$ to $+3$ would represent small alterations in function, changes of -4 to -5 or $+4$ to $+5$ would represent moderate changes, and changes of -6 to -7 or $+6$ to $+7$ would represent large changes.[276]

Expected outcomes

Based on the current best evidence supporting this approach, we would expect that this patient would experience a 50% reduction in disability in 7 days or less. Given that he has all five criteria matching him to the manipulation classification, his prognosis is excellent. Based on the 3 studies investigating the CPR that included 314 subjects,[84,86,124] patients that were positive on the rule and received high velocity manipulation experienced significant reductions in pain and disability in the short term, and, in 2 of the studies,[86,124] these excellent results were maintained out to 6 months for the majority of subjects. Patients that were positive on the rule and received high velocity manipulation, averaged a final score of 10% (out of a 0–100% scale) on the ODI and an average pain score of 1/10 on the NPRS at 6 months.

Based on our clinical experience and some data from research studies, we would expect to see this patient 6–10 times.[86,124] It is our opinion that researchers tend to undertreat in clinical trials, and it is common for patients to receive further care following the cessation of the clinical trial. We think that 10 visits, at most, would be sufficient to treat this patient, reduce his pain and disability, address work and recreational activities in a functional context, and attempt to reduce the likelihood of recurrence.[152,277,278] We believe strongly in equipping the patient with a comprehensive self management program, including patient education,[242,243,279,280] exercise to address length and strength impairments,[281] proper lifting techniques and biomechanical counseling to address any potential risks for recurrence.[281,282]

REFERENCES

1. Delitto A, Erhard RE, Bowling RW. A treatment-based classification approach to low back syndrome: identifying and staging patients for conservative treatment. *Phys Ther.* 1995;75 (6):470–485.
2. Deyo RA, Rainville J, Kent DL. What can the history and physical examination tell us about low back pain? *JAMA.* 1992;268(6):760–765.
3. Jarvik JG, Deyo RA. Diagnostic evaluation of low back pain with emphasis on imaging. *Ann Intern Med.* 2002;137(7):586–597.
4. Waddell G. 1987 Volvo award in clinical sciences. A new clinical model for the treatment of low-back pain. *Spine.* 1987;12(7):632–644.
5. Beattie PF, Meyers SP, Stratford P, Millard RW, Hollenberg GM. Associations between patient report of symptoms and anatomic impairment visible on lumbar magnetic resonance imaging. *Spine.* 2000;25(7):819–828.
6. Boden SD, Davis DO, Dina TS, Patronas NJ, Wiesel SW. Abnormal magnetic-resonance scans of the lumbar spine in asymptomatic subjects. A prospective investigation. *J Bone Joint Surg Am.* 1990;72(3):403–408.
7. Borenstein DG, O'Mara JW, Jr., Boden SD, et al.. The value of magnetic resonance imaging of the lumbar spine to predict low-back pain in asymptomatic subjects : a seven-year follow-up study. *J Bone Joint Surg Am.* 2001;83-A(9):1306–1311.
8. Jensen MC, Brant-Zawadzki MN, Obuchowski N, Modic MT, Malkasian D, Ross JS. Magnetic resonance imaging of the lumbar spine in people without back pain. *N Engl J Med.* 1994;331(2):69–73.
9. Moffroid MT, Haugh LD, Henry SM, Short B. Distinguishable groups of musculoskeletal low back pain patients and asymptomatic control subjects based on physical measures of the NIOSH Low Back Atlas. *Spine.* 1994;19(12):1350–1358.
10. The Accident Compensation Corporation. *New Zealand Acute Low Back Pain Guide.* Wellington, New Zealand: ACC and National Health Committee; 1997.
11. Schafer A, Hall T, Briffa K. Classification of low back-related leg pain—a proposed pathomechanism-based approach. *Man Ther.* 2009;14(2):222–230.
12. Walsh J, Hall T. Classification of low back-related leg pain: do subgroups differ in disability and psychosocial factors? *J Man Manip Ther.* 2009;17(2):118–123.
13. Currie SR, Wang J. Chronic back pain and major depression in the general Canadian population. *Pain.* 2004;107(1–2):54–60.
14. Sullivan MJ, Reesor K, Mikail S, Fisher R. The treatment of depression in chronic low back pain: review and recommendations. *Pain.* 1992;50(1):5–13.
15. Haggman S, Maher CG, Refshauge KM. Screening for symptoms of depression by physical therapists managing low back pain. *Phys Ther.* 2004;84(12):1157–1166.
16. Arroll B, Khin N, Kerse N. Screening for depression in primary care with two verbally asked questions: cross sectional study. *BMJ.* 2003;327(7424):1144–1146.
17. Lethem J, Slade PD, Troup JD, Bentley G. Outline of a fear-avoidance model of exaggerated pain perception--I. *Behav Res Ther.* 1983;21(4):401–408.

18. Vlaeyen JW, Crombez G. Fear of movement/(re)injury, avoidance and pain disability in chronic low back pain patients. *Man Ther.* 1999;4(4):187–195.

19. Vlaeyen JW, Kole-Snijders AM, Boeren RG, van Eek H. Fear of movement/(re)injury in chronic low back pain and its relation to behavioral performance. *Pain.* 1995;62(3):363–372.

20. Waddell G, Newton M, Henderson I, Somerville D, Main CJ. A Fear-Avoidance Beliefs Questionnaire (FABQ) and the role of fear-avoidance beliefs in chronic low back pain and disability. *Pain.* 1993;52(2):157–168.

21. Fritz JM, George SZ. Identifying psychosocial variables in patients with acute work-related low back pain: the importance of fear-avoidance beliefs. *Phys Ther.* 2002;82(10):973–983.

22. Fritz JM, George SZ, Delitto A. The role of fear-avoidance beliefs in acute low back pain: relationships with current and future disability and work status. *Pain.* 2001;94(1):7–15.

23. George SZ, Bialosky JE, Donald DA. The centralization phenomenon and fear-avoidance beliefs as prognostic factors for acute low back pain: a preliminary investigation involving patients classified for specific exercise. *J Orthop Sports Phys Ther.* 2005;35(9):580–588.

24. George SZ, Fritz JM, Childs JD. Investigation of elevated fear-avoidance beliefs for patients with low back pain: a secondary analysis involving patients enrolled in physical therapy clinical trials. *J Orthop Sports Phys Ther.* 2008;38(2):50–58.

25. Grotle M, Brox JI, Vollestad NK. Reliability, validity and responsiveness of the fear-avoidance beliefs questionnaire: methodological aspects of the Norwegian version. *J Rehabil Med.* 2006;38(6):346–353.

26. Hart DL, Werneke MW, George SZ, et al. Screening for elevated levels of fear-avoidance beliefs regarding work or physical activities in people receiving outpatient therapy. *Phys Ther.* 2009;89(8):770–785.

27. Jacob T, Baras M, Zeev A, Epstein L. Low back pain: reliability of a set of pain measurement tools. *Arch Phys Med Rehabil.* 2001;82(6):735–742.

28. Staerkle R, Mannion AF, Elfering A, et al. Longitudinal validation of the fear-avoidance beliefs questionnaire (FABQ) in a Swiss-German sample of low back pain patients. *Eur Spine J.* 2004;13(4):332–340.

29. Swinkels-Meewisse EJ, Swinkels RA, Verbeek AL, Vlaeyen JW, Oostendorp RA. Psychometric properties of the Tampa Scale for kinesiophobia and the fear-avoidance beliefs questionnaire in acute low back pain. *Man Ther.* 2003;8(1):29–36.

30. Al-Obaidi SM, Beattie P, Al-Zoabi B, Al-Wekeel S. The relationship of anticipated pain and fear avoidance beliefs to outcome in patients with chronic low back pain who are not receiving workers' compensation. *Spine.* 2005;30(9):1051–1057.

31. Cleland JA, Fritz JM, Brennan GP. Predictive validity of initial fear avoidance beliefs in patients with low back pain receiving physical therapy: is the FABQ a useful screening tool for identifying patients at risk for a poor recovery? *Eur Spine J.* 2008;17(1):70–79.

32. Korkmaz N, Akinci A, Yorukan S, Surucu HS, Saracbasi O, Ozcakar L. Validation and reliability of the Turkish version of the fear avoidance beliefs questionnaire in patients with low back pain. *Eur J Phys Rehabil Med.* 2009;45(4):527–535.

33. Crombez G, Vlaeyen JW, Heuts PH, Lysens R. Pain-related fear is more disabling than pain itself: evidence on the role of pain-related fear in chronic back pain disability. *Pain.* 1999;80(1–2):329–339.

34. George SZ, Bialosky JE, Fritz JM. Physical therapist management of a patient with acute low back pain and elevated fear-avoidance beliefs. *Phys Ther.* 2004;84(6):538–549.

35. Ostelo RW, van Tulder MW, Vlaeyen JW, Linton SJ, Morley SJ, Assendelft WJ. Behavioural treatment for chronic low-back pain. *Cochrane Database Syst Rev.* 2005;(1).

36. Smeets RJ, Vlaeyen JW, Hidding A, Kester AD, van der Heijden GJ, Knottnerus JA. Chronic low back pain: physical training, graded activity with problem solving training, or both? The one-year post-treatment results of a randomized controlled trial. *Pain.* 2008;134(3): 263–276.

37. Staal JB, Hlobil H, Koke AJ, Twisk JW, Smid T, van Mechelen W. Graded activity for workers with low back pain: who benefits most and how does it work? *Arthritis Rheum.* 2008; 59(5):642–649.

38. Brox JI, Sorensen R, Friis A, et al. Randomized clinical trial of lumbar instrumented fusion and cognitive intervention and exercises in patients with chronic low back pain and disc degeneration. *Spine.* 2003;28(17):1913–1921.

39. Linton SJ, Andersson T. Can chronic disability be prevented? A randomized trial of a cognitive-behavior intervention and two forms of information for patients with spinal pain. *Spine.* 2000;25(21):2825–2831; discussion 2824.

40. Pincus T, Vlaeyen JW, Kendall NA, Von Korff MR, Kalauokalani DA, Reis S. Cognitive-behavioral therapy and psychosocial factors in low back pain: directions for the future. *Spine.* 2002;27(5):E133–E138.

41. Smeets RJ, Vlaeyen JW, Hidding A, et al. Active rehabilitation for chronic low back pain: cognitive-behavioral, physical, or both? First direct post-treatment results from a randomized controlled trial. *BMC Musculoskelet Disord.* 2006;7:5.

42. Vlaeyen JW, de Jong J, Geilen M, Heuts PH, van Breukelen G. The treatment of fear of movement/(re)injury in chronic low back pain: further evidence on the effectiveness of exposure in vivo. *Clin J Pain.* 2002;18(4):251–261.

43. Vlaeyen JW, de Jong J, Geilen M, Heuts PH, van Breukelen G. Graded exposure in vivo in the treatment of pain-related fear: a replicated single-case experimental design in four patients with chronic low back pain. *Behav Res Ther.* 2001;39(2):151–166.

44. Vlaeyen JW, Haazen IW, Schuerman JA, Kole-Snijders AM, van Eek H. Behavioural rehabilitation of chronic low back pain: comparison of an operant treatment, an operant-cognitive treatment and an operant-respondent treatment. *Br J Clin Psychol.* 1995;34 (Pt 1): 95–118.

45. George SZ, Fritz JM, Bialosky JE, Donald DA. The effect of a fear-avoidance-based physical therapy intervention for patients with acute low back pain: results of a randomized clinical trial. *Spine.* 2003;28(23):2551–2560.

46. Sullivan MJ, Thorn B, Haythornthwaite JA, et al. Theoretical perspectives on the relation between catastrophizing and pain. *Clin J Pain.* 2001;17(1):52–64.

47. Picavet HS, Vlaeyen JW, Schouten JS. Pain catastrophizing and kinesiophobia: predictors of chronic low back pain. *Am J Epidemiol.* 2002;156(11):1028–1034.

48. Burton AK, Tillotson KM, Main CJ, Hollis S. Psychosocial predictors of outcome in acute and subchronic low back trouble. *Spine.* 1995;20(6):722–728.

49. Sullivan MJL, Bishop SR, J: P. The Pain Catastrophizing Scale: development and validation. *Psychological Assessment* 1995;7:524–532.

50. Severeijns R, van den Hout MA, Vlaeyen JWS, Picavet HSJ. Pain catastrophizing and general health status in a large Dutch community sample. *Pain.* 2002;99(1–2):367–376.

51. Woolf CJ. Central sensitization: uncovering the relation between pain and plasticity. *Anesthesiology.* 2007;106(4):864–867.

52. Woolf CJ. A new strategy for the treatment of inflammatory pain. Prevention or elimination of central sensitization. *Drugs.* 1994;47(S5):1–9.

53. Croft PR, Papageorgiou AC, Ferry S, Thomas E, Jayson MI, Silman AJ. Psychologic distress and low back pain. Evidence from a prospective study in the general population. *Spine.* 1995;20(24):2731–2737.

54. Woolf CJ. Pain. *Neurobiol Dis.* 2000;7(5):504–510.

55. Shevel E, Spierings EH. Cervical muscles in the pathogenesis of migraine headache. *J Headache Pain.* 2004;5(1):12–14.

56. Woolf CJ, Salter MW. Neuronal plasticity: increasing the gain in pain. *Science.* 2000;288 (5472):1765–1769.

57. Woolf CJ, Shortland P, Sivilotti LG. Sensitization of high mechanothreshold superficial dorsal horn and flexor motor neurones following chemosensitive primary afferent activation. *Pain.* 1994;58(2):141–155.

58. Butler DS. *The Sensitive Nervous System.* Adelaide, Australia: Noigroup Publications; 2000.

59. Barry SR. Clinical implications of basic neuroscience research. I: protein kinases, ionic channels, and genes. *Arch Phys Med Rehabil.* 1991;72(12):998–1008.

60. Devor M. Centralization, central sensitization and neuropathic pain. Focus on "sciatic chronic constriction injury produces cell-type-specific changes in the electrophysiological properties of rat substantia gelatinosa neurons". *J Neurophysiol.* 2006;96(2):522–523.

61. Devor M. Sodium channels and mechanisms of neuropathic pain. *J Pain.* 2006;7(1): S3–S12.

62. Devor M. Chapter 19 Pathophysiology of nerve injury. *Handb Clin Neurol.* 2006;81:261–264.

63. Devor M, Govrin-Lippmann R, Angelides K. Na+ channel immunolocalization in peripheral mammalian axons and changes following nerve injury and neuroma formation. *J Neurosci.* 1993;13(5):1976–1992.

64. Devor M, Seltzer Z. Pathophysiology of damaged nerves in relation to chronic pain. In: Wall PD, Melzack R, eds. *Textbook of Pain.* 4th ed. Edinburgh: Churchill Livingstone; 1999.

65. Chen Y, Devor M. Ectopic mechanosensitivity in injured sensory axons arises from the site of spontaneous electrogenesis. *Eur J Pain.* 1998;2(2):165–178.

66. Devor M. Nerve pathophysiology and mechanisms of pain in causalgia. *J Auton Nerv Syst.* 1983;7(3–4):371–384.

67. Papir-Kricheli D, Devor M. Abnormal impulse discharge in primary afferent axons injured in the peripheral versus the central nervous system. *Somatosens Mot Res.* 1988;6(1):63–77.

68. Sugawara O, Atsuta Y, Iwahara T, Muramoto T, Watakabe M, Takemitsu Y. The effects of mechanical compression and hypoxia on nerve root and dorsal root ganglia. An analysis of ectopic firing using an in vitro model. *Spine.* 1996;21(18):2089–2094.

69. Nijs J, Van Houdenhove B, Oostendorp RA. Recognition of central sensitization in patients with musculoskeletal pain: Application of pain neurophysiology in manual therapy practice. *Man Ther.* 2010;15(2):135–141.

70. Butler DS. *Mobilization of the Nervous System.* London: Churchill Livingstone; 1991.

71. Butler D. *Explain Pain.* Adelaide, Australia: Noigroup Publications; 2003.

72. Fritz JM, Cleland JA, Childs JD. Subgrouping patients with low back pain: evolution of a classification approach to physical therapy. *J Orthop Sports Phys Ther.* 2007;37(6): 290–302.

73. Riddle DL. Classification and low back pain: a review of the literature and critical analysis of selected systems. *Phys Ther.* 1998;78(7):708–737.

74. Heiss DG, Fitch DS, Fritz JM, Sanchez WJ, Roberts KE, Buford JA. The interrater reliability among physical therapists newly trained in a classification system for acute low back pain. *J Orthop Sports Phys Ther.* 2004;34(8):430–439.

75. Fritz JM, George S. The use of a classification approach to identify subgroups of patients with acute low back pain. Interrater reliability and short-term treatment outcomes. *Spine.* 2000;25(1):106–114.

76. Delitto A, Cibulka MT, Erhard RE, Bowling RW, Tenhula JA. Evidence for use of an extension-mobilization category in acute low back syndrome: a prescriptive validation pilot study. *Phys Ther.* 1993;73(4):216–222.

77. Fritz JM, Delitto A, Erhard RE. Comparison of classification-based physical therapy with therapy based on clinical practice guidelines for patients with acute low back pain: a randomized clinical trial. *Spine.* 2003;28(13):1363–1371.

78. George SZ, Delitto A. Clinical examination variables discriminate among treatment-based classification groups: a study of construct validity in patients with acute low back pain. *Phys Ther.* 2005;85(4):306–314.

79. Brennan GP, Fritz JM, Hunter SJ, Thackeray A, Delitto A, Erhard RE. Identifying subgroups of patients with acute/subacute "nonspecific" low back pain: results of a randomized clinical trial. *Spine.* 2006;31(6):623–631.

80. Erhard RE, Delitto A, Cibulka MT. Relative effectiveness of an extension program and a combined program of manipulation and flexion and extension exercises in patients with acute low back syndrome. *Phys Ther.* 1994;74(12):1093–1100.

81. Paris SV. A history of manipulative therapy through the ages and up to the current controversy in the United States. *Journal of Manual and Manipulative Therapy.* 2000;8(2): 66–77.

82. Aure OF, Nilsen JH, Vasseljen O. Manual therapy and exercise therapy in patients with chronic low back pain: a randomized, controlled trial with 1-year follow-up. *Spine.* 2003; 28(6):525–531.

83. Childs JD, Fritz JM, Flynn TW, et al. A clinical prediction rule to identify patients with low back pain most likely to benefit from spinal manipulation: a validation study. *Ann Intern Med.* 2004;141(12):920–928.

84. Flynn T, Fritz J, Whitman J, et al. A clinical prediction rule for classifying patients with low back pain who demonstrate short-term improvement with spinal manipulation. *Spine.* 2002;27(24):2835–2843.

85. Delitto A, Cibulka MT, Erhard RE, Bowling RW, Tenhula JA. Evidence for use of an extension-mobilization category in acute low back syndrome: a prescriptive validation pilot study. *Phys Ther.* 1993;73(4):216–222.

86. Cleland JA, Fritz JM, Kulig K, et al. Comparison of the effectiveness of three manual physical therapy techniques in a subgroup of patients with low back pain who satisfy a clinical prediction rule: a randomized clinical trial. *Spine.* 2009;34(25):2720–2729.

87. United Kingdom back pain exercise and manipulation (UK BEAM) randomised trial: effectiveness of physical treatments for back pain in primary care. *BMJ.* 2004;329(7479):1377.

88. Cherkin DC, Deyo RA, Battie M, Street J, Barlow W. A comparison of physical therapy, chiropractic manipulation, and provision of an educational booklet for the treatment of patients with low back pain. *N Engl J Med.* 1998;339(15):1021–1029.

89. Godfrey CM, Morgan PP, Schatzker J. A randomized trial of manipulation for low-back pain in a medical setting. *Spine.* 1984;9(3):301–304.

90. Hancock MJ, Maher CG, Latimer J, Herbert RD, McAuley JH. Independent evaluation of a clinical prediction rule for spinal manipulative therapy: a randomised controlled trial. *Eur Spine J.* 2008;17(7):936–943.

91. Hancock MJ, Maher CG, Latimer J, et al. Assessment of diclofenac or spinal manipulative therapy, or both, in addition to recommended first-line treatment for acute low back pain: a randomised controlled trial. *Lancet.* 2007;370(9599):1638–1643.

92. Assendelft WJ, Morton SC, Yu EI, Suttorp MJ, Shekelle PG. Spinal manipulative therapy for low back pain. *Cochrane Database Syst Rev.* 2004(1).

93. Assendelft WJ, Morton SC, Yu EI, Suttorp MJ, Shekelle PG. Spinal manipulative therapy for low back pain. A meta-analysis of effectiveness relative to other therapies. *Ann Intern Med.* 2003;138(11):871–881.

94. Assendelft WJJ, Morton SC, Yu EI, Suttorp MJ, Shekelle PG. Spinal manipulative therapy for low back pain. *Cochrane Database Syst Rev.* 2004(1).

95. Bronfort G, Haas M, Evans RL, Bouter LM. Efficacy of spinal manipulation and mobilization for low back pain and neck pain: a systematic review and best evidence synthesis. *Spine J.* 2004;4(3):335–356.

96. Cherkin DC, Sherman KJ, Deyo RA, Shekelle PG. A review of the evidence for the effectiveness, safety, and cost of acupuncture, massage therapy, and spinal manipulation for back pain. *Ann Intern Med.* 2003;138(11):898–906.

97. Ernst E, Canter PH. A systematic review of systematic reviews of spinal manipulation. *J R Soc Med.* 2006;99(4):192–196.

98. Haas M, Sharma R, Stano M. Cost-effectiveness of medical and chiropractic care for acute and chronic low back pain. *J Manipulative Physiol Ther.* 2005;28(8):555–563.

99. Koes BW, Assendelft WJ, van der Heijden GJ, Bouter LM. Spinal manipulation for low back pain. An updated systematic review of randomized clinical trials. *Spine.* 1996;21(24):2860–2871.

100. van Tulder MW, Koes BW, Bouter LM. Conservative treatment of acute and chronic non-specific low back pain. A systematic review of randomized controlled trials of the most common interventions. *Spine.* 1997;22(18):2128–2156.

101. Greenman P. *Principles of Manual Medicine.* 2nd ed. Baltimore: Williams and Wilkins; 1996.

102. Cyriax J. *Textbook of Orthopaedic Medicine, Volume I.* London: Bailliere Tindall; 1982.

103. Cyriax J. *Textbook of Orthopaedic Medicine, Volume II.* Vol II. London: Bailliere Tindall; 1982.

104. Fryette HH. Physiologic Movements of the Spine. 1959 AAO Yearbook. 91st ed; 1959.

105. Freburger JK, Riddle DL. Measurement of sacroiliac joint dysfunction: a multicenter inter-tester reliability study. *Phys Ther.* 1999;79(12):1134–1141.

106. Potter NA, Rothstein JM. Intertester reliability for selected clinical tests of the sacroiliac joint. *Phys Ther.* 1985;65(11):1671–1675.

107. Riddle DL, Freburger JK. Evaluation of the presence of sacroiliac joint region dysfunction using a combination of tests: a multicenter intertester reliability study. *Phys Ther.* 2002;82(8):772–781.

108. Huijbregts PA. Spinal motion palpation: a review of reliability studies. *J Man Manip Ther.* 2002;10(1):24–39.

109. Huijbregts PA. Chiropractic legal challenges to the physical therapy scope of practice: anybody else taking the ethical high ground? *J Man Manip Ther.* 2007;15(2):69–80.

110. Huijbregts PA. Evidence-based diagnosis and treatment of the painful sacroiliac joint. *J Man Manip Ther.* 2008;16(3):153–154.

111. Cook C. Coupling behavior of the lumbar spine: a literature review. *J Man Manip Ther.* 2003;11(3):137–145.

112. Levangie PK. Four clinical tests of sacroiliac joint dysfunction: the association of test results with innominate torsion among patients with and without low back pain. *Phys Ther.* 1999;79(11):1043–1057.

113. Levangie PK. The association between static pelvic asymmetry and low back pain. *Spine.* 1999;24(12):1234–1242.

114. McGinn TG, Guyatt GH, Wyer PC, Naylor CD, Stiell IG, Richardson WS. Users' guides to the medical literature: XXII: how to use articles about clinical decision rules. Evidence-Based Medicine Working Group. *JAMA.* 2000;284(1):79–84.

115. Fritz JM, Childs JD, Flynn TW. Pragmatic application of a clinical prediction rule in primary care to identify patients with low back pain with a good prognosis following a brief spinal manipulation intervention. *BMC Fam Pract.* 2005;6(1):29.

116. Fritz JM, Brennan GP, Leaman H. Does the evidence for spinal manipulation translate into better outcomes in routine clinical care for patients with occupational low back pain? A case-control study. *Spine J.* 2006;6(3):289–295.

117. Fritz JM, Whitman JM, Flynn TW, Wainner RS, Childs JD. Factors related to the inability of individuals with low back pain to improve with a spinal manipulation. *Phys Ther.* 2004;84(2):173–190.

118. Cleland JA, Fritz JM, Whitman JM, Childs JD, Palmer JA. The use of a lumbar spine manipulation technique by physical therapists in patients who satisfy a clinical prediction rule: a case series. *J Orthop Sports Phys Ther.* 2006;36(4):209–214.

119. Wright A. Hypoalgesia post-manipulative therapy: a review of a potential neurophysiological mechanism. *Manual Therapy.* 1995;1(1):11–16.

120. Bialosky JE, Bishop MD, Robinson ME, Barabas JA, George SZ. The influence of expectation on spinal manipulation induced hypoalgesia: an experimental study in normal subjects. *BMC Musculoskelet Disord.* 2008;9:19.

121. Bialosky JE, Bishop MD, Robinson ME, Zeppieri G, Jr., George SZ. Spinal manipulative therapy has an immediate effect on thermal pain sensitivity in people with low back pain: a randomized controlled trial. *Phys Ther.* 2009;89(12):1292–1303.

122. Bialosky JE, George SZ, Bishop MD. How spinal manipulative therapy works: why ask why? *J Orthop Sports Phys Ther.* 2008;38(6):293–295.

123. George SZ, Bishop MD, Bialosky JE, Zeppieri G, Jr., Robinson ME. Immediate effects of spinal manipulation on thermal pain sensitivity: an experimental study. *BMC Musculoskelet Disord.* 2006;7:68.

124. Childs JD, Fritz JM, Flynn TW, et al. A clinical prediction rule to identify patients with low back pain most likely to benefit from spinal manipulation: a validation study. *Ann Intern Med.* 2004;141(12):920–928.

125. Skargren EI, Carlsson PG, Oberg BE. One-year follow-up comparison of the cost and effectiveness of chiropractic and physiotherapy as primary management for back pain. Subgroup analysis, recurrence, and additional health care utilization. *Spine.* 1998;23(17):1875–1883.

126. Axen I, Jones JJ, Rosenbaum A, et al. The Nordic Back Pain Subpopulation Program: validation and improvement of a predictive model for treatment outcome in patients with low back pain receiving chiropractic treatment. *J Manipulative Physiol Ther.* 2005;28(6):381–385.

127. Maitland G. *Vertebral Manipulation.* 5th ed. Sydney, New South Wales, Australia: Butterworths; 1986.

128. Chiradejnant A, Latimer J, Maher CG, Stepkovitch N. Does the choice of spinal level treated during posteroanterior (PA) mobilisation affect treatment outcome? *Physiother Theory Pract.* 2002;18(4):165–174.

129. Chiradejnant A, Maher CG, Latimer J, Stepkovitch N. Efficacy of "therapist-selected" versus "randomly selected" mobilisation techniques for the treatment of low back pain: a randomised controlled trial. *Aust J Physiother.* 2003;49(4):233–241.

130. Cleland JA, Fritz JM, Whitman JM, Childs JD, Palmer JA. The use of a lumbar spine manipulation technique by physical therapists in patients who satisfy a clinical prediction rule: a case series. *J Orthop Sports Phys Ther.* 2006;36(4):209–214.

131. Beffa R, Mathews R. Does the adjustment cavitate the targeted joint? An investigation into the location of cavitation sounds. *J Manipulative Physiol Ther.* 2004;27(2).

132. Haas M, Groupp E, Panzer D, Partna L, Lumsden S, Aickin M. Efficacy of cervical endplay assessment as an indicator for spinal manipulation. *Spine.* 2003;28(11):1091–1096.

133. Kent P, Marks D, Pearson W, Keating J. Does clinician treatment choice improve the outcomes of manual therapy for nonspecific low back pain? A metaanalysis. *J Manipulative Physiol Ther.* 2005;28(5):312–322.

134. Frymoyer JW, Selby DK. Segmental instability. Rationale for treatment. *Spine.* 1985;10(3):280–286.

135. Nachemson A. Lumbar spine instability. A critical update and symposium summary. *Spine.* 1985;10(3):290–291.

136. Nachemson AL. Lumbar spine instability: outcome and randomized controlled trials. *Bull Hosp Jt Dis.* 1996;55(3):166.

137. Dupuis PR, Yong-Hing K, Cassidy JD, Kirkaldy-Willis WH. Radiologic diagnosis of degenerative lumbar spinal instability. *Spine.* 1985;10(3):262–276.
138. Hayes MA, Howard TC, Gruel CR, Kopta JA. Roentgenographic evaluation of lumbar spine flexion-extension in asymptomatic individuals. *Spine.* 1989;14(3):327–331.
139. Boden SD, Wiesel SW. Lumbosacral segmental motion in normal individuals. Have we been measuring instability properly? *Spine.* 1990;15(6):571–576.
140. Panjabi MM. The stabilizing system of the spine. Part I. Function, dysfunction, adaptation, and enhancement. *J Spinal Disord.* 1992;5(4):383–389; discussion 397.
141. Hodges PW, Richardson CA. Altered trunk muscle recruitment in people with low back pain with upper limb movement at different speeds. *Arch Phys Med Rehabil.* 1999;80(9): 1005–1012.
142. Koumantakis GA, Watson PJ, Oldham JA. Trunk muscle stabilization training plus general exercise versus general exercise only: randomized controlled trial of patients with recurrent low back pain. *Phys Ther.* 2005;85(3):209–225.
143. Goldby LJ, Moore AP, Doust J, Trew ME. A randomized controlled trial investigating the efficiency of musculoskeletal physiotherapy on chronic low back disorder. *Spine.* 2006;31(10):1083–1093.
144. Lewis JS, Hewitt JS, Billington L, Cole S, Byng J, Karayiannis S. A randomized clinical trial comparing two physiotherapy interventions for chronic low back pain. *Spine.* 2005;30 (7):711–721.
145. Cairns MC, Foster NE, Wright C. Randomized controlled trial of specific spinal stabilization exercises and conventional physiotherapy for recurrent low back pain. *Spine.* 2006;31(19):E670–E681.
146. Kwon BK, Fisher CG, Boyd MC, et al. A prospective randomized controlled trial of anterior compared with posterior stabilization for unilateral facet injuries of the cervical spine. *J Neurosurg Spine.* 2007;7(1):1–12.
147. Hodges P, Richardson C, Jull G. Evaluation of the relationship between laboratory and clinical tests of transversus abdominis function. *Physiother Res Int.* 1996;1(1):30–40.
148. Hodges PW, Richardson CA. Relationship between limb movement speed and associated contraction of the trunk mucles. *Ergonomics.* 1997;40(11):1220–1230.
149. Hodges PW, Richardson CA. Contraction of the abdominal muscles associated with movement of the lower limb. *Phys Ther.* 1997;77(2):132–144.
150. Hodges PW, Richardson CA. Inefficient muscular stabilization of the lumbar spine associated with low back pain: a motor control evaluation of transversus abdominis. *Spine.* 1996;21(22):2640–2650.
151. Richardson CA, Hodges PW, Hides JA. *Therapeutic Exercise for Spinal Segmental Stabilization in Low Back Pain.* Edinburgh, London, New York, Philadelphia, Sydney, Toronto: Churchill Livingstone; 2004.
152. Hides JA, Jull GA, Richardson CA. Long-term effects of specific stabilizing exercises for first-episode low back pain. *Spine.* 2001;26(11):E243–E248.
153. Hides JA, Richardson CA, Jull GA. Multifidus muscle recovery is not automatic after resolution of acute, first-episode low back pain. *Spine.* 1996;21(23):2763–2769.
154. Hides JA, Stokes MJ, Saide M, Jull GA, Cooper DH. Evidence of lumbar multifidus muscle wasting ipsilateral to symptoms in patients with acute/subacute low back pain. *Spine.* 1994;19(2):165–172.
155. Richardson CA, Snijders CJ, Hides JA, Damen L, Pas MS, Storm J. The relation between the transversus abdominis muscles, sacroiliac joint mechanics, and low back pain. *Spine.* 2002;27(4):399–405.
156. Shaughnessy M, Caulfield B. A pilot study to investigate the effect of lumbar stabilisation exercise training on functional ability and quality of life in patients with chronic low back pain. *Int J Rehabil Res.* 2004;27(4):297–301.

157. O'Sullivan PB, Phyty GD, Twomey LT, Allison GT. Evaluation of specific stabilizing exercise in the treatment of chronic low back pain with radiologic diagnosis of spondylolysis or spondylolisthesis. *Spine.* 1997;22(24):2959–2967.

158. Stuge B, Laerum E, Kirkesola G, Vollestad N. The efficacy of a treatment program focusing on specific stabilizing exercises for pelvic girdle pain after pregnancy: a randomized controlled trial. *Spine* . 2004;29(4):351–359.

159. Bereznick DE, Ross JK, McGill SM. The frictional properties at the thoracic skin-fascia interface: implications in spine manipulation. *Clin Biomech.* 2002;17(4):297–303.

160. Hicks GE, Fritz JM, Delitto A, McGill SM. Preliminary development of a clinical prediction rule for determining which patients with low back pain will respond to a stabilization exercise program. *Arch Phys MedRehabi.* 2005;86(9):1753–1762.

161. Hough E, Stephenson R, Swift L. A comparison of manual therapy and active rehabilitation in the treatment of nonspecific low back pain with particular reference to a patient's Linton & Hallden psychological screening score: a pilot study. *BMC Musculoskelet Disord.* 2007;8:106.

162. McGill SM. Low back stability: from formal description to issues for performance and rehabilitation. *Exerc Sport Sci Rev.* 2001;29(1):26–31.

163. McGill SM. Low back exercises: evidence for improving exercise regimens. *Phys Ther.* 1998;78(7):754–765.

164. Stuge B, Hilde G, Vollestad N. Physical therapy for pregnancy-related low back and pelvic pain: a systematic review. *Acta Obstet Gynecol Scand.* 2003;82(11):983–990.

165. Vleeming A, Albert HB, Ostgaard HC, Sturesson B, Stuge B. European guidelines for the diagnosis and treatment of pelvic girdle pain. *Eur Spine J.* 2008;17(6):794–819.

166. Vollestad NK, Stuge B. Prognostic factors for recovery from postpartum pelvic girdle pain. *Eur Spine J.* 2009;18(5):718–726.

167. Donelson R. The McKenzie approach to evaluating and treating low back pain. *Orthop Rev.* 1990;19(8):681–686.

168. McKenzie R. *The Lumbar Spine: Mechanical Diagnosis and Therapy.* Waikanae, New Zealand: Spinal Publications; 2003.

169. Donelson R, Silva G, Murphy K. Centralization phenomenon. Its usefulness in evaluating and treating referred pain. *Spine.* 1990;15(3):211–213.

170. Fritz JM, Delitto A, Vignovic M, Busse RG. Interrater reliability of judgments of the centralization phenomenon and status change during movement testing in patients with low back pain. *Arch Phys Med Rehabi.* 2000;81(1):57–61.

171. Laslett M, Oberg B, Aprill CN, McDonald B. Centralization as a predictor of provocation discography results in chronic low back pain, and the influence of disability and distress on diagnostic power. *Spine J.* 2005;5(4):370–380.

172. Long AL. The centralization phenomenon. Its usefulness as a predictor or outcome in conservative treatment of chronic law back pain (a pilot study). *Spine.* 1995;20(23):2513–2520.

173. Skytte L, May S, Petersen P. Centralization: its prognostic value in patients with referred symptoms and sciatica. *Spine.* 2005;30(11):E293–E299.

174. Sufka A, Hauger B, Trenary M, et al. Centralization of low back pain and perceived functional outcome. *J Orthop Sports Phys Ther.* 1998;27(3):205–212.

175. Werneke M, Hart DL. Centralization phenomenon as a prognostic factor for chronic low back pain and disability. *Spine.* 2001;26(7):758–764.

176. Werneke M, Hart DL, Cook D. A descriptive study of the centralization phenomenon. A prospective analysis. *Spine.* 1999;24(7):676–683.

177. Werneke M, May S. The centralization phenomenon and fear-avoidance beliefs as prognostic factors for acute low back pain. *J Orthop Sports Phys Ther.* 2005;35(12):844–845.

178. Werneke MW, Hart DL. Centralization: association between repeated end-range pain responses and behavioral signs in patients with acute non-specific low back pain. *J Rehabil Med.* 2005;37(5):286–290.

179. Werneke MW, Hart DL, Resnik L, Stratford PW, Reyes A. Centralization: prevalence and effect on treatment outcomes using a standardized operational definition and measurement method. *J Orthop Sports Phys Ther.* 2008;38(3):116–125.

180. Kilpikoski S, Airaksinen O, Kankaanpaa M, Leminen P, Videman T, Alen M. Interexaminer reliability of low back pain assessment using the McKenzie method. *Spine.* 2002;27(8):E207–E214.

181. Long A, Donelson R, Fung T. Does it matter which exercise? A randomized control trial of exercise for low back pain. *Spine.* 2004;29(23):2593–2602.

182. Dettori JR, Bullock SH, Sutlive TG, Franklin RJ, Patience T. The effects of spinal flexion and extension exercises and their associated postures in patients with acute low back pain. *Spine.* 1995;20(21):2303–2312.

183. Indahl A, Velund L, Reikeraas O. Good prognosis for low back pain when left untampered. A randomized clinical trial. *Spine.* 1995;20(4):473–477.

184. Machado LA, de Souza MS, Ferreira PH, Ferreira ML. The McKenzie method for low back pain: a systematic review of the literature with a meta-analysis approach. *Spine.* 2006;31(9): E254–E262.

185. Moffett JK, Jackson DA, Gardiner ED, et al. Randomized trial of two physiotherapy interventions for primary care neck and back pain patients: 'McKenzie' vs brief physiotherapy pain management. *Rheumatology.* 2006;45(12):1514–1521.

186. Nwuga G, Nwuga V. Relative therapeutic efficacy of the Williams and McKenzie protocols in back pain management. *Physiotherapy Practice.* 1985;1(2):99–105.

187. Malmivaara A, Hakkinen U, Aro T, et al. The treatment of acute low back pain—bed rest, exercises, or ordinary activity? *N Engl J Med.* 1995;332(6):351–355.

188. Donelson R, Aprill C, Medcalf R, Grant W. A prospective study of centralization of lumbar and referred pain. A predictor of symptomatic discs and anular competence. *Spine.* 1997;22(10):1115–1122.

189. Wetzel FT, Donelson R. The role of repeated end-range/pain response assessment in the management of symptomatic lumbar discs. *Spine J.* 2003;3(2):146–154.

190. Long A, May S, Fung T. Specific directional exercises for patients with low back pain: a case series. *Physiother Can.* 2008;60(4):307–317.

191. Werneke MW, Hart DL, George SZ, Stratford PW, Matheson JW, Reyes A. Clinical outcomes for patients classified by fear-avoidance beliefs and centralization phenomenon. *Arch Phys Med Rehabil.* 2009;90(5):768–777.

192. Fritz JM, Brennan GP. Preliminary examination of a proposed treatment-based classification system for patients receiving physical therapy interventions for neck pain. *Phys Ther.* 2007;87(5):513–524.

193. Fritz JM, Brennan GP, Clifford SN, Hunter SJ, Thackeray A. An examination of the reliability of a classification algorithm for subgrouping patients with low back pain. *Spine.* 2006;31(1):77–82.

194. Karas R, McIntosh G, Hall H, Wilson L, Melles T. The relationship between nonorganic signs and centralization of symptoms in the prediction of return to work for patients with low back pain. *Phys Ther.* 1997;77(4):354–360.

195. Young S, Aprill C, Laslett M. Correlation of clinical examination characteristics with three sources of chronic low back pain. *Spine J.* 2003;3(6):460–465.

196. Razmjou H, Kramer JF, Yamada R. Intertester reliability of the McKenzie evaluation in assessing patients with mechanical low-back pain. *J Orthop Sports Phys Ther.* 2000;30(7):368–383.

197. Browder DA, Childs JD, Cleland JA, Fritz JM. Effectiveness of an extension-oriented treatment approach in a subgroup of subjects with low back pain: a randomized clinical trial. *Phys Ther.* 2007;87(12):1608–1618.

198. Petersen T, Kryger P, Ekdahl C, Olsen S, Jacobsen S. The effect of McKenzie therapy as compared with that of intensive strengthening training for the treatment of patients with

subacute or chronic low back pain: A randomized controlled trial. *Spine.* 2002;27(16): 1702–1709.

199. Petersen T, Larsen K, Jacobsen S. One-year follow-up comparison of the effectiveness of McKenzie treatment and strengthening training for patients with chronic low back pain: outcome and prognostic factors. *Spine.* 2007;32(26):2948–2956.

200. Fritz JM, Delitto A, Welch WC, Erhard RE. Lumbar spinal stenosis: a review of current concepts in evaluation, management, and outcome measurements. *Arch Phys Med Rehabil.* 1998;79(6):700–708.

201. Whitman JM, Flynn TW, Childs JD, et al. A comparison between two physical therapy treatment programs for patients with lumbar spinal stenosis: a randomized clinical trial. *Spine.* 2006;31(22):2541–2549.

202. Fritz JM, Erhard RE, Vignovic M. A nonsurgical treatment approach for patients with lumbar spinal stenosis. *Phys Ther.* 1997;77(9):962–973.

203. Murphy DR, Hurwitz EL, Gregory AA, Clary R. A non-surgical approach to the management of lumbar spinal stenosis: a prospective observational cohort study. *BMC Musculoskelet Disord.* 2006;7:16.

204. Rittenberg JD, Ross AE. Functional rehabilitation for degenerative lumbar spinal stenosis. *Phys Med Rehabil Clin N Am.* 2003;14(1):111–120.

205. Fritz JM, Erhard RE, Delitto A, Welch WC, Nowakowski PE. Preliminary results of the use of a two-stage treadmill test as a clinical diagnostic tool in the differential diagnosis of lumbar spinal stenosis. *J Spinal Disord.* 1997;10(5):410–416.

206. Whitman JM, Flynn TW, Fritz JM. Nonsurgical management of patients with lumbar spinal stenosis: a literature review and a case series of three patients managed with physical therapy. *Phys Med Rehabil Clin N Am.* 2003;14(1):77–101.

207. Apeldoorn AT, Ostelo RW, van Helvoirt H, Fritz JM, de Vet HC, van Tulder MW. The cost-effectiveness of a treatment-based classification system for low back pain: design of a randomised controlled trial and economic evaluation. *BMC Musculoskelet Disord.* 2010;11 (1):58.

208. Gillan MG, Ross JC, McLean IP, Porter RW. The natural history of trunk list, its associated disability and the influence of McKenzie management. *Eur Spine J.* 1998;7(6):480–483.

209. Harrison DE, Cailliet R, Betz JW, et al. A non-randomized clinical control trial of Harrison mirror image methods for correcting trunk list (lateral translations of the thoracic cage) in patients with chronic low back pain. *Eur Spine J.* 2005;14(2):155–162.

210. Beurskens AJ, de Vet HC, Koke AJ, et al. Efficacy of traction for non-specific low back pain: a randomised clinical trial. *Lancet.* 1995;346(8990):1596–1600.

211. Beurskens AJ, de Vet HC, Koke AJ, et al. Efficacy of traction for nonspecific low back pain. 12-week and 6-month results of a randomized clinical trial. *Spine.* 1997;22(23): 2756–2762.

212. Clarke JA, van Tulder MW, Blomberg SE, et al. Traction for low-back pain with or without sciatica. *Cochrane Database Syst Rev.* 2007(2).

213. Harte AA, Baxter GD, Gracey JH. The efficacy of traction for back pain: a systematic review of randomized controlled trials. *Arch Phys Med Rehabil.* 2003;84(10):1542–1553.

214. Pellecchia GL. Lumbar traction: a review of the literature. *J Orthop Sports Phys Ther.* 1994;20(5):262–267.

215. van Tulder MW, Koes BW, Assendelft WJ, Bouter LM, Maljers LD, Driessen AP. Chronic low back pain: exercise therapy, multidisciplinary programs, NSAID's, back schools and behavioral therapy effective; traction not effective; results of systematic reviews. *Ned Tijdschr Geneeskd.* 2000;144(31):1489–1494.

216. Fritz JM, Lindsay W, Matheson JW, et al. Is there a subgroup of patients with low back pain likely to benefit from mechanical traction? Results of a randomized clinical trial and subgrouping analysis. *Spine.* 2007;32(26):E793–800.

217. Cai C, Pua YH, Lim KC. A clinical prediction rule for classifying patients with low back pain who demonstrate short-term improvement with mechanical lumbar traction. *Eur Spine J.* 2009;18(4):554–561.

218. Beurskens AJ, van der Heijden GJ, de Vet HC, et al. The efficacy of traction for lumbar back pain: design of a randomized clinical trial. *J Manipulative Physiol Ther.* 1995;18(3): 141–147.

219. Fritz JM, Piva SR, Childs JD. Accuracy of the clinical examination to predict radiographic instability of the lumbar spine. *Eur Spine J.* 2005;14(8):743–750.

220. Kiesel KB, Underwood FB, Mattacola CG, Nitz AJ, Malone TR. A comparison of select trunk muscle thickness change between subjects with low back pain classified in the treatment-based classification system and asymptomatic controls. *J Orthop Sports Phys Ther.* 2007; 37(10):596–607.

221. Whitman JM, Fritz JM, Childs JD. The influence of experience and specialty certifications on clinical outcomes for patients with low back pain treated within a standardized physical therapy management program. *J Orthop Sports Phys Ther.* 2004;34(11):662–672.

222. Donahue MS, Riddle DL, Sullivan MS. Intertester reliability of a modified version of McKenzie's lateral shift assessments obtained on patients with low back pain. *Phys Ther.* 1996;76(7):706–716.

223. Ng JK, Kippers V, Richardson CA, Parnianpour M. Range of motion and lordosis of the lumbar spine: reliability of measurement and normative values. *Spine.* 2001;26(1):53–60.

224. Waddell G, Somerville D, Henderson I, Newton M. Objective clinical evaluation of physical impairment in chronic low back pain. *Spine.* 1992;17(6):617–628.

225. Hicks GE, Fritz JM, Delitto A, Mishock J. Interrater reliability of clinical examination measures for identification of lumbar segmental instability. *Arch Phys Med Rehabil.* 2003; 84(12):1858–1864.

226. Abbott JH, Flynn TW, Fritz JM, Hing WA, Reid D, Whitman JM. Manual physical assessment of spinal segmental motion: intent and validity. *Man Ther.* 2009;14(1):36–44.

227. Fritz JM, Whitman JM, Childs JD. Lumbar spine segmental mobility assessment: an examination of validity for determining intervention strategies in patients with low back pain. *Arch Phys Med Rehabil.* 2005;86(9):1745–1752.

228. Smedmark V, Wallin M, Arvidsson I. Inter-examiner reliability in assessing passive intervertebral motion of the cervical spine. *Manual Ther.* 2000;5(2):97–101.

229. Abbott JH, Fritz JM, McCane B, et al. Lumbar segmental mobility disorders: comparison of two methods of defining abnormal displacement kinematics in a cohort of patients with non-specific mechanical low back pain. *BMC Musculoskelet Disord.* 2006;7:45.

230. Binkley J, Stratford PW, Gill C. Interrater reliability of lumbar accessory motion mobility testing. *Phys Ther.* 1995;75(9):786–792.

231. Gill NW, Teyhen DS, Lee IE. Improved contraction of the transversus abdominis immediately following spinal manipulation: a case study using real-time ultrasound imaging. *Man Ther.* 2007;12(3):280–285.

232. Raney NH, Teyhen DS, Childs JD. Observed changes in lateral abdominal muscle thickness after spinal manipulation: a case series using rehabilitative ultrasound imaging. *J Orthop Sports Phys Ther.* 2007;37(8):472–479.

233. American Physical Therapy Association. *Guide to Physical Therapist Practice.* 2nd ed. Alexandria, VA: APTA; 2001.

234. Fairbank JC, Pynsent PB. The Oswestry Disability Index. *Spine.* 2000;25(22):2940–2952.

235. Mintken PE, Derosa C, Little T, Smith B. A model for standardizing manipulation terminology in physical therapy practice. *J Man Manip Ther.* 2008;16(1):50–56.

236. Mintken PE, DeRosa C, Little T, Smith B. AAOMPT clinical guidelines: a model for standardizing manipulation terminology in physical therapy practice. *J Orthop Sports Phys Ther.* 2008;38(3):A1–A6.

237. Bialosky JE, Bishop MD, Robinson ME, George SZ. The relationship of the audible pop to hypoalgesia associated with high-velocity, low-amplitude thrust manipulation: a secondary analysis of an experimental study in pain-free participants. *J Manipulative Physiol Ther.* 2010;33(2):117–124.

238. Cleland JA, Flynn TW, Childs JD, Eberhart S. The audible pop from thoracic spine thrust manipulation and its relation to short-term outcomes in patients with neck pain. *J Man Manip Ther.* 2007;15(3):143–154.

239. Flynn TW, Childs JD, Fritz JM. The audible pop from high-velocity thrust manipulation and outcome in individuals with low back pain. *J Manipulative Physiol Ther.* 2006;29(1):40–45.

240. Flynn TW, Fritz JM, Wainner RS, Whitman JM. The audible pop is not necessary for successful spinal high-velocity thrust manipulation in individuals with low back pain. *Arch Phys Med Rehabil.* 2003;84(7):1057–1060.

241. Burton AK, Waddell G, Burtt R, Blair S. Patient educational material in the management of low back pain in primary care. *Bull Hosp Jt Dis.* 1996;55(3):138–141.

242. Burton AK, Waddell G, Tillotson KM, Summerton N. Information and advice to patients with back pain can have a positive effect. A randomized controlled trial of a novel educational booklet in primary care. *Spine.* 1999;24(23):2484–2491.

243. Coudeyre E, Tubach F, Rannou F, et al. Effect of a simple information booklet on pain persistence after an acute episode of low back pain: a non-randomized trial in a primary care setting. *PLoS One.* 2007;2(1):e706.

244. Maluf KS, Sahrmann SA, Van Dillen LR. Use of a classification system to guide nonsurgical management of a patient with chronic low back pain. [see comment]. *Phys Ther.* 2000;80(11):1097–1111.

245. Modic MT, Obuchowski NA, Ross JS, et al. Acute low back pain and radiculopathy: MR imaging findings and their prognostic role and effect on outcome. *Radiology.* 2005;237(2):597–604.

246. Hides JA, Stanton WR, McMahon S, Sims K, Richardson CA. Effect of stabilization training on multifidus muscle cross-sectional area among young elite cricketers with low back pain. *J Orthop Sports Phys Ther.* 2008;38(3):101–108.

247. Hodges P, Richardson C, Jull G. Evaluation of the relationship between laboratory and clinical tests of transversus abdominis function.[see comment]. *Physiother Res Int.* 1996; 1(1):30–40.

248. Hodges PW, Richardson CA. Transversus abdominis and the superficial abdominal muscles are controlled independently in a postural task. *Neurosci Lett.* 1999;265(2):91–94.

249. Richardson CA, Hides JA, Wilson S, Stanton W, Snijders CJ. Lumbo-pelvic joint protection against antigravity forces: motor control and segmental stiffness assessed with magnetic resonance imaging. *J Gravit Physiol.* 2004;11(2):P119–P122.

250. Richardson CA, Jull GA. Muscle control-pain control. What exercises would you prescribe? *Man Ther* 1995;1(1):2–10.

251. Grenier SG, McGill SM. Quantification of lumbar stability by using 2 different abdominal activation strategies. *Arch Phys Med Rehabil.* 2007;88(1):54–62.

252. McGill SM. Electromyographic activity of the abdominal and low back musculature during the generation of isometric and dynamic axial trunk torque: implications for lumbar mechanics. *J Orthop Res.* 1991;9(1):91–103.

253. McGill SM. Distribution of tissue loads in the low back during a variety of daily and rehabilitation tasks. *J Rehabil Res Dev.* 1997;34(4):448–458.

254. Koppenhaver SL, Hebert JJ, Fritz JM, Parent EC, Teyhen DS, Magel JS. Reliability of rehabilitative ultrasound imaging of the transversus abdominis and lumbar multifidus muscles. *Arch Phys Med Rehabil.* 2009;90(1):87–94.

255. Ng JK, Richardson CA, Jull GA. Electromyographic amplitude and frequency changes in the iliocostalis lumborum and multifidus muscles during a trunk holding test. *Phys Ther.* 1997;77(9):954–961.

256. Koppenhaver SL, Parent EC, Teyhen DS, Hebert JJ, Fritz JM. The effect of averaging multiple trials on measurement error during ultrasound imaging of transversus abdominis and lumbar multifidus muscles in individuals with low back pain. *J Orthop Sports Phys Ther.* 2009;39(8):604–611.

257. Teyhen DS, Bluemle LN, Dolbeer JA, et al. Changes in lateral abdominal muscle thickness during the abdominal drawing-in maneuver in those with lumbopelvic pain. *J Orthop Sports Phys Ther.* 2009;39(11):791–798.

258. Teyhen DS, Rieger JL, Westrick RB, Miller AC, Molloy JM, Childs JD. Changes in deep abdominal muscle thickness during common trunk-strengthening exercises using ultrasound imaging. *J Orthop Sports Phys Ther.* 2008;38(10):596–605.

259. Childs JD. *Validation of a clinical prediction rule to identify patients likely to benefit from spinal manipulation: a randomized clinical trial* [dissertation]. Pittsburgh, PA: School of Health and Rehabilitation Sciences, University of Pittsburgh; 2003.

260. Akuthota V, Ferreiro A, Moore T, Fredericson M. Core stability exercise principles. *Curr Sports Med Rep.* 2008;7(1):39–44.

261. Fairbank JC, Couper J, Davies JB, O'Brien JP. The Oswestry Low Back Pain Disability Questionnaire. *Physiotherapy.* 1980;66(8):271–273.

262. Fritz JM, Irrgang JJ. A comparison of a modified Oswestry Low Back Pain Disability Questionnaire and the Quebec Back Pain Disability Scale. *Phys Ther.* 2001;81(2):776–788.

263. Beurskens AJ, de Vet HC, Koke AJ, van der Heijden GJ, Knipschild PG. Measuring the functional status of patients with low back pain. Assessment of the quality of four disease-specific questionnaires. *Spine.* 1995;20(9):1017–1028.

264. Kopec JA, Esdaile JM, Abrahamowicz M, et al. The Quebec Back Pain Disability Scale. Measurement properties. *Spine.* 1995;20(3):341–352.

265. Downie WW, Leatham PA, Rhind VM, Wright V, Branco JA, Anderson JA. Studies with pain rating scales. *Ann Rheum Dis.* 1978;37(4):378–381.

266. Jensen MP, Karoly P, Braver S. The measurement of clinical pain intensity: a comparison of six methods. *Pain.* 1986;27(1):117–126.

267. Jensen MP, Miller L, Fisher LD. Assessment of pain during medical procedures: a comparison of three scales. *Clin J Pain.* 1998;14(4):343–349.

268. Jensen MP, Turner JA, Romano JM. What is the maximum number of levels needed in pain intensity measurement? *Pain.* 1994;58(3):387–392.

269. Katz J, Melzack R. Measurement of pain. *Surg Clin North Am.* 1999;79(2):231–252.

270. Price DD, Bush FM, Long S, Harkins SW. A comparison of pain measurement characteristics of mechanical visual analogue and simple numerical rating scales. *Pain.* 1994;56(2):217–226.

271. Chan CW, Goldman S, Ilstrup DM, Kunselman AR, O'Neill PI. The pain drawing and Waddell's nonorganic physical signs in chronic low-back pain. *Spine.* 1993;18(13):1717–1722.

272. Mann NH, 3rd, Brown MD, Hertz DB, Enger I, Tompkins J. Initial-impression diagnosis using low-back pain patient pain drawings. *Spine.* 1993;18(1):41–53.

273. Uden A, Astrom M, Bergenudd H. Pain drawings in chronic back pain. *Spine.* 1988;13(4):389–392.

274. Uden A, Landin LA. Pain drawing and myelography in sciatic pain. *Clin Orthop.* 1987;(216):124–130.

275. Werneke MW, Harris DE, Lichter RL. Clinical effectiveness of behavioral signs for screening chronic low-back pain patients in a work-oriented physical rehabilitation program. *Spine.* 1993;18(16):2412–2418.

276. Jaeschke R, Singer J, Guyatt GH. Measurement of health status. Ascertaining the minimal clinically important difference. *Control Clin Trials.* 1989;10(4):407–415.

277. Flynn TW, Wainner RS, Fritz JM. Spinal manipulation in physical therapist professional degree education: A model for teaching and integration into clinical practice. *J Orthop Sports Phys Ther.* 2006;36(8):577–587.

278. Fritz JM, Cleland JA, Brennan GP. Does adherence to the guideline recommendation for active treatments improve the quality of care for patients with acute low back pain delivered by physical therapists? *Med Care.* 2007;45(10):973–980.

279. Cheatle MD, Brady JP, Ruland T. Chronic low back pain, depression, and attributional style. *Clin J Pain.* 1990;6(2):114–117.

280. Liddle SD, Gracey JH, Baxter GD. Advice for the management of low back pain: a systematic review of randomised controlled trials. *Man Ther.* 2007;12(4):310–327.

281. Bach SM, Holten KB. Guideline update: what's the best approach to acute low back pain? *J Fam Pract.* 2009;58(12):E1.

282. George SZ, Childs JD, Teyhen DS, et al. Rationale, design, and protocol for the prevention of low back pain in the military (POLM) trial. *BMC Musculoskelet Disord.* 2007;8:92.

appendix one

Treatment-Based Classification Stage I Examination Form (Short Version)

Source: Phyllis Clapis.

TREATMENT-BASED CLASSIFICATION LBP EXAM FORM (SHORT)

DEMOGRAPHICS (Initial Only)

Status ☐ Licensed PT ☐ Student PT Date (Initial) _____

Patient ID _____ Age _____ Gender ☐ Male ☐ Female

HISTORY (Initial Only)

Location (check one)
☐ LBP
☐ LBP and buttock/thigh symptoms (not distal to knee)
☐ LBP and leg symptoms distal to knee

Duration
☐ ≤15 Days
☐ > 15 Days

Location of other symptoms (check all that apply)
☐ N/A
☐ Head/Neck
☐ Thoracic Spine
☐ Upper Extremity (ies)
☐ Hip (s)
☐ Knee (s)
☐ Foot/Feet

FABQ	Post Surgical	Sought medical care for this same episode in the past?
PA _____	☐ Yes	
WK _____	☐ No	☐ Yes ☐ No

Previous episodes of LBP ☐ 0 ☐ 1-2 ☐ 3-5 ☐ > 5

Frequency
Increasing ☐ Yes ☐ No

PHYSICAL EXAM: ☐ Initial ☐ Follow-up (Date: _____ Visit #: _____)

Avg SLR
☐ ≥91
☐ <91

Prone Instability Test
☐ Positive
☐ Negative

Mobility Testing
☐ Hypo
☐ Normal
☐ Hyper

Directional Preference
☐ Extension
☐ Flexion
☐ No Directional Preference

Aberrant Movements
☐ Yes
☐ No

Hip IR ROM: Lt _____; Rt _____

Pain (worst): _____ Flexion ROM: _____ Oswestry:_____

TREATMENT CLASSIFICATION (Initial & Weekly)

Stage I (check one)
☐ Thrust Manipulation (Grade V)
☐ Nonthrust Manipulation (Grade I–IV)
☐ Stabilization
☐ Flexion Directional Preference
☐ Extension Directional Preference
☐ Traction
Stage II (check all that apply)
☐ Aerobic
☐ General Conditioning

FABQ-W Status (check one)
☐ Negative (<29)
☐ "At Risk" (29-34)
☐ Positive (> 34)

FABQ-PA Status
☐ Positive (>14)
☐ Negative (≤14)

NOTE: You must check

1. One stage I category _or_ one or more stage II categories _and_
2. One FABQ status (initial only; weekly optional)

INTERVENTIONS (Initial & Weekly) (check all that apply)

☐ Patient Education/Instruction
☐ Flexion Exercises
☐ Extension Exercises
☐ Flexibility Exercises
☐ Stabilization Exercises
☐ General Conditioning Exercises
☐ Thrust Manipulation (Grade V)
☐ Nonthrust Manipulation (Grave I–IV)

☐ Aerobic Exercise
☐ Functional Training
☐ Heat Modalities
☐ Cold Modalities
☐ Traction – Mechanical
☐ Traction – Autotraction
☐ De-weighting / Unloading
☐ Behavioral Exercise Approach

☐ NMES (Strengthening)
☐ NMES (Pain Control)
☐ Soft Tissue Massage
☐ Myofacial Release
☐ Craniosacral Therapy
☐ Other

FILL OUT AT FINAL VISIT: Examined by (circle): Licensed PT / SPT / Both Treated by: Licensed PT / SPT / Both

Is the last visit recorded a discharge visit? Yes / No Total number of visits: _____ Total duration care (wks): _____

chapter twelve

Synthesis and Conclusions

Julia Chevan, PT, PhD, MPH, OCS
Phyllis A. Clapis, PT, DHSc, OCS

Conceptually, any one chapter in this book could provide you with the background you would need to manage a patient with acute low back pain (LBP). We, however, have asked that you read nine chapters, each with a different approach. At this point, we would anticipate that you, like our own students, might be feeling overwhelmed by the amount of information presented in this text. In this chapter, we will mitigate any uncertainty by synthesizing the information and providing our own insights into the similarities and differences among the approaches. Many of these approaches are related in their theoretical and applied derivations. Thus, we divide this chapter into a comparative analysis first by theoretical background, and then by clinical application.

THEORETICAL COMPARISONS

Basis of Classification

We began this book with a brief overview of how the practice of physical therapy in the United States has evolved over the years. In the 1980s, shortly after physical therapists were given the green light to evaluate their patients and develop a diagnostic label, Sahrmann[1] urged clinicians to avoid using those labels that they could not confirm through tests and measures that were within the scope of physical therapy practice. For example, a diagnosis of "herniated lumbar disc" would not be appropriate for two reasons: 1) The tests required to make this diagnosis are outside the scope of practice of physical therapists and 2) The diagnosis "herniated lumbar disc" does not sufficiently guide our treatment. Unless a specific impairment was identified, it would be difficult to direct one form of treatment to this diagnosis. Furthermore, we know that the identification of a specific source of LBP is a futile endeavor; hence as mentioned earlier in this book, the term "nonspecific low back pain" has been coined.[2,3]

The recognition that most LBP is best termed nonspecific has prompted a shift away from diagnosing patients on the basis of pathoanatomy and toward diagnosing them on the basis of clustering signs and symptoms. *The Guide to Physical Therapist Practice*[4] dictates that the goal of the diagnostic process is to classify patients into subgroups based on signs and symptoms rather than on specific anatomical sources. The formation of subgroups based on these signs and symptoms enables us to guide the decision-making process to the most effective strategies for intervention. Today, the majority of orthopedic physical therapist clinical specialists use diagnostic classification systems that are distinct from medical diagnoses when managing patients with LBP.[5]

Many approaches presented in this text utilize a system of subgroup classification. Table 12–1 compares the approaches by their use of diagnostic classification systems. It is important to note not only which approaches use classification but, also, the differences in *how* these classifications are categorized. The Cyriax approach, which has historically followed a traditional medical model of pathoanatomic classification, has evolved to include four clinical categories that are based more on the patient's signs and symptoms and less on the identification of the specific pathology. The McKenzie approach classifies patients into syndromes that are based on the patient's response to repeated movements and sustained postures. The diagnostic classifications identified in the osteopathic approach are based on alterations in structural relationships, whereas the Movement System Impairment Syndromes (MSIS) approach organizes patients into syndromes that are based on the movement directions that most consistently cause symptoms and that are associated with movement impairments. One of the more recently developed approaches is the Treatment-Based Classification (TBC) approach, which attempts to link specific treatments to specific patient characteristics and subgroups that are best responders.[6] The Paris approach is somewhat unique in that it is the only model that categorizes patients into syndromes that are based on pathoanatomy and disease.

The Maitland, Mulligan, and Kaltenborn-Evjenth approaches do not use subgroup classifications. These models place less value on diagnostic or pathological labels and place more emphasis on the process of reexamination in order to monitor treatment effectiveness.

It is important to note that while subgrouping patients is used to better guide the decision-making process, it is not an absolute prerequisite for

Table 12–1 Comparison of the Diagnostic Classifications and Etiology of Pain Across the Approaches

Approach	What Are the Diagnostic Classifications?	What Cause Is Attributed to Pain Generation?	What Is the Anatomic Source of Pain Generation?
Cyriax	Model 1 Model 2 Model 3 Model 4	Tissue stress	Historically disc, now acknowledges structural source not clear
Kalteborn-Evjenth	None used	Joint hypo/hypermobility	No pathoanatomic structure identified
Maitland	None used	Joint hypomobility	No pathoanatomic structure identified
McKenzie	1. Derangement 2. Dysfunction 3. Posture 4. Other	Repeated and prolonged tissue stress	Historically disc, now acknowledges structural source not clear
Mulligan	None used	Positional fault and subsequent faulty movement patterns	No pathoanatomic structure identified
Paris	1. Myofascial states 2. Facet dysfunction 3. Sacroiliac dysfunction 4. Ligamentous weakness 5. Instability 6. Disc dysfunction 7. Spondylolisthesis 8. Lumbar spine stenosis (central spine stenosis, and lateral foraminal stenosis) 9. The lesion complex 10. Lumbar spine: Kissing spines (Baastrap's disease) 11. Thoracolumbar syndrome	Joint hypo/hypermobility	No pathoanatomic structure identified

(continued)

Table 12–1 Comparison of the Diagnostic Classifications and Etiology of Pain Across the Approaches (continued)

Approach	What Are the Diagnostic Classifications?	What Cause Is Attributed to Pain Generation?	What Is the Anatomic Source of Pain Generation?
Osteopathic	1. ERS dysfunction 2. FRS dysfunction 3. Rotated sacrum 4. Flexed sacrum 5. Extended sacrum 6. Anterior innominate rotation 7. Posterior innominate rotation 8. Inferior pubic shear 9. Superior pubic shear	Structural dysfunction of position or joint hypo/ hypermobility	No pathoanatomic structure identified
MSIS	1. Rotation-extension 2. Extension 3. Rotation 4. Flexion-rotation 5. Flexion	Altered precision of joint motion that is causing accessory motion hyper- mobility	No pathoanatomic structure identified
TBC	1. Manipulation 2. Stabilization 3. Specific exercise 4. Traction	Not determined through this model	No pathoanatomic structure identified

diagnosis, especially if the examination process is built around individual patient responses to trial treatments. We acknowledge that the development of classification systems is a dynamic process and we expect this process to continue to evolve as new evidence emerges.

Etiology of Symptom Generation

The traditional medical model for management of LBP is based on identifying the exact pathoanatomic source of a patient's symptoms, often through costly tests and imaging studies. Over the years, more and more evidence has emerged that supports the notion that determining the exact pathoanatomical source of LBP is a problem.[7–9] Still, physical therapists place a strong value on identification of an anatomical cause of pain. In a recent study[5] 88% of orthopedic clinical specialists surveyed felt that identification of a tissue source of pain was an important factor in determining appropriate treatment. Nearly all of the models presented in this text represent a shift away from attempting to identify a relevant pathological structure or condition. The Cyriax and the McKenzie approaches were originally based on models of disc pathology, but those who practice these approaches now acknowledge that identification of the anatomic source of pain is less important than the ability to cluster patients according to their signs and symptoms. The Paris approach is unique again in that it names specific pathological conditions such as facet dysfunction, spinal stenosis, and spondylolisthesis.

While there has been broad consistency between approaches in terms of identifying the *source* of pain, three primary categories have emerged with regard to the factors that contribute to the *cause* of pain. These are not exclusive—some overlap between them exists. The first is joint hyper- or hypo-mobility, to which the Kaltenborn, Paris, and Maitland models subscribe. Paris also recognizes deficits in motor performance that could also contribute to symptoms. The second is faulty positions and movement patterns under which the Mulligan, osteopathic, and MSIS approach belong. While the MSIS model states that faulty movement patterns are the underlying cause of pain, the sequela to this is accessory motion hypermobility. The third category is related to abnormal tissue stress, which are the causative factors identified in the Cyriax and McKenzie models. The TBC model is exempt from either of these categories, as this model is not concerned with the cause of symptoms, rather the response of identified patient subgroups to specific treatments. Again, take a look at Table 12–1 where the comparison has been more fully developed.

Philosophies and Hallmarks of Assessment

While the differences in classification schemes between the approaches have already been highlighted, it is important to appreciate the underlying philosophies on which these diagnoses are based (Table 12–2). Cook described three distinct philosophies of assessment that underlie many manual therapy models.[10] The first is the *biomechanical-pathological assessment method,* which is grounded in principles of biomechanics and arthrokinematics. This method uses selected biomechanical theories for assessment of abnormal position and movement, and treatments that incorporate similar biomechanical constructs. The Cyriax, Kaltenborn-Evjenth (KE), Paris, MSIS, and

Table 12–2 Comparison of the Philosophies and Unique Components of Assessment Across the Approaches

Approach	What Is the Underlying Assessment Philosophy?	Unique Examination Components
Cyriax	Biomechanical-pathological	Examination of symptom response to selective tension by using active, passive, and resistive movements. Loss of motion analyzed as capsular or non-capsular.
Kaltenborn-Evjenth	Biomechanical-pathological	Symptom-localization testing and passive intervertebral motion testing using small amplitude translatoric motions.
Maitland	Patient response	Identification of a patient's comparable sign through active, passive, and accessory movement testing.
McKenzie	Mixed	Examination of symptom response to repeated movement with specific consideration given to centralization and peripheralization of symptoms.
Mulligan	Mixed	Use of trial intervention to direct treatment.
Paris	Biomechanical-pathological	14-step process that includes palpation for condition, position, and mobility.
Osteopathic	Biomechanical-pathological	Structural examination to determine if there are bony positional faults with particular focus on spine and pelvic girdle.
MSIS	Biomechanical-pathological	Tests of trunk motion and limb motions performed in various positions. In addition, the precision of motion; the effect on symptoms; and the muscle performance, length, stiffness, and functional activities are also assessed.
TBC	Not identified	Selection of tests and measures based on best evidence in empirical literature that results in an exam that integrates components from many other approaches.

osteopathic approaches follow this model. The Cyriax examination incorporates end-feel, capsular patterns, and selective tension tests, with treatments that are based on anatomical principles. The Kaltenborn-Evjenth approach aims to identify hyper- or hypomobile segments, with treatment directed to either stabilizing or restoring joint motion via arthrokinematically-based techniques. Key features of this approach include symptom localization testing and the use of passive angular and translatoric intervertebral motion testing. The Paris approach shares similarities with Kaltenborn-Evjenth in attempting to identify and treat segmental hyper- and hypomobility. This approach relies heavily on palpation for condition, position, and mobility. MSIS approach is based on the premise that there is a kinesiopathological relationship to the pain, with the goal of examination being the identification of the offending movement direction through assessment of patient-generated movements. Finally, one of the tenets of the osteopathic model is that structure dictates function and that an abnormality in structure can lead to abnormal function. The examination then is based on the identification of abnormal structural relationships, with heavy emphasis on palpation of position and movement, specifically of the lumbar spine, pelvis, and sacrum.

The second method is the *patient-response model*, which places less emphasis on biomechanics and more on the symptom response of the patient. With this method, selected treatments are based on movements that either reduce the patient's pain and/or restore their movement. The Maitland approach seems to be guided by this method of assessment as evidenced by the goal of finding a comparable sign through assessment of active, passive, and accessory motion testing. Learman and Showalter described the benefits of the patient-response model in Chapter 5:

> *"Using a patient response model liberates the clinician from applying theories of biomechanics, protocols, or assessment and treatment algorithms in situations where their use may complicate the clinical reasoning process or be fundamentally flawed."*

The third method is a *mixed model*, in which assessment and treatment strategies are both biomechanical-pathological–based and patient response-based. The Mulligan and McKenzie model seem to follow this method. The Mulligan approach is based on the positional fault theory and examination is guided by the patient's response to a trial intervention. In a similar manner, the McKenzie model is based on biomechanical principles, but the examination and treatment selection are both guided by the patient's symptom response (e.g., centralization) and mechanical response (e.g., increased motion) to *repeated* movements. The TBC model stands alone in that it does not fall into any of the three aforementioned models. Instead, the goal of the examination in this approach is to use current evidence to identify subgroups of patients who will best respond to specific interventions.

PRACTICAL COMPARISONS

Diagnosis

If symptom generation is the area of greatest similarity among the models, the diagnoses assigned to Joe would be the area of the greatest difference. Table 12–3 illustrates the wide range in diagnoses among the models. Of interest, the models that rely on palpation findings had the most in common with each other. The Kaltenborn-Evjenth model specifically identified hypomobility at the L4-L5 segment; similarly the Paris and Mulligan models identified the same segment as containing a dysfunction. The Osteopathic model named dysfunctions at L5 and the sacrum. While we recognize the differences in diagnoses, perhaps we should place less emphasis on labeling the problem and more emphasis on the process of arriving at treatment decisions.[5]

Intervention

Probably of greatest interest to the reader is not how each model examined Joe or diagnosed him, but rather the selection of interventions. Joe (hypothetically) was seen by nine different clinicians who examined him and diagnosed him in their own unique ways. Just how different were the treatment plans? We have summarized the approaches used for Joe in Tables 12–3 and 12–4 and find that there is a great deal of similarity among the models with regard to treatment interventions. With the exception of the MSIS approach, which is centered on correction of faulty movement patterns, all of the models incorporated some type of spinal mobilization or manipulation techniques. Not surprising, since the majority of these approaches are classified as manual therapy approaches. The Kaltenborn-Evjenth, Paris, Maitland, Mulligan, McKenzie, and osteopathic models employ techniques that are segment-specific whereas the techniques used in the Cyriax and TBC approach are more general, placing less credence on isolation of a specific spinal segment. Muscle energy technique was unique to the osteopathic model, but this technique could be classified as a type of mobilization. More

Table 12–3 Comparison of the Specific Diagnoses, Interventions and Prognoses for Joe Lores

Approach	Diagnosis	Intervention	Prognosis
Cyriax	Cyriax Model 2 Annular lesion of sudden onset	Manipulation sequence • Distraction manipulation technique • Rotation manipulation techniques • Unilateral extension thrust technique • 'Pretzel' technique	Complete recovery in 2–3 sessions
Kaltenborn-Evjenth	Hypomobile and painful L5 > L4 Impaired muscle length and strength of the right lumbar paraspinal; Decreased right iliopsoas muscle length	Translatoric mobilizations and manipulation • Grade I–II "slack zone" mobilizations for pain relief • Grade I–II mobilizations for relaxation • Grade III mobilization and manipulation to increase mobility at L5 • Traction manipulation of L5 spinal segment Functional massage Manual muscle stretching Therapeutic exercise (K-E categories 3 and 4) Self mobilization, self stretching	"Good prognosis" but no time frame stated
Maitland	Mechanical LBP that is exacerbated by the comparable movements of flexion, extension, and right sidebending. Most comparable signs: 1. Unilateral PA glide on L4-L5 for treatment 2. Active forward flexion for functional reassessment Discogenic disorder may be "surmised"	Grade III or IV R unilateral UPAs at L4-L5 Grade III or IV Physiologic Lumbar rotations Grade V lumbar manipulation Extension exercises Self-mobilization	Resolution of symptoms expected over the next 3 weeks

(continued)

Table 12–3 Comparison of the Specific Diagnoses, Interventions and Prognoses for Joe Lores (continued)

Approach	Diagnosis	Intervention	Prognosis
McKenzie	Derangement with a directional preference to extension	Extension in standing and extension in lying exercises • Progression of forces that includes therapist technique only if symptoms do not fully centralize or do not improve Postural correction	Resolution of symptoms expected over the next 3–4 weeks
Mulligan	Dysfunction of the L4-L5 segment	Trial intervention: • Right L4 SNAG during seated flexion Intervention progression for nonresponse: • Right L5 SNAG during seated flexion Extension exercises Self SNAGS	Resolution of symptoms expected within 2 weeks or 6 visits
Paris	Paris category 2 facet dysfunction Facet synovitis/restriction with hypertonic muscle guarding	Lumbar extension exercise program Manipulation to restore facet joint mobility Myofascial manipulation Passive hip stretching Lumbar stabilization exercise program Functional training Education/back school	Resolution of symptoms expected within 10 visits over 6 weeks
Osteopathic	Somatic dysfunction Myofascial dysfunction, right gluteus medius, piriformis and quadratus lumborum Flexed rotated sidebent right (FRSR) at L5; Limited extension side bending and rotation left at L5	Lengthening and softening of the piriformis, psoas, quadrates lumborum Muscle energy techniques for FRSR L5 and L/R BST (possibly for type I dysfunction as well) Home exercise program	Resolution of symptoms expected within 6–8 visits

(continued)

Table 12–3 Comparison of the Specific Diagnoses, Interventions and Prognoses for Joe Lores (continued)

Approach	Diagnosis	Intervention	Prognosis
Osteopathic	Type I side bent left, rotated right in the lumbar spine; limited right side bending, left rotation Sacral left rotation on a right oblique axis backward sacral torsion (L/R BST); limited right forward sacral rotation (limited forward rotation of left base)		
MSIS	Lumbar rotation-flexion syndrome	Exercises that stress proper alignment during performance of forward bending, side bending, rotation, rolling and walking Correction of proper sitting posture Avoidance of lumbar flexion Conditioning exercises (e.g., walking) Functional Training	Resolution of symptoms expected within 6 visits over 3 months
TBC	Manipulation classification	High velocity low amplitude thrust manipulation directed to lumbar spine Range of motion exercises for the lumbar spine	50% improvement expected in 7 days, 6–10 total visits

than half of the approaches included extension exercises and only one-third included soft tissue mobilization. Stabilization exercises were a component of the Paris, Kaltenborn-Evjenth, and TBC approaches. While many approaches supplemented their treatment plans with stretching, strengthening, and conditioning exercises and all of them incorporated some form of patient education and home exercise.

Table 12-4 Comparison of Interventions Used for Joe Lores Across the Approaches

Approach	Manipulation/ Mobilization	Soft Tissue Mobilization	Extension Exercises	Strengthening, Stretching, and Conditioning Exercises	Stabilization Exercises	Corrective Exercises	Home Exercises / Patient Education
Cyriax	X			X			X
Kaltenborn-Evjenth	X	X		X	X		X
Maitland	X		X				X
McKenzie	X (if needed in progression of treatment)		X				X
Mulligan	X		X				X
Paris	X	X	X	X	X		X
Osteopathic	X (via muscle energy technique	X		X			X
MSIS				X		X	X
TBC	X		X	X	X		X

Prognosis

Table 12–3 outlines the anticipated recovery time frames for Joe. Each model identified Joe as having a good prognosis but we can see that the range of anticipated treatments visits spanned between 3 and 10 visits. This number falls within the *Guide to Physical Therapist Practice*[4] recommendation for patients in pattern 4F "Impaired Joint Mobility, Motor Function, Muscle Performance, Range of Motion, and Reflex Integrity Associated with Spinal Disorders" that provides an estimate of an acceptable number of visits as 8–24 and a restoration of function within 1–6 months.

AN INTEGRATED APPROACH TO TREATING JOE LORES

While the aim of this book was to present the reader with an overview of the common approaches used in the treatment of LBP, we are aware that many therapists use an integrated approach to treating a LBP case that presents similar to Joe. The selection of approaches might be dependent on the therapist's education and experience, their reliance on evidence to inform treatment, and an analysis of patient outcomes. An integrated approach to treating Joe can take many shapes, but what we feel is important is that the therapist be able to acknowledge the models from which they are "borrowing" and be able to justify the rationale behind the history, examination, and selected interventions. The following is just one example of how the approaches presented in this book might be integrated:

The patient's history clearly pointed to a directional preference of extension (McKenzie), however the onset of symptoms was less than 16 days and he had no pain below his knee (TBC and Cyriax). Based on his history alone, the therapist might consider an extension-oriented treatment approach (McKenzie and TBC) or spinal manipulation (TBC and Cyriax).

In terms of examination, using a biomechanical-pathological model the therapist would have identified hypomobility at the L4-L5 segment as well as concordant myofascial restrictions (Paris, Kaltenborn-Evjenth). In addition, a left on right backward sacral torsion and an FRSR dysfunction at L5 would have been identified (osteopathic). All of these dysfunctions would limit the patient's ability to fully extend due to the left sacral base being unable to rotate anteriorly (nutate) and L5 being unable to "close." Examination of specific active movements would have revealed faulty movement patterns as well as patterns of movement that eliminated or reduced symptoms (MSIS). Looking through the lens of a patient-response model, the therapist would have found that repeated UPAs and CPAs directed at L4 and L5 decreased stiffness and symptoms (Maitland). Finally, the mixed-model assessment would have revealed that the patient's symptoms improved with the application of repeated extension (McKenzie) and SNAGs to L4 and L5 (Mulligan).

It is evident that each model has provided a guide for clinical decision making with regard to treatment interventions and the evidence to support these interventions is included in the specific chapters. The TBC model supports two initial treatment approaches: Manipulation (nonspecific) and an extension-oriented treatment approach. (The Cyriax approach would also suggest a nonspecific manipulation). In the absence of contraindications, which Joe did not have, manipulation would be among the first approaches for this patient, followed by an extension-oriented treatment approach. It would be imperative to educate this patient with regard to correct movement patterns (MSIS) and postural education (all models). Early on the therapist would perform muscle energy techniques to correct the backward sacral torsion and dysfunction at L5 (osteopathic). In addition, the therapist would incorporate soft tissue mobilization (Kaltenborn-Evjenth, Paris, and osteopathic) and segment-specific spinal mobilizations and manipulations, including SNAGs (Mulligan), oscillatory techniques (Maitland), sustained techniques (Kaltenborn-Evjenth and McKenzie), and mid-range and end-range mobilizations (Paris).

Once the patient demonstrated improved structural alignment, centralization of symptoms and improved segmental mobility, the therapist would begin a stabilization program, which would eventually progress to an overall conditioning program (Cyriax, Paris, MSIS, TBC, and Kaltenborn-Evjenth.) Concomitant with the exercise program would be a movement training approach, in which the patient will be trained to perform correct movement patterns during all functional activities (MSIS). The prognosis for this patient would be that he would achieve a modified Oswestry score of 5% or lower within 8–10 visits, over the course of 8 weeks.

SUMMARY

In this book we have presented nine different approaches commonly used in the management of a patient with nonspecific LBP. We have made no judgments about which model is the best or the correct model to follow, rather, we have endeavored to provide a resource to students and clinicians to understand the underpinnings and decisions made in each model. Over time some of the dividing lines among these models have and are still likely to become more blurred.[11] We encourage our students and our readers to consider each approach with care and to appraise and understand the supporting evidence. Ultimately we ask ourselves, nine approaches and nine intervention plans, just how far have we come from that "One Bum Knee" article? Considering the supportive evidence and the considerable similarities among approaches, we would argue that we've come far—very far.

REFERENCES

1. Sahrmann S. Diagnosis by the physical therapist—a prerequisite for treatment. *Phys Ther.*1988;11:1703–1706.
2. Beattie PF. Current understanding of lumbar intervertebral disc degeneration: a review with emphasis upon etiology, pathophysiology, and lumbar magnetic resonance imaging findings. *J Orthop Sports Phys Ther.* 2008;38(6):329–340.
3. Beattie PF. The relationship between symptoms and abnormal magnetic resonance images of lumbar intervertebral disks. *Phys Ther.* 1996;76:601–608.
4. American Physical Therapy Association. *Guide to Physical Therapist Practice.* 2nd ed. Alexandria, VA: APTA; 2001.
5. Spoto MM, Collins J. Physiotherapy diagnosis in clinical practice: a survey of orthopaedic certified specialists in the USA. *Physiother Res Int.* 2008;13:31–41.
6. Delitto A, Erhard RE, Bowling RW. A treatment based classification approach to low back syndrome: identifying and staging patients for conservative treatment. *Phys Ther.* 1995;75: 470–485.
7. Deyo RA, Rainville J, Kent DL. What can the history and physical examination tell us about low back pain? *JAMA.*1992;268(6):760–765.
8. Jarvik JG, Deyo RA. Diagnostic evaluation of low back pain with emphasis on imaging. *Ann Intern Med.* 2002;137(7):586–597.
9. Haldeman S. Presidential Address, North American Spine Society: Failure of the pathology model to predict back pain. *Spine.* 1990;15:718–724.
10. Cook CE. *Orthopedic Manual Therapy an Evidenced-based Approach.* Upper Saddle River, NJ: Pearson Prentice Hall; 2007.
11. Farrell JP, Jensen GM. Manual therapy: a critical assessment of role in the profession of physical therapy. *Phys Ther.*72;12:11–20.

index